Lecture Notes in Artificial Intelligence 9105

Subseries of Lecture Notes in Computer Science

More information about this series at http://www.springer.com/series/1244

John H. Holmes · Riccardo Bellazzi
Lucia Sacchi · Niels Peek (Eds.)

Artificial Intelligence in Medicine

15th Conference on Artificial Intelligence
in Medicine, AIME 2015
Pavia, Italy, June 17–20, 2015
Proceedings

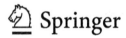 Springer

Editors
John H. Holmes
University of Pennsylvania
Philadelphia
Pennsylvania
USA

Lucia Sacchi
University of Pavia
Pavia
Italy

Riccardo Bellazzi
University of Pavia
Pavia
Italy

Niels Peek
University of Manchester
Manchester
UK

ISSN 0302-9743   ISSN 1611-3349   (electronic)
Lecture Notes in Artificial Intelligence
ISBN 978-3-319-19550-6   ISBN 978-3-319-19551-3   (eBook)
DOI 10.1007/978-3-319-19551-3

Library of Congress Control Number: 2015940570

LNCS Sublibrary: SL7 – Artificial Intelligence

Springer Cham Heidelberg New York Dordrecht London

Printed on acid-free paper

Springer International Publishing AG Switzerland is part of Springer Science+Business Media
(www.springer.com)

Preface

The European Society for Artificial Intelligence in Medicine (AIME) was established in 1986 following a very successful workshop held in Pavia, Italy, the year before. The principal aims of AIME are to foster fundamental and applied research in the application of artificial intelligence (AI) techniques to medical care and medical research, and to provide a forum at biennial conferences for discussing any progress made. For this reason the main activity of the society was the organization of a series of biennial conferences, held in Marseilles, France (1987), London, UK (1989), Maastricht, The Netherlands (1991), Munich, Germany (1993), Pavia, Italy (1995), Grenoble, France (1997), Aalborg, Denmark (1999), Cascais, Portugal (2001), Protaras, Cyprus (2003), Aberdeen, UK (2005), Amsterdam, The Netherlands (2007), Verona, Italy (2009), Bled, Slovenia (2011), and Murcia, Spain (2013). This volume contains the proceedings of AIME 2015, the 15th Conference on Artificial Intelligence in Medicine, held in Pavia, Italy, June 17–20, 2015.

The AIME 2015 goals were to present and consolidate the international state of the art of AI in biomedical research from the perspectives of theory, methodology, systems, and applications. AIME 2015 focused on AI methods and approaches to address big biomedical data challenges. The conference included two invited lectures, full and short papers, tutorials, workshops, and a doctoral consortium.

In the conference announcement, authors were invited to submit original contributions regarding the development of theory, methods, systems, and applications for solving problems in the biomedical field, including AI approaches in biomedical informatics, molecular medicine, and health-care organizational aspects. Authors of papers addressing theory were requested to describe the properties of novel AI models potentially useful for solving biomedical problems. Authors of papers addressing theory and methods were asked to describe the development or the extension of AI methods, to address the assumptions and limitations of the proposed techniques, and to discuss their novelty with respect to the state of the art. Authors of papers addressing systems and applications were asked to describe the development, implementation, or evaluation of new AI-inspired tools and systems in the biomedical field. They were asked to link their work to underlying theory, and either analyze the potential benefits to solve biomedical problems or present empirical evidence of benefits in clinical practice.

AIME 2015 received 110 abstract submissions, 99 thereof were eventually submitted as complete papers. Submissions came from 25 countries, including five outside Europe. All papers were carefully peer-reviewed by experts from the Program Committee with the support of additional reviewers. Each submission was reviewed by at least two, and in most cases three reviewers. The reviewers judged the overall quality of the submitted papers, together with their relevance to the AIME conference, technical correctness, novelty with respect to state of the art, scholarship, and quality of presentation. In addition, the reviewers provided detailed written comments on each paper, and stated their confidence in the subject area.

A small committee consisting of the AIME 2015 Scientific Chair John H. Holmes, the Local Organization Co-chairs Riccardo Bellazzi and Lucia Sacchi, and Niels Peek, Doctoral Consortium Chair and AIME 2013 Scientific Chair, made the final decisions regarding the AIME 2015 scientific program. This process began with virtual meetings held weekly starting in January 2015. The process ended with a face-to-face meeting of the committee in Pavia to assemble the final program.

As a result, 19 long papers (with an acceptance rate of 25%) and 24 short papers were accepted. Each long paper was presented in a 25-minute oral presentation during the conference. Each short paper was presented in a 5-minute presentation and by a poster. The papers were organized according to their topics in the following main themes: (1) Data Mining and Machine Learning; (2) Knowledge Representation and Guidelines; (3) Prediction in Clinical Practice; (4) Process Mining and Phenotyping; (5) Temporal Data Mining; (6) Text Mining; and (7) Uncertainty and Bayesian Methods.

AIME 2015 had the privilege of hosting two invited speakers: George M. Hripcsak, from Columbia University, USA, and Goran Nenadic, from the University of Manchester, UK. George Hripcsak discussed the importance of dealing with the temporal nature of the electronic medical record in using these data for studies. He called for further study of the "physics of the medical record," health-care processes, and new methods for analyzing electronic medical record data. Goran Nenadic's keynote focused on the use of and challenges presented by text mining of health data from a variety of sources, including the medical record as well as patient-generated data. He called for the integration of spatiotemporal and reasoning under uncertainly models to be incorporated into the text mining paradigm.

The Doctoral Consortium provided an opportunity for six PhD students to present their research goals, proposed methods, and preliminary results. A scientific panel consisting of experienced researchers in the field (Ameen Abu-Hanna, John Holmes, José Juarez, Goran Nenadic, David Riaño, Lucia Sacchi, Stephen Swift, Annette ten Teije, and Blaz Zupan) provided constructive feedback to the students in an informal atmosphere. The Doctoral Consortium was chaired by Niels Peek.

Three full-day workshops were organized after the AIME 2015 main conference. These included the 7th International Workshop on Knowledge Representation for Health Care (KRH4C) and the 8th International Workshop on Process-oriented Information Systems in Healthcare (ProHealth), joined together for the first time at AIME 2015. This workshop included a keynote address presented by Robert Greenes from Arizona State University, "Evolution and Revolution in Knowledge-Driven Health IT: A 50-Year Perspective and a Look Ahead." This workshop was chaired by Richard Lenz, Silvia Miksch, Mor Peleg, Manfred Reichert, David Riaño, and Annette ten Teije. A second full-day workshop was the First Workshop on Matrix Computations for Biomedical Informatics, chaired by Riccardo Bellazzi, Jimeng Sun, and Ping Zhang. The third workshop was the 4th International Workshop on Artificial Intelligence and Assistive Medicine, chaired by Constantine Spyropoulos and Aldo Franco Dragoni.

In addition to the workshops, three interactive tutorials were presented prior to the AIME 2015 main conference: "Data Fusion of Everything" (Marinka Zitnik and Blaz Zupan, University of Ljubljana, Slovenia); "Big Data Analytics for Healthcare" (Jimeng Sun, Georgia Institute of Technology); and "Evaluation of Prediction Models in Medicine" (Ameen Abu-Hanna, Academic Medical Center, Amsterdam, and Niels Peek, University of Manchester).

We would like to thank everyone who contributed to AIME 2015. First of all, we would like to thank the authors of the papers submitted and the members of the Program Committee together with the additional reviewers. Thanks are also due to the invited speakers as well as to the organizers of the workshops and the tutorial and doctoral consortium. Many thanks go to the local Organizing Committee, who managed all the work making this conference possible. The free EasyChair conference system (http://www.easychair.org/) was an important tool supporting us in the management of submissions, reviews, selection of accepted papers, and preparation of the overall material for the final proceedings. We would like to thank the University of Pavia, which hosted AIME 2015, and our sponsors, who so generously supported the conference.

Finally, we thank the Springer team for helping us in the final preparation of this LNCS book.

June 2015   John H. Holmes
                                                                        Riccardo Bellazzi
                                                                        Lucia Sacchi
                                                                        Niels Peek

Organization

Program Committee

Syed Sibte Raza Abidi	Dalhousie University, Canada
Ameen Abu-Hanna	Academic Medical Center, University of Amsterdam, The Netherlands
Klaus Peter Adlassnig	Medical University of Vienna, Austria
Riccardo Bellazzi	University of Pavia, Italy
Brian Chapman	University of Utah, USA
Carlo Combi	Università degli Studi di Verona, Italy
Amar Das	Dartmouth Institute, USA
Michel Dojat	INSERM, France
Paulo Felix	USC, Spain
Catherine Garbay	CNRS - LIG, France
Adela Grando	Arizona State University, USA
Milos Hauskrecht	University of Pittsburgh, USA
John Holmes	University of Pennsylvania, USA
Arjen Hommersom	University of Nijmegen, The Netherlands
Val Jones	University of Twente, The Netherlands
Jose M. Juarez	University of Murcia, Spain
Katharina Kaiser	University of Applied Sciences St. Poelten, Austria
Elpida Keravnou-Papailiou	University of Cyprus, Cyprus
Pedro Larranaga	University of Madrid, Spain
Nada Lavrač	Jozef Stefan Institute, Slovenia
Helena Lindgren	Umeå University, Sweden
Peter Lucas	Radboud University Nijmegen, The Netherlands
Mar Marcos	Universitat Jaume I, Spain
Michael Marschollek	Peter L. Reichertz Instituts für Medizinische Informatik, Germany
Roque Marín	University of Murcia, Spain
Paola Mello	University of Bologna, Italy
Silvia Miksch	Vienna University of Technology, Austria
Stefania Montani	University Piemonte Orientale, Italy
Barbara Oliboni	University of Verona, Italy
Niels Peek	Centre for Health Informatics
Mor Peleg	University of Haifa, Israel
Christian Popow	Medical University of Vienna, Austria
Silvana Quaglini	University of Pavia, Italy

David Riaño	Universitat Rovira i Virgili, Spain
Pedro Rodrigues	University of Porto, Portugal
Lucia Sacchi	University of Pavia, Italy
Stefan Schulz	Medical University of Graz, Austria
Brigitte Seroussi	Assistance Publique - Hôpitaux de Paris, France
Yuval Shahar	Ben Gurion University, Israel
Brett South	University of Utah, USA
Constantine Spyropoulos	NCSR Demokritos, Greece
Gregor Stiglic	University of Maribor, Slovenia
Annette Ten Teije	Vrije Universiteit Amsterdam, The Netherlands
Paolo Terenziani	University of Turin, Italy
Samson Tu	Stanford University, USA
Allan Tucker	Brunel University, UK
Frank Van Harmelen	Vrije Universiteit Amsterdam, The Netherlands
Alfredo Vellido	Universitat Politecnica de Catalunya, Spain
Dongwen Wang	Biomedical Informatics Program
Szymon Wilk	Poznan University of Technology, Poland
Blaz Zupan	University of Ljubljana, Slovenia
Pierre Zweigenbaum	LIMSI-CNRS, France

Additional Reviewers

Anselma, Luca	Krithara, Anastasia
Bacelar-Silva, Gustavo	Liu, Manxia
Bohanec, Marko	Liu, Zitao
Bonfietti, Alessio	Lombardi, Michele
Bottrighi, Alessio	Martinez-Salvador, Begoña
Bueno, Marcos Luiz De Paula	Mowery, Danielle
Büsching, Felix	Orphanou, Kalia
Campos, Manuel	Riguzzi, Fabrizio
Chapman, Wendy	Sa-Couto, Carla
Chesani, Federico	Sarker, Abeed
Dias, Claudia Camila	Sernani, Paolo
Dragoni, Aldo Franco	Seyfang, Andreas
Ferrandez, Oscar	Skeppstedt, Maria
Fung, Nick	Smailovic, Jasmina
Gamberger, Dragan	Stassopoulou, Athena
Giannakopoulos, George	Teijeiro, Tomás
Giannakopoulos, Theodoros	Torres-Sospedra, Joaquín
Haarbrandt, Birger	van der Heijden, Maarten
Hong, Charmgil	Vavpetic, Anze
Huang, Zhisheng	Wenzina, Reinhardt
Jiang, Guoqian	

Contents

Temporal Data Mining

Uncertainty and Bayesian Networks

Text Mining

Prediction in Clinical Practice

Knowledge Representation and Guidelines

Keynote Presentations

Physics of the Medical Record:
Handling Time in Health Record Studies

George Hripcsak[✉]

Department of Biomedical Informatics, Columbia University Medical Center,
New York, NY, USA
hripcsak@columbia.edu

The rapid increase in adoption of electronic health records (EHRs) creates the possibility of tracking billions of patient visits per year and exploiting them for clinical research. The international observational research collaboration, Observational Health Data Sciences and Informatics (OHDSI), has counted 682 million patient records that have been converted to a common format known at the OMOP Common Data Model [1]. While this number includes duplicates and records that have not been made broadly available to researchers, its scale demonstrates that converting the world population to a common format is feasible.

Yet even with massive amounts of data available and even in a common format, a number of challenges exist. Data can be inaccurate, complex, and missing, and the health care process affects the measurement and recording of information to cause bias [2]. For example, tests from the middle of the night are more likely to be abnormal because patients will most likely be tested then only because they are very ill. Previous work demonstrated some of the human factors that can affect recording, such as not entering symptoms for deceased patients [3] with a consequent large effect on outcomes studies. Not surprisingly, clinical variables are correlated with variables related to health care processes like admission, and they each do so in ways that are distinctive but follow patterns such that related concepts have similar patterns [4]. The result of these challenges is that existing statistical and machine learning data analysis methods, if used naïvely on EHR data, will produced biased results.

Therefore, as both a source of information—e.g., to tease out causality—and as a source of bias to be avoided, time is pervasive in EHR studies. Time has been studied since the creation of the field of biomedical informatics and the use of artificial intelligence in medicine. The remainder of this paper covers topics in the collection and analysis of temporal data, with an emphasis on correcting bias associated with the temporal data. The term, "physics of the medical record," refers to the study of the record as an object of interest in itself (as opposed to the study of the patient) to better understand the health care processes that create the record and the resulting biases associated with the recording of data. It also refers to the general method of building and testing models, aggregating across units, and in some cases employing methods drawn from non-linear time series analysis.

The first challenge is collecting the temporal information. Structured clinical data are usually associated with one or more timestamps, and one of them is often identifiable as a primary time of interest [5]. Narrative clinical data, which today provide a deeper view of the patient in terms of symptoms and clinicians' motivation, require natural language

© Springer International Publishing Switzerland 2015
J.H. Holmes et al. (Eds.): AIME 2015, LNAI 9105, pp. 3–6, 2015.
DOI: 10.1007/978-3-319-19551-3_1

processing, and assessing the time of events abstracted from narrative reports is complex. For example, the time that an event really occurred differs from the time that a patient reports it to a clinician or the time that the clinician writes a note about it. Progress has been made in temporal processing [6] with surprisingly good performance both on predefined tasks [7] and even on general tasks for which the system was not optimized [8,9]. More research is required, however, including understanding how temporal concepts are used. It was previously found, for example, that the uncertainty of temporal declarations is predictable and can be modeled with a regression equation [10] to supply information to downstream analysis.

Temporal data may be analyzed in many ways. The literature is filled with a diverse set of techniques to include time in analyses. This includes machine-learning approaches during phenotyping [11,12], pattern discovery [13,14,15], temporal abstraction over intervals [16,17], and dynamic Bayesian networks [18,19]. Several of these directly handle the irregularity of time [12,13,18,19].

In keeping with the "physics of the medical record" theme, it may be useful to step back and better understand the temporal properties of the EHR. As noted above, data are collected irregularly and in a biased fashion such that patients are sampled more often when they are more ill. Thus they are not at all sampled at random. Furthermore, physiology is by its nature non-stationary—we hope so because our goal is ultimately to change a person's state from ill to healthy. This non-stationarity can affect algorithms. For example, predictive algorithms generally assume that the distributions of data and model parameters remain constant over the prediction period. It was previously demonstrated that the predictability of clinical data is better correlated with sampling frequency than with actual time [20]. Further analysis showed that sequential measurements have roughly constant variability over a broad range of time scales [21]. That is, it appears that clinicians sample patients at a rate commensurate with the change in variability, sampling more often when patients are more ill and generally more variable. It was recently shown that clinicians sometimes over- and sometimes under-correct for changes in variability [22]. By parameterizing a problem not by actual time, but by units of sampling—i.e., arbitrarily define the time between sequential measurements as one—one can achieve greater stationarity and at least in one example improve predictive power [21].

While an EHR may have many health records, the data available for any given patient is often limited, especially once one selects variables relevant to some specific task. The result is a large number of short time series. Combining the information from these disparate patients is challenging because there may be too few measurements in each patient to draw reliable conclusions about each one's time series. Instead, the information implicit in the short time series must be aggregated. In a study of predictability [23], as quantified by the mutual information between different time points within a patient, which was referred to as time-delayed mutual information (TDMI), it was shown that such aggregation could produce interpretable results. A method was developed to decide when such aggregation is warranted [24], how to assess baseline mutual information and therefore excess information, and bias. [25].

Similar work outside of biomedicine [26] demonstrates the generalizability of such research and the benefit of looking broadly outside of biomedicine for new methods.

Given the ability to aggregate time series, one can exploit health record data to uncover correlations among variables, carrying out tasks like pharmacovigilance. A relatively simple algorithm using only lagged linear correlation, linear temporal interpolation, and within-patient normalization, produced informative results about temporal processes based on definitional, physiologic, and intentional associations [27] despite being applied blindly to all health record data regardless of source or clinical context.

With advances in understanding and applying time series methods to health record data, we will be better able to exploit health record data. For example, one study revealed whether seizures in the setting of intracerebral bleed are merely symptoms or whether they cause further morbidity [28]. Further work is needed studying the EHR, studying the health care processes that underlie it, and developing new methods to analyze it.

References

1. Hripcsak, G., Duke, J.D., Shah, N.H., Reich, C.G., Huser, V., Schuemie, M.J., Suchard, M.A., Park, R.W., Wong, I.C.K., Rijnbeek, P.R., van der Lei, J., Pratt, N., Norén, G.N., Lim, Y.C., Stang, P.E., Madigan, D., Ryan, P.B.: Observational Health Data Sciences and Informatics (OHDSI): opportunities for observational researchers. In: MEDINFO 2015, São Paulo, Brazil, August 19-23 (2015)
2. Hripcsak, G., Albers, D.J.: Next-generation phenotyping of electronic health records. J. Am. Med. Inform. Assoc. 20, 117–121 (2013), doi:10.1136/amiajnl-2012-001145.
3. Hripcsak, G., Knirsch, C., Zhou, L., Wilcox, A., Melton, G.B.: Bias associated with mining electronic health records. J. Biomed. Discov. Collab. 6, 48–52 (2011), PMC3149555
4. Hripcsak, G., Albers, D.J.: Correlating electronic health record concepts with health care process events. J. Am. Med. Inform. Assoc. 20(e2), e311-e318 (2013), doi:10.1136/amiajnl-2013-001922.
5. Hripcsak, G., Ludemann, P., Pryor, T.A., Wigertz, O.B., Clayton, P.D.: Rationale for the Arden Syntax. Comput. Biomed. Res. 27, 291–324 (1994)
6. Zhou, L., Hripcsak, G.: Temporal reasoning with medical data - A review with emphasis on medical natural language processing. J. Biomed. Inform. 40, 183–202 (2007)
7. Uzuner, Ö., Stubbs, A., Sun, W.: Chronology of your health events: Approaches to extracting temporal relations from medical narratives. J. Biomed. Inform. 46, S1–S4 (2013)
8. Zhou, L., Parsons, S., Hripcsak, G.: The evaluation of a temporal reasoning system in processing clinical discharge summaries. J. Am. Med. Inform. Assoc. 15, 99–106 (2008), PMC2274869
9. Sun, W., Rumshisky, A., Uzuner, O.: Temporal reasoning over clinical text: the state of the art. J. Am. Med. Inform. Assoc. 20, 814–819 (2013)
10. Hripcsak, G., Elhadad, N., Chen, C., Zhou, L., Morrison, F.P.: Using empirical semantic correlation to interpret temporal assertions in clinical texts. J. Am. Med. Inform. Assoc. 16, 220–227 (2009), PMC2649319
11. Lasko, T.A., Denny, J.C., Levy, M.: Computational phenotype discovery using unsupervised feature learning over noisy, sparse, and irregular clinical data. PLoS One 8, e66341 (2013)

12. Liu, Z., Hauskrecht, M.: Sparse linear dynamical system with its application in multivariate clinical time series. In: NIPS 2013 Workshop on Machine Learning for Clinical Data Analysis and Healthcare (December 2013)
13. Wang, F., Lee, N., Hu, J., Sun, J., Ebadollahi, S.: Towards heterogeneous temporal clinical event pattern discovery: a convolutional approach. In: KDD 2012, Beijing, China, August 12-16, pp. 453–461 (2012)
14. Batal, I., Valizadegan, H., Cooper, G.F., Hauskrecht, M.: A pattern mining approach for classifying multivariate temporal data. In: Proceedings IEEE Int. Conf. Bioinformatics Biomed., pp. 358–365 (2011)
15. Noren, G.N., Hopstadius, J., Bate, A., Star, K., Edwards, I.R.: Temporal pattern discovery in longitudinal electronic patient records. Data Min. Knowl. Discov. 20, 361–387 (2010)
16. Shahar, Y.: A framework for knowledge-based temporal abstraction. Artificial Intelligence 90(1-2), 79–133 (1997)
17. Moskovitch, R., Shahar, Y.: Medical temporal-knowledge discovery via temporal abstraction. In: AMIA Annu. Symp. Proc., pp. 452–456 (2009)
18. Sebastiani, P., Mandl, K.D., Szolovits, P., Kohane, I.S., Ramoni, M.F.: A Bayesian dynamic model for influenza surveillance. Stat. Med. 25(11), 1803–1816 (2006)
19. Ramati, M., Shahar, Y.: Irregular-time Bayesian networks. In: Proceedings of the 26th Conference on Uncertainty in Artificial Intelligence (UAI 2010), Catalina Island, CA, USA (2010)
20. Albers, D.J., Hripcsak, G.: An information-theoretic approach to the phenome (abstract). In: AMIA Summit on Translational Bioinformatics, March 15-17, San Francisco, CA (2009)
21. Hripcsak, G., Albers, D.J., Perotte, A.: Parameterizing time in electronic health record studies. J. Am. Med. Inform. Assoc. (February 26, 2015), pii: ocu051, doi: 10.1093/jamia/ocu051.
22. Lasko, T.A.: Nonstationary Gaussian process regression for evaluating repeated clinical laboratory tests. In: Proceedings of the Twenty-Ninth AAAI Conference on Artificial Intelligence, Austin, TX, January 25-30 (2015)
23. Albers, D.J., Hripcsak, G.: A statistical dynamics approach to the study of human health data: resolving population scale diurnal variation in laboratory data. Physics Letters A 374, 1159–1164 (2010), PMC2882798
24. Albers, D.J., Hripcsak, G.: Using time-delayed mutual information to discover and interpret temporal correlation structure in complex populations. Chaos 22, 013111 (2012), doi:10.1063/1.3675621
25. Albers, D.J., Hripcsak, G.: Estimation of time-delayed mutual information and bias for irregularly and sparsely sampled time-series. Chaos, Solitons & Fractals 45, 853–860 (2012), PMC3332129
26. Komalapriya, C., Thiel, M., Ramano, M.C., Marwan, N., Schwarz, U., Kurths, J.: Reconstruction of a system's dynamics from short trajectories. Phys. Rev. E 78, 066217 (2008)
27. Hripcsak, G., Albers, D.J., Perotte, A.: Exploiting time in electronic health record correlations. J. Am. Med. Inform. Assoc. 18(suppl. 1), i109–i115 (2011)
28. Claassen, J., Albers, D., Schmidt, J.M., De Marchis, G.M., Pugin, D., Falo, C.M., Mayer, S.A., Cremers, S., Agarwal, S., Elkind, M.S.V., Connolly, E.S., Dukic, V., Hripcsak, G., Badjatia, N.: Nonconvulsive seizures in subarachnoid hemorrhage link inflammation and outcome. Annals of Neurology (in press)

Contextualisation of Biomedical Knowledge Through Large-Scale Processing of Literature, Clinical Narratives and Social Media

Goran Nenadic[1,2](✉)

[1] The Farr Institute of Health Informatics Research, Health eResearch Centre, Manchester, UK
[2] School of Computer Science, University of Manchester, Manchester, UK
g.nenadic@manchester.ac.uk

Medicine is often pictured as one of the main examples of "big data science" with a number of challenges and successful stories where *data have saved lives* [1]. In addition to structured databases that store expert-curated information, unstructured and semi-structured data is a huge and often most up-to-date resource of medical knowledge. These include scientific literature, clinical narratives and social media, which typically capture findings, knowledge and experience of the three main "stakeholder" communities: researchers, clinicians and patients/carers. The ability to harness such data is essential for the integration of medical information to support clinical decision making and medical research.

To identify key biomedical information from text, automated text mining has been used for over 30 years [2]. Specific foci in recent years were on mining mentions of clinical *episodes* and *events* (e.g. specific treatments and problems [3]), molecular *interactions* (e.g. profiling diseases [4]), and adverse drug reactions from patient-generated reports [5], in particular capturing *temporal* links and relations between them [6]. Results – despite numerous challenges – have demonstrated the potential in supporting curation of medical knowledge bases, generation and prioritisation of hypotheses for research, reducing the risk of medical errors, inferring clinical care pathways and enhancing medical understanding [1]. For example, state-of-the art text mining has been used to reliably catalogue pain-specific molecular interactions from the literature and identify possible drug targets [4]; extract details of a patient's medication chronology from electronic health records [3]; harvest social media data to support pharmacovigilance [5].

In addition to the extraction of "raw" data, text mining has been used to *contextualise* existing facts. For example, information extracted about the molecular basis of pain can be contextualised with related biological pathways and known drug targets, the patient's disease status, severity and type of pain, anatomical location, etc. [4]. Further, the information can be augmented by provenance, including, for example, recentness of the finding and its "popularity" (e.g. the number of citations), "trustworthiness" of the source, whether it has been disputed or is conflicting with other data etc. Such *contextualised* data aggregated from multiple articles can be then used as detailed 'prior knowledge' to input into medical knowledge systems.

While literature is typically reporting more generic findings, clinical notes and narratives are often the primary and richest source of patient-level information, providing

© Springer International Publishing Switzerland 2015
J.H. Holmes et al. (Eds.): AIME 2015, LNAI 9105, pp. 7–9, 2015.
DOI: 10.1007/978-3-319-19551-3_2

various type of context (e.g. social/family history) and details that are necessary to understand specific patient conditions. For example, free text medication directions often contain detailed information that is not coded elsewhere (e.g. an option to take a tablet when needed up to a maximum number of times a day); extracting such information is key for allowing healthcare data analysts to study the impact of different prescription options and plans (on a large-scale), as well as for personalised "rewiring" of knowledge models (on a "small"-scale, e.g. in clinical decision support).

Complementary to clinical records, patient-led healthcare data co-production (e.g. patient reported outcomes, well-being measures, impact on quality of life or side effects; pre-consultation self-reports, etc.) provide an opportunity to harness the personalised subjective experience that further contextualises knowledge about medical issues.

Extraction and integration of data from all types of medical text are characterised by typical big data issues since the data is complex, heterogeneous, longitudinal, and voluminous, often with partial, missing and "bad" data. Specific challenges include:

- **Conceptual and lexical dynamics**: medical knowledge and clinical practice are constantly changing, which is reflected in the conceptual space represented in literature and clinical notes; the social media space has its own laymen sublanguage that needs to be mapped to the medical knowledge space [5].
- **Variety of forms**: in addition to unstructured text, valuable information is often represented in tables, graphs and figures, requiring multi-modal processing.
- Identification and representation of **modality** and **uncertainty** of extracted research and clinical findings on one hand, and **subjectivisation** of patient-generated data on the other hand is key for contextualisation of knowledge [2].

Similarly to other domains, a critical aspect of medical text mining is ensuring *reproducibility* and *transparency* of the methods to ensure fidelity of extracted data, which can be achieved through development and sharing of digital **research objects** with sufficient details to represent methods, data and knowledge (e.g. http://www.farrcommons.org/). Specifically, given the quality and sensitivity of medical information, *data provenance*, *veracity* and *availability* need to be considered, with details on data collection methods, possible data loss due to personal de-identification of clinical text on one, and possible disclosure risks, on the other hand.

Despite the challenges, text mining is now widely considered as an integral part of medical knowledge management systems, in particular when combined with other semantic technologies (e.g. ontologies and linked data). For example, text mining is widely used as part of clinical decision support systems, typically pointing to related clinical cases (e.g. similar context/history), or supporting monitoring and evaluation of healthcare processes. Either on its own or combined with other resources, text-mined data can also provide a large, dynamic and often most up-to-date base for data analytics and reasoning. Importantly, such data can reflect the three aspects of medicine (clinical practice, science, patients) and can provide necessary meta-data and context for medical/clinical models that are used for disease outcome prediction and/or treatment planning. Text mining is also useful for semi-automated updates of knowledge bases. However, the nature of knowledge extracted from text often requires further consolidation e.g. by identification of conflicting and contrasting facts through application of spatial/temporal analyses and reasoning under uncertainty.

References

1. Jensen, P.B., Jensen, L.J., Brunak, S.: Mining electronic health records: towards better research applications and clinical care. Nat. Rev. Genet. 13(6), 395–405 (2012)
2. Spasic, I., Livsey, J., Keane, J.A., Nenadic, G.: Text mining of cancer-related information: Review of current status and future directions. Int. J. Med. Inform. 83(9), 605–623 (2014)
3. Kovacevic, A., Dehghan, A., Filannino, M., Keane, J., Nenadic, G.: Combining rules and machine learning for extraction of temporal expressions and events from clinical narratives. J. Am. Med. Inform. Assn. 20(5), 859–866 (2013)
4. Jamieson, D.G., Moss, A., Kennedy, M., Jones, S., Nenadic, G., Robertson, D.L., Sidders, B.: The pain interactome: connecting pain specific protein interactions. Pain 155(11), 2243–2252 (2014)
5. Sarker, A., Ginn, R., Nikfarjam, A., O'Connor, K., Smith, K., Jayaraman, S., Upadhaya, T., Gonzalez, G.: Utilizing social media data for pharmacovigilance: A review. J. Biomed. Inf. 54, 202–212 (2015)
6. Sun, W., Rumshisky, A., Uzuner, O.: Evaluating temporal relations in clinical text: 2012 i2b2 Challenge. J. Am. Med. Inform. Assoc. 20(5), 806–813 (2013)

Process Mining and Phenotyping

An Active Learning Framework for Efficient Condition Severity Classification

Nir Nissim[1(✉)], Mary Regina Boland[2], Robert Moskovitch[2], Nicholas P. Tatonetti[2], Yuval Elovici[1], Yuval Shahar[1], and George Hripcsak[2]

[1] Department of Information Systems Engineering, Ben-Gurion University, Beer-Sheva, Israel
nirni.n@gmail.com
[2] Department of Biomedical Informatics, Columbia University, New York, USA

Abstract. Understanding condition severity, as extracted from Electronic Health Records (EHRs), is important for many public health purposes. Methods requiring physicians to annotate condition severity are time-consuming and costly. Previously, a passive learning algorithm called CAESAR was developed to capture severity in EHRs. This approach required physicians to label conditions manually, an exhaustive process. We developed a framework that uses two Active Learning (AL) methods (Exploitation and Combination_XA) to decrease manual labeling efforts by selecting only the most informative conditions for training. We call our approach CAESAR-Active Learning Enhancement (CAESAR-ALE). As compared to passive methods, CAESAR-ALE's first AL method, Exploitation, reduced labeling efforts by 64% and achieved an equivalent true positive rate, while CAESAR-ALE's second AL method, Combination_XA, reduced labeling efforts by 48% and achieved equivalent accuracy. In addition, both these AL methods outperformed the traditional AL method (SVM-Margin). These results demonstrate the potential of AL methods for decreasing the labeling efforts of medical experts, while achieving greater accuracy and lower costs.

Keywords: Active-learning · Condition · Electronic health records · Phenotyping

1 Introduction

Connected health is increasingly becoming an important framework for improving health. A crucial aspect of this includes labeling condition severity for prioritization purposes. Many national and international organizations study medical conditions and their clinical outcomes. The Observational Medical Outcomes Partnership standardized condition/phenotype identification and extraction from electronic data sources, including Electronic Health Records (EHRs) [1]. The Electronic Medical Records and Genomics Network [2] successfully extracted over 20 phenotypes from EHRs [3]. However, defining phenotypes from EHRs is a complex process because of definition discrepancies [4], data sparseness, data quality [5], bias [6], and healthcare process effects [7]. Currently, around 100 conditions/phenotypes have been successfully defined and extracted from

© Springer International Publishing Switzerland 2015
J.H. Holmes et al. (Eds.): AIME 2015, LNAI 9105, pp. 13–24, 2015.
DOI: 10.1007/978-3-319-19551-3_3

EHRs out of the approximately $401,200^1$ conditions they contain. To utilize all data available in EHRs, a prioritized list of conditions classified by severity at the condition-level is needed. Condition-level severity classification can distinguish acne (mild condition) from myocardial infarction (severe condition). In contrast, patient-level severity determines whether a given patient has a mild or severe form of a condition (e.g., acne). The bulk of the literature focuses on patient-level severity. Patient-level severity generally requires individual condition metrics [8-11], although whole-body methods exist [12]. We defined as "severe conditions" those conditions that are life-threatening or permanently disabling, and thus, would have a high priority for generating phenotype definitions for tasks such as pharmacovigilance.

In this paper, we describe the development and validation of a specially designed Active Learning (AL) approach, an approach to learning, the objective of which is to minimize the number of training instances that need to be labeled by experts (see Section 2.3) for classifying condition severity from EHRs. This builds on our previous work using passive learning, called CAESAR (Classification Approach for Extracting Severity Automatically from Electronic Health Records) [13]. We call our algorithm the CAESAR Active Learning Enhancement, or CAESAR-ALE. We show that CAESAR-ALE can reduce the burden on medical experts by minimizing the number of conditions requiring manual severity assignment. Our AL methods, integrated in CAESAR-ALE, actively select during the classification-model training phase only those conditions that both add new informative knowledge to the classification model and improve its classification performance. This focused, informed selection contrasts with the randomly selected, poorly informative conditions that are selected by a passive learning method.

2   Background and Significance

Our previous algorithm, CAESAR, used passive learning to capture condition severity from EHRs [13]. This method required medical experts to review conditions manually and assign a severity status (severe or mild) to each. The resulting reference-standard contained 516-labeled conditions. Because of the significant effort involved, only a relatively small number of conditions was labeled by a group of human experts in the original CAESAR study [13]. These severity assignments were then used to evaluate the quality of CAESAR.

2.1   SNOMED-CT

The Systemized Nomenclature of Medicine-Clinical Terms (SNOMED-CT) is a specialized ontology developed for conditions obtained during the clinical encounter and recorded in EHRs [14, 15]. SNOMED-CT is the terminology of choice of the World Health Organization and the International Health Terminology Standards Development Organization and satisfies the Meaningful Use requirements of the Health Information Technology component of the American Recovery and Reinvestment Act

---

[1] The number of SNOMED-CT codes as of September 9, 2014. Accessed via: http://bioportal.bioontology.org/ontologies/SNOMEDCT

of 2009 [16]. We used SNOMED-CT, because clinical ontologies are useful for retrieval [17]. Each coded clinical event is considered a "condition" or "phenotype," knowing that this is a broad definition [4].

2.2 Classification of Conditions

In biomedicine, condition classification follows two main approaches: 1) manual approaches, where experts manually assign labels to conditions [18-22]; and 2) passive classification approaches that require a labeled training set and are based on machine learning approaches and text classification [23-24].

2.3 Active Learning

AL approaches are learning methods useful for selecting, during the learning process, the most discriminative and informative conditions from the entire dataset, thus minimizing the number of instances that experts need to review manually. Studies in several domains have successfully applied AL to reduce the time and money required for labeling examples [25-27]. The two major AL approaches are *membership queries* [28], in which examples are artificially generated from the problem space, and *selective-sampling* [29], in which examples are selected from a pool (a method used in this paper). Applications in the biomedical domain remain limited. Liu described a method similar to relevance feedback for cancer classification [30]. Warmuth et al. used a similar approach to separate compounds for drug discovery [31]. More recently, AL was applied in biomedicine for text [32] and radiology report classification [33].

3 Materials and Methods

3.1 Dataset

The development and evaluation of CAESAR-ALE used the CAESAR dataset developed previously [13], which contains 516 conditions (SNOMED-CT codes) labeled as mild and severe. These 516 conditions were randomly selected out a total of 4683 unlabeled conditions. The gold-standard labeling of the 516 conditions used in the current study was manual, following an automated filtering phase that significantly reduced the labeling expert's effort (e.g., all malignant cancers and accidents were labeled as "severe"), as described elsewhere [13]. The dataset contains six severity features for each condition: the number of comorbidities, procedures, and medications; cost; treatment time; and a proportion term. Each one of these features describing a specific condition was aggregated as an average value for all the records of the same condition in the EHR system.

3.2 The CAESAR-ALE Framework

The purpose of CAESAR-ALE is to decrease experts' labeling efforts. Utilizing AL methods, CAESAR-ALE directs only informative conditions to experts for labeling. Informative conditions are defined as those that improve the classification model's predictive capabilities when added to the training set. Figure 1 illustrates the process of labeling and acquiring new conditions by maintaining the updatability of the classification model within CAESAR-ALE. Conditions are introduced to the classification model, which is based on the SVM algorithm and AL methods, using both of which the informative conditions are selected and sent to medical expert for annotation. We can maintain an accurate model and decrease labeling efforts by adding only two types of informative conditions: 1) those identified by the classifier as low confidence (similar probability that the condition is mild and severe) and 2) those conditions that are at a maximal distance from the separating hyper-plane (see **Equation 1**). These conditions are deep within the "severe" instances sub-space of the SVM's separating hyper-plane. Adding the mild conditions that exist within this space of otherwise severe conditions greatly informs and improves the classification model. The overall CAESAR-ALE framework integrates two main phases. **Training:** The model is trained using an initial set of severe and mild conditions and evaluated against a test set consisting of conditions not used during training. **Classification and updating:** The AL method ranks how informative each condition is using the classification model's prediction. Only the most informative are selected and labeled by the expert. These conditions are added to the training set and removed from the pool. The model is then retrained using the updated training set. This process is repeated until all conditions in the pool have been added to the training set. We employed the SVM classification algorithm using the radial basis function (RBF) kernel in a supervised learning approach, because it has proven to be very efficient when combined with AL methods [26], [27]. We used the Lib-SVM implementation [34] because it supports multiclass classification.

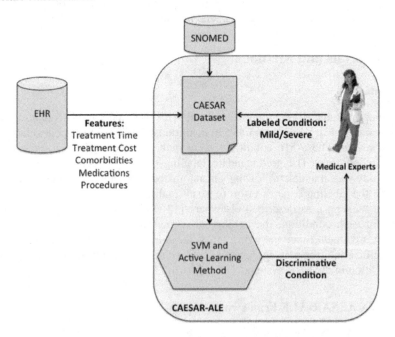

Fig. 1. Process of using AL methods to detect discriminative conditions requiring medical expert annotation

3.3   Active Learning Methods

CAESAR-ALE uses two AL methods (Exploitation and Combination_XA), described below, together with the SVM-margin and random method.

3.3.1   Random Selection or Passive Learning (Random)

Random selection, machine learning's default case/"lower bound," involves adding conditions randomly selected from the pool to the training set.

3.3.2   The SVM-Simple-Margin AL Method (SVM-Margin)

The SVM-Simple-Margin method [35] (or SVM-Margin) is directly related to the SVM classifier. SVM-Margin selects examples to explore and acquire informative conditions according to their distance from the separating hyper-plane, disregarding their classified label. Examples that lie closest to the separating hyper-plane (inside the margin) are more likely to be informative and therefore are acquired and labeled. SVM-Margin is fast and yet has significant limitations [35] based on assumptions that have been shown to fail [36].

3.3.3   Exploitation

Exploitation, one of CAESAR-ALE's AL methods, efficiently detects malicious contents, files, and documents [37-41]. Exploitation is based on SVM classifier principles, selecting examples more likely to be severe lying further from the separating hyper-plane. Thus, this method supports the goal of boosting the classification capabilities of the model by acquiring as many new severe conditions as possible. Exploitation rates the distance of every condition X from the separating hyper-plane using **Equation 1** based on the Normal of the separating hyper-plane of the SVM classifier that serves as the classification model. Accordingly, the distance in **Equation 1** is calculated between example X and W (**Equation 2**), the Normal that represents the separating hyper-plane.

$$Dist(X) = \left(\sum_{1}^{n} \alpha_i y_i K(x_i \, x) \right) \tag{1}$$

$$w = \sum_{1}^{n} \alpha_i y_i \Phi(x_i) \tag{2}$$

To optimally enhance the training set, we also checked the similarity among selected conditions using the kernel farthest-first (KFF) method, suggested by Baram et al. [42], enabling us to avoid acquiring similar conditions, which would waste manual analysis resources.

3.3.4   Combination_XA: A Combined Active Learning Method

The "Combination_XA" method is a hybrid of SVM-Margin and Exploitation. It conducts a cross acquisition (XA) of informative conditions, meaning that during the first trial (and all odd-numbered trials) it acquires conditions according to SVM-Margin criteria and during the next trial (and all even-numbered trials) it selects conditions using Exploitation's criteria. This strategy alternates between the exploration phases (conditions acquired using SVM-margin) and the exploitation phase (conditions acquired using Exploitation) to select the most informative conditions, both mild and severe, while boosting the classification model with severe conditions or very informative mild conditions that lie deep inside the severe side of the SVM's hyper-plane.

4   Evaluation

The objective of our experiments was to evaluate the performance of CAESAR-ALE's two new AL methods and compare it with that of the existing AL method, SVM-Margin, for two tasks:

(1) To update the predictive capabilities (Accuracy) of the classification model that serves as the knowledge store of AL methods and improve its ability to identify efficiently the most informative new conditions.

(2) To identify the method that best improves the capabilities of the classification model by correctly classifying conditions according to the accuracy measure and also specifically severe conditions as assessed by the *true positive rate* (TPR), with minimal errors as measured by the *false positive rate* (FPR). This task is of particular importance, given the need to identify severe conditions from the outset.

In our first acquisition experiment, we used 516 conditions (372 mild, 144 severe) in our repository and created 10 randomly selected datasets, with each dataset containing three elements: an initial set of six conditions that were used to induce the initial classification model, a test set of 200 conditions on which the classification was tested and evaluated after every trial in which it was updated, and a pool of 310 unlabeled conditions. Informative conditions were selected according to each method's criteria and then sent to a medical expert for labeling. Conditions were later acquired by the training set for enrichment with an additional five new informative conditions. The process was repeated over the next trials until the entire pool was acquired. The performance of the classification model was averaged for 10 runs over the 10 different datasets that were created.

The experiment's steps (below) are repeated until the entire pool is acquired:

(1) Induce the initial classification model from the initial training set.

(2) Evaluate the classification model's initial performance using the test set.

(3) Introduce unlabeled conditions to the pool for the selective sampling method. The five most informative conditions are selected according to each method's criteria and then sent to the medical expert for labeling.

(4) Add acquired conditions to the training set (removing them from the pool).

(5) Induce an updated classification model by using the updated training set and applying the updated model on the pool (now containing fewer conditions).

5   Results

Results are presented for the core evaluation measures used in this study: accuracy and TPR. We also measured the number of new severe conditions discovered and acquired into the training set at each trial.

Figure 2 presents accuracy levels and their trends in the 62 trials with an acquisition level of 5 conditions per trial (62*5=310 conditions in pool). In most trials, the AL methods outperformed Random selection, illustrating that using AL methods can reduce the number of conditions required to achieve accuracy similar to that of passive learning (i.e., random). The classification model had an initial accuracy of 0.72, and all methods converged at an accuracy of 0.975 after the pool was fully acquired. Combination_XA reached a 0.95 rate of accuracy first, requiring 23 acquisition trials (115/310 conditions), while the other AL methods required 26 trials. Furthermore, Combination_XA required only approximately half the number of conditions required by the random acquisition method (23 vs. 44 trials), while achieving the same accuracy of 0.95.

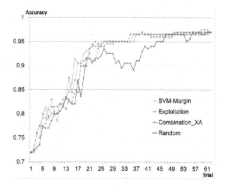

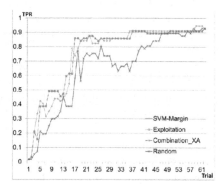

Fig. 2. The accuracy of CAESAR-ALE AL methods versus SVM-Margin and Random over 62 trials (five conditions acquired during each trial)

Fig. 3. TPR for active and passive learning methods over 62 trials

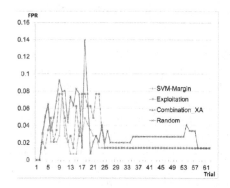

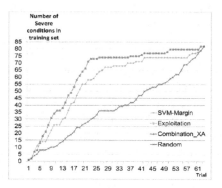

Fig. 4. FPR for active and passive learning methods over 62 trials

Fig. 5. Number of acquired severe conditions for active and passive learning methods over 62 trials

Figure 3 shows TPR levels and their trends over 62 trials. Exploitation outper-formed the other selection methods, achieving a TPR rate of 0.85 after only 17 trials (85/310 conditions). This was much better than random selection (TPR=0.85 after 47 trials), and performance improved as additional conditions were acquired. After 36 trials, all AL methods converged to TPR rates around 0.92. Our results demonstrate that using AL methods for condition selection can reduce the number of trials re-quired in training the classifier, thereby reducing the total number of conditions re-quired for medical expert labeling, and correspondingly reducing the training costs.

Figure 4 shows FPR levels and their trends over 62 trials. It can be seen that throughout the trials, the random selection method had the highest FPR values, as compared to the AL methods. Furthermore, its FPR levels were mostly unstable until the end of the trials. In contrast, from trial 23 onward, all the AL methods displayed a low and stable FPR of 1.3%. Considering the TPR and FPR measures together, we can see how efficient the AL methods were, in spite of the unbalanced mix of condi-tion severities in our data set.

The cumulative number of severe conditions acquired for each trial is shown in Figure 5. By the fifth trial, Exploitation and Combination_XA outperformed the other selection methods (both lines overlap in **Figure 5**). We observed that after 23 trials (115 conditions) both of CAESAR-ALE's methods acquired 73 out of 82 severe con-ditions in the pool, as compared to 42 trials (210 conditions) for SVM-Margin and 60 trials (300 conditions) for random. This represents a 46% reduction as compared to SVM-margin and a 62% reduction as compared to random. After 23 trials **(Figure 5),** we observed the largest difference between CAESAR-ALE's methods and random, a difference of 43 severe conditions.

6   Discussion

We present CAESAR-ALE, an AL framework for identifying informative conditions for medical expert labeling. CAESAR-ALE was evaluated based on accuracy and TPR. Traditional passive learning approaches require large amounts of training data to achieve a satisfactory performance. Exploitation achieved a TPR of 0.85 after only 17 trials (a scenario in which only 85 conditions would require manual expert label-ing), whereas random selection required 47 trials or 235 conditions to achieve the same TPR, representing a 64% reduction in labeling efforts. This would reduce costs by almost two-thirds, allowing medical experts to focus their energy elsewhere. In terms of accuracy, Combination_XA performed best with a reduction in the number of trials from 44 to 23, as compared to the random acquisition method. Therefore, the Combination_XA method required 115 vs. 220 conditions (representing a 48% reduc-tion) to achieve equivalent accuracy. The Exploitation and Combination_XA methods have an exploitation phase during which they attempt to acquire more severe condi-tions. They both acquire mild conditions when they are thought to be severe, and this contributes to the methods' strong acquisition performance. These mild conditions are very informative to the classification model, because they lead to a major modifica-tion of the SVM margin and its separating hyper-plane. Consequently, acquisition of these conditions improves the performance of the model.

In contrast, traditional AL methods (e.g., SVM-Margin) focus on acquiring conditions that lead to only small changes in its separating hyper-plane and contribute less to the improvement of the classification model. Our research points to the existence of noisy "mild" conditions lying deep within what seems to be the sub-space of the "severe" conditions. This is explained in a recent study focused on the detection of PC worms [38] that mentioned "surprising" cases that are very informative and valuable to the improvement of the classification model, and helpful in acquiring severe conditions that eventually update and enrich the knowledge store. These conditions are more informative than severe conditions, because they provide relevant information that was previously not considered (they were initially classified tentatively as severe by the classifier when they are mild). SVM-Margin acquires examples that the classification model determines to be low confidence. Consequently, they are informative but not necessarily severe. In contrast, the CAESAR-ALE framework is oriented toward acquiring the most informative severe conditions by obtaining conditions from the severe side of the SVM margin. As a result, more new severe conditions are acquired in earlier trials. Additionally, if an acquired condition that lies deep within the supposedly severe side of the margin is found to be mild, it is still informative (perhaps even more so) and can be used to improve the iteratively modified classifier's classification capabilities in the next trials.

In our future work, we hope to develop an online tool that medical experts can use to label condition severity. This should further reduce the workload on busy clinicians, and offer an easy to use method for condition-level severity labeling. Using several different labelers for subsets of conditions, we would like to scrutinize and analyze the difference between the different labelers and understand how AL methods can handle these differences. The presented approach is general and not domain-dependent; therefore, it can be applied to and provide a solution for every medical domain (and even non-medical domains) in which it is beneficial to reduce the costly or time-consuming labeling efforts at training time. In addition, we will consider applying our AL framework to the publicly available MIMIC II intensive care domain database, to understand better the benefits of applying active learning methods to various medical domains.

7   Conclusions

We presented the CAESAR-ALE framework, which uses AL to identify important conditions for labeling. AL methods are based on the predictive capabilities of the classification model; thus, an updated classification model directly affects the AL method's ability to select the most informative conditions and thereby decreases labeling efforts. CAESAR-ALE reduced labeling efforts by 48%, while achieving equivalent accuracy. Overall, CAESAR-ALE demonstrates the strength and utility of employing AL methods that are specially designed for the biomedical domain. In addition, both our AL methods (Exploitation and Combination_XA) outperformed the traditional AL method (SVM-Margin). These results demonstrate the potential of AL methods for decreasing the labeling efforts of medical experts, while achieving greater accuracy and lower costs.

References

1. Stang, P.E., Ryan, P.B., Racoosin, J.A., et al.: Advancing the science for active surveillance: rationale and design for the Observational Medical Outcomes Partnership. Ann. Intern. Med. 153(9), 600–606 (2010)
2. Kho, A.N., Pacheco, J.A., Peissig, P.L., et al.: Electronic medical records for genetic research: results of the eMERGE consortium. Science Translational Medicine 3(79), 79re1 (2011)
3. Denny, J.C., Ritchie, M.D., Basford, M.A., et al.: PheWAS: demonstrating the feasibility of a phenome-wide scan to discover gene–disease associations. Bioinformatics 26(9), 1205–1210 (2010)
4. Boland, M.R., Hripcsak, G., Shen, Y., Chung, W.K., Weng, C.: Defining a comprehensive verotype using electronic health records for personalized medicine. J. Am. Med. Inform. Assoc. 20(e2), e232–e238 (2013)
5. Weiskopf, N.G., Weng, C.: Methods and dimensions of electronic health record data quality assessment: enabling reuse for clinical research. J. Am. Med. Inform. Assoc. 20(1), 144–151 (2013)
6. Hripcsak, G., Knirsch, C., Zhou, L., Wilcox, A., Melton, G.B.: Bias associated with mining electronic health records. Journal of Biomedical Discovery and Collaboration 6, 48 (2011)
7. Hripcsak, G., Albers, D.J.: Correlating electronic health record concepts with healthcare process events. J. Am. Med. Inform. Assoc. 20(e2), e311–e318 (2013)
8. Rich, P., Scher, R.K.: Nail psoriasis severity index: a useful tool for evaluation of nail psoriasis. Journal of the American Academy of Dermatology 49(2), 206–212 (2003)
9. Bastien, C.H., Vallières, A., Morin, C.M.: Validation of the Insomnia Severity Index as an outcome measure for insomnia research. Sleep Medicine 2(4), 297–307 (2001)
10. McLellan, A.T., Kushner, H., Metzger, D., et al.: The fifth edition of the Addiction Severity Index. Journal of Substance Abuse Treatment 9(3), 199–213 (1992)
11. Rockwood, T.H., Church, J.M., Fleshman, J.W., et al.: Patient and surgeon ranking of the severity of symptoms associated with fecal incontinence. Diseases of the Colon & Rectum 42(12), 1525–1531 (1999)
12. Horn, S.D., Horn, R.: Reliability and validity of the severity of illness index. Medical Care 24(2), 159–178 (1986)
13. Boland, M.R., Tatonetti, N., Hripcsak, G.: CAESAR: A classification approach for extracting severity automatically from electronic health records. In: Intelligent Systems for Molecular Biology Phenotype Day, Boston, MA, pp. 1–8 (2014) (in Press)
14. Elkin, P.L., Brown, S.H., Husser, C.S., et al.: Evaluation of the content coverage of SNOMED CT: ability of SNOMED clinical terms to represent clinical problem lists. In: Mayo Clinic Proceedings, pp. 741–748. Elsevier (2006)
15. Stearns, M.Q., Price, C., Spackman, K.A., Wang, A.: SNOMED clinical terms: overview of the development process and project status. In: Proceedings of the AMIA Symposium 2001, p. 662. American Medical Informatics Association (2001)
16. Elhanan, G., Perl, Y., Geller, J.: A survey of SNOMED CT direct users, 2010: impressions and preferences regarding content and quality. Journal of the American Medical Informatics Association 18(suppl. 1), i36–i44 (2011)
17. Moskovitch, R., Shahar, Y.: Vaidurya–a concept-based, context-sensitive search engine for clinical guidelines. American Medical Informatics Association (2004)

18. HCUP Chronic Condition Indicator for ICD-9-CM. Healthcare Cost and Utilization Project (HCUP) (2011), http://www.hcup-us.ahrq.gov/toolssoftware/chronic/chronic.jsp (accessed on February 25, 2014)
19. Hwang, W., Weller, W., Ireys, H., Anderson, G.: Out-of-pocket medical spending for care of chronic conditions. Health Affairs 20(6), 267–278 (2001)
20. Chi, M.-J., Lee, C.-Y., Wu, S.-C.: The prevalence of chronic conditions and medical expenditures of the elderly by chronic condition indicator (CCI). Archives of Gerontology and Geriatrics 52(3) (2011)
21. Perotte, A., Pivovarov, R., Natarajan, K., Weiskopf, N., Wood, F., Elhadad, N.: Diagnosis code assignment: models and evaluation metrics. Journal of the American Medical Informatics Association 21(2), 231–237 (2014)
22. Perotte, A., Hripcsak, G.: Temporal properties of diagnosis code time series in aggregate. IEEE Journal of Biomedical and Health Informatics 17(2), 477–483 (2013)
23. Torii, M., Wagholikar, K., Liu, H.: Using machine learning for concept extraction on clinical documents from multiple data sources. Journal of the American Medical Informatics Association (June 27, 2011)
24. Nguyen, A.N., Lawley, M.J., Hansen, D.P., et al.: Symbolic rule-based classification of lung cancer stages from free-text pathology reports. Journal of the American Medical Informatics Association 17(4), 440–445 (2010)
25. Nissim, N., Moskovitch, R., Rokach, L., Elovici, Y.: Novel active learning methods for enhanced PC malware detection in windows OS. Expert Systems with Applications 41(13), 5843–5857 (2014)
26. Nissim, N., Moskovitch, R., Rokach, L., Elovici, Y.: Detecting unknown computer worm activity via support vector machines and active learning. Pattern Analysis and Applications 15, 459–475 (2012)
27. Nissim, N., Cohen, A., Glezer, C., Elovici, Y.: Detection of malicious PDF files and directions for enhancements: A state-of-the art survey. Computers & Security 48, 246–266 (2015)
28. Angluin, D.: Queries and concept learning. Machine Learning 2, 319–342 (1988)
29. Lewis, D., Gale, W.: A sequential algorithm for training text classifiers. In: Proceedings of the Seventeenth Annual International ACM-SIGIR Conference on Research and Development in Information Retrieval, pp. 3–12. Springer (1994)
30. Liu, Y.: Active learning with support vector machine applied to gene expression data for cancer classification. Journal of Chemical Information and Computer Sciences 44(6), 1936–1941 (2004)
31. Warmuth, M.K., Liao, J., Rätsch, G., Mathieson, M., Putta, S., Lemmen, C.: Active learning with support vector machines in the drug discovery process. Journal of Chemical Information and Computer Sciences 43(2), 667–673 (2003)
32. Figueroa, R.L., Zeng-Treitler, Q., Ngo, L.H., Goryachev, S., Wiechmann, E.P.: Active learning for clinical text classification: is it better than random sampling? Journal of the American Medical Informatics Association (2011), 2012:amiajnl-2011-000648
33. Nguyen, D.H., Patrick, J.D.: Supervised machine learning and active learning in classification of radiology reports. Journal of the American Medical Informatics Association (2014)
34. Chang, C.C., Lin, C.J.: LIBSVM: a library for support vector machines. ACM Transactions on Intelligent Systems and Technology (TIST) 2(3), 27 (2011)
35. Tong, S., Koller, D.: Support vector machine active learning with applications to text classification. Journal of Machine Learning Research 2, 45–66 (2000-2001)
36. Ralf, H., Graepel, T., Campbell, C.: Bayes point machines. The Journal of Machine Learning Research 1, 245–279 (2001)

37. Nissim, N., Moskovitch, R., Rokach, L., Elovici, Y.: Novel active learning methods for enhanced pc malware detection in Windows OS. Expert Systems With Applications 41(13) (2014)
38. Nissim, N., Moskovitch, R., Rokach, L., Elovici, Y.: Detecting unknown computer worm activity via support vector machines and active learning. Pattern Analysis and Applications 15(4), 459–475 (2012)
39. Moskovitch, R., Nissim, N., Elovici, Y.: Malicious code detection using active learning. In: ACM SIGKDD Workshop in Privacy, Security and Trust in KDD, Las Vegas (2008)
40. Moskovitch, R., Stopel, D., Feher, C., Nissim, N., Japkowicz, N., Elovici, Y.: Unknown malcode detection and the imbalance problem. Journal in Computer Virology 5(4) (2009)
41. Nissim, N., Cohen, A., Moskovitch, R., et al.: ALPD: Active learning framework for enhancing the detection of malicious PDF files aimed at organizations. In: Proceedings of JISIC (2014)
42. Baram, Y., El-Yaniv, R., Luz, K.: Online choice of active learning algorithms. Journal of Machine Learning Research 5, 255–291 (2004)
43. Herman R. 72 Statistics on Hourly Physician Compensation (2013), http://www.beckershospitalreview.com/compensation-issues/72-statistics-on-hourly-physician-compensation.html

Predictive Monitoring of Local Anomalies in Clinical Treatment Processes

Zhengxing Huang[1], Jose M. Juarez[2], Wei Dong[3], Lei Ji[4], Huilong Duan[1(✉)]

[1] College of Biomedical Engineering and Instrument Science,
Zhejiang University, Hangzhou, China
`zhengxing.h@gmail.com, duanhl@zju.edu.cn`
[2] Department of Information and Communication Engineering,
University of Murcia, Murcia, Spain
[3] Cardiology Department of Chinese PLA General Hospital, Beijing, China
[4] IT Department of Chinese PLA General Hospital, Beijing, China

Abstract. Local anomalies are small outliers that exist in some sub-segments of clinical treatment processes (CTPs). They provide crucial information to medical staff and hospital managers for determining the efficient medical service delivered to individual patients, and for promptly handling unusual treatment behaviors in CTPs. Existing studies mainly focused on the detection of large deviations of CTPs, called of global anomalous inpatient traces. However, local anomalies in inpatient traces are easily overlooked by existing approaches. In some medical problems, such as unstable angina, local anomalies are important since they may indicate unexpected changes of patients' physical conditions. In this work, we propose a predictive monitoring service on local anomalies using a Latent Dirichlet Allocation (LDA)-based probabilistic model. The proposal was evaluated in the study of unstable angina CTP, testing 12,152 patient traces from the Chinese PLA General Hospital.

1 Introduction

Clinical treatment processes (CTPs), being affected by many factors and uncertainties, are unpredictable by nature. Many concepts, such as clinical practical guidelines, or clinical pathways, have been adopted by health-care organizations to standardize CTPs, normalize treatment behaviors, reduce variations, decrease costs and improve quality, etc [1,2]. Unfortunately, patient traces may not go well towards the expected direction, and they have deviations with the predefined CTPs. In fact, the uncertainties, resulting from inter-observer variability, inaccurate evaluation of the patient and some deficiencies in grading scales [3,4], make the organization of clinical work corresponding challenging, and lead to breakdowns such as delays, waste of resources and cancelations on the day of surgery, etc [1]. In such cases, local anomalies happen inevitably.

Unlike global anomalous patient traces of CTPs, which are largely deviated from normal ones, local anomalies are unusual treatment events existing in some subsegments in patient traces of CTPs [5]. They may occur occasionally in regular patient traces, although in which normal treatment behaviors are frequently

J.H. Holmes et al. (Eds.): AIME 2015, LNAI 9105, pp. 25–34, 2015.
DOI: 10.1007/978-3-319-19551-3_4

and consistently present. For CTP analysis, it is imperative to predict potential local anomalies from observations in a maximally-informative manner. Once these unusual events are timely predicted, a health-care organization can either update its CTP specifications to cover the respective case, or it can adjust an ongoing patient trace to enforce best clinical practice execution. In this way, local anomaly prediction is a central piece in the puzzle of advancing health-care organizations towards effective and efficient CP management and health service delivery.

In many applications, local anomalies are detected only after they have occurred in CTPs. Alternatively, this work presents a new approach to provide predictive monitoring of local anomalies in CPs. In detail, we employ a probabilistic topic model to disclose essential features of CTPs from clinical event logs. The generated probabilistic topic model provides an accurate description of CTPs by combining different classes of distributions. In particular, it recognizes patient traces as a probabilistic combination of underlying treatment patterns, and describes treatment patterns as a probabilistic combination of various clinical events [6]. Based on the derived topic model, a predictive monitoring service of local anomalies in CTPs is provided on ongoing patient traces, which looks insight into CTPs to map the prediction task to a classification task such that unusual variant execution of clinical activities can be timely predicted in an ongoing patient trace. The proposed approach is evaluated via real-world data set consisting of 12,152 patient traces and collected from the Cardiology department of Chinese PLA General Hospital.

2   Preliminary

Formally, let A be the treatment activity domain, and T the time domain. A clinical event e is represented as $e = (a, t)$, where a is the clinical activity type of e ($a \in A$), and t is the occurring time of e ($t \in T$). For convenience, let $e.a$ and $e.t$ be the activity type and the occurring time stamp of e, respectively. A clinical event is a performed treatment activity at a particular time stamp. A patient trace is represented by $\sigma = id : \langle e_1, e_2, \ldots, e_n \rangle$, where id is the patient identifier, and $\langle e_1, e_2, \ldots, e_n \rangle$ ($n \geq 2$) is a finite non-empty sequence of clinical events such that $e_1.a = admission$, $e_n.a = discharged$, and each event appears only once, and time is non-decreasing, i.e., for $1 \leq i \leq j \leq n : e_i \neq e_j$ and $e_i.t \leq e_j.t$. A clinical event log $\mathcal{L}$ is a set of patient traces, i.e., $\mathcal{L} = \{\sigma\}$.

For example, Figure 1(A) shows an example patient trace (patient id: 476104-3) of the Unstable Angina (UA) CTP in the hospital. The trace contains a set of clinical activities, and spread along the observed time period of the patient's length of stay, i.e., $\langle (admission, 1), (xray, 1), \cdots, (discharge, 12) \rangle$.

3   Methodology

In this study, we use an extension of Latent Dirichlet Allocation (LDA) to model patient traces, named clinical pathway model (CPM) that we presented in our

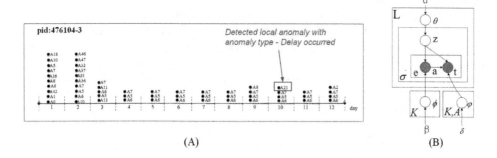

Fig. 1. (A) An example patient trace of the Unstable Angina clinical treatment process. (B) Graphical representation of Clinical Pathway Model (CPM)[6].

previous work [6]. As shown in Figure 1(B), using CPM, each patient trace is modeled as a multinomial distribution of treatment patterns, and each treatment pattern is modeled as a multinomial distribution of clinical events. CPM assumes a Dirichlet prior distribution on the treatment pattern mixture parameters θ, ϕ, and φ, to provide a complete generative model for patient traces. θ is an $|\mathcal{L}| \times K$ matrix of patient trace-specific mixture weights for the K treatment patterns, each drawn from a Dirichlet (α) prior. ϕ is an $A \times K$ matrix of clinical activity-specific mixture weights over A activity types for the K treatment patterns, each drawn from a Dirichlet (β) prior. φ is an $T \times A \times K$ matrix of occurring time stamp-specific mixture weights over T time instants for V activity types and K treatment patterns, each drawn from a Dirichlet (γ) prior. Fitting the proposed CPM is equivalent to finding parameters α, β, and γ that maximize the likelihood of the data for patient traces in an event log:

$$\text{Likelihood}(\alpha, \beta, \gamma) = \prod_{\sigma \in \mathcal{L}} \int P(\theta_\sigma | \alpha)$$

$$\times (\prod_{e \in \sigma} \sum_{z=1}^{K} P(e.t | z, e.a, \gamma) P(e.a | z, \beta) P(z | \theta_\sigma)) d\theta_\sigma \qquad (1)$$

where K is the number of treatment patterns and each patient trace σ consists of a set of clinical events **e**. For a more detailed description of the learning process, please refer to [6]. The general idea in this study is based on the hypothesis that a patient trace σ can be represented as a mixture of treatment patterns. To perform a particular treatment pattern then means to conduct a clinical event e with a certain probability from the pool of clinical events of that pattern. Equation (1) describes how to employ CPM to calculate the likelihood of a particular clinical event e given a particular patient trace σ:

$$P(e | \sigma) = \sum_{z \in K} P(e | z) P(z | \sigma) = \sum_{z \in K} P(e.t | z, e.a) P(e.a | z) P(z | \sigma) \qquad (2)$$

where $P(e|z)$ is the probability of e within the treatment pattern z, and $P(z|\sigma)$ is the probability of performing a clinical event from z in the whole patient trace σ. Note that the number of latent treatment patterns K has to be defined in advance and allows to adjust the degree of specialization of the latent patterns. The derived CPM estimates the pattern-event distribution $P(e|z) = P(e.t|z, e.a)P(e.a|z)$ and the trace-pattern distribution $P(z|\sigma)$ from a clinical event log using Dirichlet priors for the distributions and a fixed number of treatment patterns [6]:

$$P(e|\sigma) = \sum_{z \in K} P(e.t|z, e.a)P(e.a|z)P(z|\sigma) = \varphi_{e.t,e.a,z}\phi_{e.a,z}\theta_{\sigma,z} \qquad (3)$$

Equation (2) can be used to detect whether a clinical event is normal or abnormal with respect to the host patient trace. To this end, we define the normality measure of a particular clinical event e given a particular patient trace σ as follows:

$$\Xi(e, \sigma) = \frac{P(e|\sigma)}{\max_{e' \in \sigma', \sigma' \in \mathcal{L}} P(e'|\sigma')} \qquad (4)$$

where e' denotes the typical clinical event in the log $\mathcal{L}$ which receives the largest probability given a particular patient trace σ'. Based on the normality measure $\Xi(e, \sigma)$, we define two specific thresholds ν_{low} and ν_{up} ($0 \leq \nu_{low} < \nu_{up} \leq 1$) for classifying an unusual clinical event e into one of the four following a local CTP anomaly types:

- **Unexpected event**: e is an unexpected clinical event to a particular patient trace σ in the observable time domain T, iff $e \in \sigma$, $\Xi(e, \sigma) < \nu_{low}$, and $\nexists t \in T$, where $t \leq \max\{e'.t|e' \in \sigma\}$ and $\Xi(\langle e.a, t \rangle, \sigma) \geq \nu_{low}$.
- **Absent event**: e is an absent event to a particular patient trace σ in the observable time domain T, iff $e \notin \sigma$, and
- $\Xi(e, \sigma) > \nu_{up}$.
- **Early event**: e is an early event to a particular patient trace σ in the observable time domain T, iff $e \in \sigma$, $\Xi(e, \sigma) < \nu_{low}$, and $\exists T_\sigma$, $T_\sigma \subseteq T$ and $T_\sigma \neq \emptyset$, where $\forall t \in T_\sigma$ satisfying $t \leq \max\{e'.t|e' \in \sigma\}$ and $\Xi(\langle e.a, t \rangle, \sigma) \geq \nu_{low}$, and $\forall t \in T_\sigma$, $e.t < t$.
- **Delay event**: e is a delay event to a particular patient trace σ in the observable time domain T, if $e \in \sigma$, $\Xi(e, \sigma) < \nu_{low}$, and $\exists T_\sigma$, $T_\sigma \subseteq T$ and $T_\sigma \neq \emptyset$, where $\forall t \in T_\sigma$ satisfying $t \leq \max\{e'.t|e' \in \sigma\}$ and $\Xi(\langle e.a, t \rangle, \sigma) \geq \nu_{low}$, and $\forall t \in T_\sigma$, $e.t > t$.

Taking the detected local anomaly $x = \langle A21, \text{delay} \rangle$ shown in Figure 1(A) as an example, it illustrates that there is a delay-occurred treatment event that relates to one (i.e., patient id: 476104-3) out of the selected patient traces. This observation, in turn, provides a starting point for the analysis of the respective CTP. The reasons for delay occurred execution of treatment activity $A21$ have to be determined as root causes for non-compliant treatment behavior in its host patient trace.

Based on the definitions above, we can detect local anomalies taking place in complete patient traces, and then use the detected anomalies to build a classification model such that ongoing patient traces can be checked if local anomalies could occur and in which type. The rationale of the proposed local anomaly prediction is described as follows: for a given clinical activity a, the execution of a (a.k.a a clinical event) in a complete patient trace can be viewed as a training sample. In particular, treatment information such as patient conditions recorded in clinical event logs can be viewed as features of this training sample. In addition, the training sample has a class label that indicates the execution state of a, i.e., normal, unexpected, absent, early, or delay. Then, supervised machine learning algorithms such as decision tree, support vector machine (SVM), etc., can take a set of training samples with known class labels as input, and generate a classifier. The generated classifier can then be used to assign a label to an unknown sample, which, in the context of CTPs, is the predicted execution state of a in an ongoing patient trace. Note that the process of creating a classifier from a set of training samples is known as training the classifier.

indent To train a classifier for predicting variant execution state of a target clinical activity, we need to provide a set of training samples to the machine learning algorithms. In this study, we consider patient-specific information represented as a set of patient feature-value pairs in constructing training samples, ensuring that each execution of the target activity in a complete patient trace correspond to a unique training sample. Using the method described above, a set of training samples to describe the executions of a target clinical activity can be constructed from complete patient traces. Based on the constructed training samples, machine learning algorithms can be applied to obtain a classifier for local anomaly prediction in CTPs. In particular, three widely used machine learning algorithms, i.e., C4.5 decision tree, Naïve Bayes, and SVM, are implemented in our framework by employing an existing tool WEKA to train the classifiers and to perform the tests.

4   Case Study

The experimental log is collected from the Cardiology department of the Chinese PLA General hospital. The CTP of unstable angina is selected in the case study. Unstable angina is angina pectoris caused by disruption of an atherosclerotic plaque with partial thrombosis and possibly embolization or vasospasm [7]. While the risk of unstable angina is high, the population of unstable angina is huge, and thus, the anomaly prediction in the unstable angina CTP will be of significant value and interest. In the case study, we extract a clinical event log consisting of 12152 patient traces following the unstable angina CTP (from 2004 to 2013) from EMR system of Chinese PLA general hospital. The collected event logs have 144 patient features, and 704004 clinical events within 606 treatment activity types. The average length of stay (LOS) recorded in the log is 10.14

days, which some patient treatment journeys take a very short time, e.g., only 1 day in the hospital, and other treatment journeys take much longer, e.g., more than 6 months in the hospital, which implicitly indicates the diversity of treatment behaviors in the unstable angina CTP.

In CTPs, some activities, e.g., nursing care, routine examinations on vital signs, etc., are trivial and regularly executed each day in CTPs. Thus, no extra monitor effort is needed for monitoring these activities. In fact, clinical activities that are suitable to be monitored should be essential/critical to CTPs such that the abnormal executions of these activities have significant impacts on the effects of CTPs. To this end, we asked our clinical collaborators to select the following 23 target clinical activities: *"Antianginal therapy"*, *"Ultrasonography examination"*, *"Radiology examination"*, *"Antiplatelet therapy"*, *"Lipid regulating therapy"*, *"Discharge"*, *"Biochemical examination"*, *"Regulate blood sugar"*, *"CT examination"*, *"ECG"*, *"Coagulation"*, *"Routine blood test"*, *"-adrenergic receptor blockers"*, *"Vasodilation"*, *"Cephalosporins"*, *"Multifunction fetal monitors"*, *"Diuretics"*, *"Troponin T"*, *"ECG monitoring oxygen"*, *"Transfer"*, *"Coronary angiography"*, *"Stenting"*, and *"Transluminal coronary angioplasty"*.

4.1 CPM Generation

The first step is to learn a CPM from the collected unstable angina event log. To this end, we choose the Dirichlet prior α, β, and δ of CPM as 0.1, 0.01, and 0.01, respectively, which are common settings in literature [8]. In addition, we applied Gibbs sampling to learn the CPM from the log. The number of iterations of the Markov chain for Gibbs sampling is set to 1000. Before generating CPM from the collected log, we first determined the number of topics (i.e., treatment patterns) using the perplexity score, which is a standard measure to evaluate the prediction power of a probabilistic model, and has been used before to determine the number of topics (i.e., treatment patterns in this work) [6]:

$$\text{Perplexity} = exp[-\frac{\sum_{\sigma \in \mathcal{L}} log P(\mathbf{e}_\sigma | \mathcal{M})}{\sum_{\sigma \in \mathcal{L}} |\sigma|}] \tag{5}$$

where $\mathcal{M}$ is the learned CPM, and $\mathbf{e}_\sigma$ are the set of unseen events in the patient trace σ.

We calculated the perplexity scores of the trained CPM over a held-out test data set with a different number of topics. Specifically, 10% samples from the collected log are randomly selected as the test. In general, the number of topics is set to the value resulting in the smallest perplexity score. However, we observed that the perplexity of CPM roughly drops with the increase of K in the experiments. If we only take into account the perplexity, we probably select the maximum K of a given range, which may make the learned model over-fitting. Thus, we balanced the above-mentioned approach by a simple way; that is, if the reducing ratio of perplexity is less than τ, we do not select a larger K. In practice, we set τ to be 10% according to experiment analysis. In this study, we empirically choose the number of patterns $K = 3$ for the experimental log, where the perplexity seems to decrease rapidly and appear to settle down.

4.2   Experiment Results on Local Nomaly Detection

The prerequisite step of our local anomaly prediction is to detect unusual clinical events from complete patient traces to generate classifiers for typical clinical activities monitoring. Based on the normality measure, local anomalies can be detected from complete patient traces. Figure 2(A) depicts the number of absent-occurred anomalies when different ν_{up} are applied. As shown in Figure 2(A), when ν_{up} is larger than 0.94, there are no detected absent-occurred anomalies. With the further decreases of ν_{up}, the absent-occurred anomalies are detected from the experimental log. When $\nu_{up} = 0.9$, there are 749 absent-occurred local anomalies detected from the log. Looking insight into these absent events, we found that the type of all 749 absent events with ν_{up}=0.9 is "Antianginal drugs", which is the most common type of treatment interventions for the unstable angina CTP such that the detection of the absent "Antianginal drugs" may indicate the omissions of the common treatment behaviors for the unstable angina patients in hospital. Figure 2(B) depicts the impact of ν_{low} on the number of anomalies detected from the experimental log. As shown in Figure 2(B), the curves of unexpected and delay events increase linearly, the curve of early events increases at first with the increase of ν_{low}, and then remain stable with the further increase of ν_{low}. When ν_{low} is set as 0.05, there are 3776 unexpected events, 986 early events, and 38825 delay events detected form the experimental log. Based on the identified local anomalies, classifiers for predic-

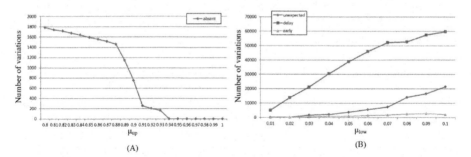

(A)   (B)

Fig. 2. Variation detection using the unstable angina data-set

tive monitoring of typical clinical activities can be generated. To this end, we selectd several significant patient features to generate samples for classification. As mentioned above, there are 144 patient features in the collected event log. But not all features are closely related with the treatment process of unstable angina, and it should select significant features for the unstable angina patients to improve the accuracy of predictive monitoring. To this end, we asked our clinical collaborators to pick up 21 patient features: *"Age"*, *"Gender"*, *"Creatine kinase"*, *"Creatinine"*, *"Angina pectoris"*, *"Hypertension"*, *"Troponin T measurement"*, *"Quantitative determination of creatine kinase"*, *"High-sensitivity C-reactive protein"*, *"Diabetes"*, *"Renal insufficiency"*, *"Cardiac insufficiency"*, *"Hyperlipidemia"*, *"History of coronary heart disease"*, *"Blood sugar"*, *"Tumor"*,

"Hypercholesterolemia", "Prostate disease", "Artery stenosis", "Arrhythmia", and "High triglycerides hyperlipidemia".

Figure 3 shows the prediction accuracy of 10-fold cross validation for the selected treatment activities of the unstable angina CTP. In order to provide a reference, we connected the pixels of SVM classifiers using dotted lines. As shown in the figure, the prediction accuracy is not the same for all the selected treatment activities. Most classifiers have achieved a prediction accuracy that is greater than 70%, and some of them are even well predicted by the generated classifier ($\geq 90\%$).

As a further investigation, we evaluated some special cases. The worst predicted activities are "Radiology Examination", and "Troponin T" as shown in Figure 3. Although these activities have been selected as target activities, they have imbalanced training samples in comparison with normal executions. The execution states of these activities are not clearly demonstrated in such an imbalanced training set, thus the classifier's performance is not quite good. In contrast, well predicted treatment activities do exist, for example, "Vasodilation", "ECG monitoring oxygen", and "Stenting". The difference is that their training samples are balanced between unusual events and normal cases, which means that the execution states of the well predicted activities exist for the balanced training samples, which is obvious for the learning algorithm to derive.

The overall prediction accuracies of the three algorithms (i.e. SVM, C4.5, and Naïve Bayes) are 82.838%, 82.533%, and 82.38%, respectively. According to the results, all three machine learning algorithms have achieved an overall prediction accuracy of well over 80% on the experimental log. Among three algorithms, SVM generally performs the best although it is marginally.

Ideally, each execution of a target treatment activity in the experimental dataset should be evaluated by clinicians such that true variations can be identified by clinicians. However, due to the burden of daily work of our clinical collaborators, we cannot ask them to validate all 12152 patient traces for local anomaly prediction. To validate the applicability of the proposed method in clinical settings, we randomly selected 100 patient traces as test data-set, and use the other 12052 traces to train the classification model. In particular, we adopt SVM to build classifiers for the variation prediction. As a result, 25 unexpected events, 3 early events, 326 delay events, and 19 absent events for the target clinical activities are predicted by the proposed method. Then, we ask three clinicians to validate the detected variations using a major voting strategy. As shown in Figure 4, almost all classifiers have achieved a precision that is greater than 70%. Some classifiers, e.g., "Antiplatelet therapy", "ECG monitoring oxygen", and "Stenting" etc., even have achieved 100% precisions. It indicates that the predicated variations of the proposed approach are well recognized by clinicians. Table 1 depicts the overall precisions. The overall precision of our approach is 83.4%, which indicates the feasibility of the proposed approach for local anomaly prediction in CTPs.

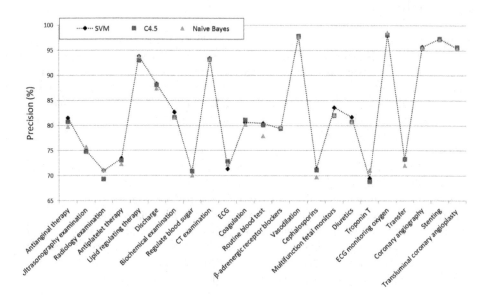

Fig. 3. Prediction accuracy of classifiers on the experimental log

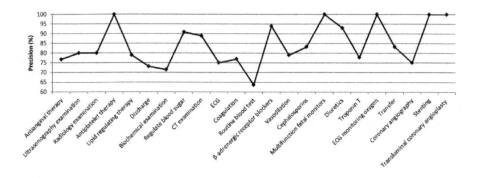

Fig. 4. Precisions achieved by the trained classifiers on the selected 100 patient traces with the efforts of human evaluation

Table 1. Overall performance of prediction accuracy on the selected 100 patient traces with the efforts of human evaluation

	Number of predictions	Number of correct predictions	Prediction accuracy (%)
Unexpected events	25	22	88
Absent events	19	15	78.9
Early events	3	3	100
Delay events	326	271	83.1
Overall	373	311	83.4

5   Conclusion

In this study, we propose a computational model for CTP anomaly prediction. In particular, we used some previous techniques from [6] to learn a probabilistic topic model to describe the general characteristics of patient traces from a clinical event log. Then we propose to predict local anomalies via fitting the normal treatment behaviors depicted in the model. We believe that the proposed approach can be used at the run-time instantiation and execution stages in CTPs to improve current state of treatment compliance checking and CTP management.

In our future work, we aim to study the merits of our framework in further clinical collaborations to investigate on additional sources of information, explore on the experiments results, and empirical study the usage of our approach in real clinical environments. As well, we plan to work with the developers on integrating the proposed approach into the EMR system, which is supposed to provide clinicians real time insights into violations of the established CP specification and support online compliance checking, to achieve high quality of health services and prevent medical errors with an adaptive mechanism for CTPs.

References

1. Lenz, R., Blaser, R., Beyer, M., Heger, O., Biber, C., Aumlein, M.B., Schnabe, M.: IT support for clinical pathways-lessons learned. International Journal of Medical Informatics 76(3), S397–S402 (2007)
2. Blaser, R., Schnabel, M., Biber, C., Baumlein, M., Heger, O., Beyer, M., Opitz, E., Lenz, R., Kuhn, K.A.: Improving pathway compliance and clinician performance by using information technology. International Journal of Medical Informatics 76(2-3), 151–156 (2007)
3. Hatiboglu, M.A., Altunkaynak, A., Ozger, M., Iplikcioglu, A.C., Cosar, M., Turgut, N.: A predictive tool by fuzzy logic for outcome of patients with intracranial aneurysm. Expert Systems with Applications 37(2), 1043–1049 (2010)
4. Peleg, M.: Computer-interpretable clinical guidelines: A methodological review. Journal of Biomedical Informatics 46(4), 744–763 (2013)
5. Cheah, J.: Development and implementation of a clinical pathway programme in an acute care general hospital in singapore. International Journal for Quality in Health Care 12, 403–412 (2000)
6. Huang, Z., Dong, W., Ji, L., Gan, C., Lu, X., Duan, H.: Discovery of clinical pathway patterns from event logs using probabilistic topic models. Journal of Biomedical Informatics 47(0), 39–57 (2014)
7. Aderson, J.L., Adams, C.D., Antman, E.M., et al.: 2012 accf/aha focused update incorporated into the accf/aha 2007 guidelines for the management of patients with unstable angina/non-st-elevation myocardial infarction. J. Am. Coll. Cardiol. 61(23), e179–e347 (2012)
8. Blei, D.M., Ng, A.Y., Jordan, M.I.: Latent Dirichlet allocation. Journal of Machine Learning Research 3, 993–1022 (2003)

Mining Surgery Phase-Related Sequential Rules from Vertebroplasty Simulations Traces

Ben-Manson Toussaint[1,2(✉)] and Vanda Luengo[1]

[1] Université Grenoble Alpes, 38406, St-Martin d'Hères, France
{ben-manson.toussaint,vanda.luengo}@imag.fr
[2] Ecole Supérieure d'Infotronique d'Haïti, Port-au-Prince, Haiti
ben-manson.toussaint@esih.edu

Abstract. We present in this paper an algorithm for extracting perceptual-gestural rules from heterogeneous multisource traces. The challenge that we address is two-fold: 1) represent traces such that they render coherently all aspect of this multimodal knowledge; 2) ensure that key tutoring services can be produced on top of represented traces. In the spirit of automatic knowledge acquisition paradigm proposed in the literature, we implemented PhARules, a modified version of an existing algorithm, CMRules, for mining surgery phase-aware sequential rules from simulated surgery traces. We demonstrated the efficiency of our algorithm as well its performance limits on traces of simulations of vertebroplasty recorded in TELEOS, an Intelligent Tutoring System dedicated to percutaneous orthopedic surgery.

Keywords: Intelligent tutoring systems · Educational data mining · Sequential rules mining · Simulated surgery · Percutaneous orthopedic surgery

1 Introduction

Knowledge involved in percutaneous orthopedic surgery is perceptual-gestural. In other words, this knowledge implies the combination of actions and gestures along with perceptions that support their execution. These perceptions are visual, auditory or haptic. It requires that the surgeons master the coordination of anatomical knowledge, visual guidance through X-rays and various progression insights provided by the instruments at different points of insertion in the body and the bones. TELEOS (Technology Enhanced Learning Environment for Orthopedic Surgery) is a simulation-based Intelligent Tutoring System (ITS) that has been designed to train interns in performing this type of surgery, specifically vertebroplasty and sacra-iliac screw fixation [7]. Capturing perceptions in such simulated learning environment requires the use of two sensing devices, namely, an eye-tracker and a haptic arm. These devices cover learner's behavior and all aspect of involved knowledge. On the other hand, they generate highly heterogeneous traces. The challenge is to represent these traces coherently considering the specificity of related knowledge as to foster the production of key tutoring services or learning analytics on top of them.

© Springer International Publishing Switzerland 2015
J.H. Holmes et al. (Eds.): AIME 2015, LNAI 9105, pp. 35–46, 2015.
DOI: 10.1007/978-3-319-19551-3_5

Further, percutaneous orthopedic surgery is ill-defined [10] as there is no complete theoretical framework of the domain and no fixed best solutions to perform a given operation or to respond to incoming situations during an operation. Traditional paradigms and approaches of the state of the art are not suitable for the implementation of tutoring services for ITSs dedicated to such domains. One proposition to addressing this issue in the literature is a hybrid paradigm including automatic knowledge acquisition from activity traces [4]. This is namely the use of artificial intelligence techniques in the modeling of tutoring services for these environments as to compensate the limits of the traditional approaches. For example, data mining techniques are applied on educational data for extracting frequent patterns of knowledge that can possibly be reused to enrich progressively the knowledge model of ITSs.

The efficiency of this proposition has been discussed in [3] and [4]. However, mining algorithms are limited for the extraction of rules on top of traces related to multiple-phases resolution exercises. A phase refers to one of the finite set of parts of an exercise. It involves possibly actions sharing common and exclusive characteristics comparing to actions from other phases; or actions that are not or less executed in other phases. For example, in vertebroplasty, all actions and gestures executed with the trocar are observable in the third phase of the procedure; the first phase is dedicated to the settings and validation of the position of the fluoroscope with respect to the targeted vertebra; and the second phase, to the cutaneous marks that spot the entry points of the trocar on the patient's skin. The phases of an exercise are not always uniform in terms of duration or number of executed actions. Hence, frequent actions within one phase can be invisible to mining algorithms if activity traces are mined as a homogeneous set. Our propositions addresses this issue. First, we propose a method for transforming multisource heterogeneous traces into coherent perceptual-gestural sequences suitable for advanced automatic treatment. Secondly, we propose a modified version of an existing algorithm, CMRules [5], to mining phase-aware sequential rules common to several sequences. We referred to this new algorithm as PhARules. We tested our proposition in two different ways. We tested the performance of the proposed algorithm compared to the existing algorithm CMRules and we evaluated the interestingness of the sequential rules that it finds for didactic purpose.

The rest of the paper is organized as follows. The 2nd section presents the background of this work as well as related works on sequential rules mining with the use of background knowledge; the 3rd section presents the simulation-based ITS TELEOS and the nature of the traces recorded from its learning environment; the 4th section describes our proposed methodology to transforming and representing these traces as perceptual-gestural sequences; the 5th section presents our proposed algorithm, PhARules that is able to mine phase-related sequential rules; the 6th section describes the evaluations conducted on PhARules performance compared to CMRules as well as the interestingness of the rules that it mines; finally, the 7th section draws our conclusion and future works.

2   Background and Related Works

Association rules are statements of the form *if/then* that uncover relationships between seemingly unrelated data in a transaction database, relational database or other types of repositories. This knowledge discovery technique has been proposed in [1] and is nowadays widely used for a very large variety of purposes. The notation of an association rule is as follows: A → B which means that if an occurrence of A is observed in a transaction then an occurrence of B will be observed with respect to a certain support and confidence.

The support and confidence [1] are user-defined thresholds that determines if a rule is important (interesting) or not: the support and the confidence of all reported rules must be greater or equal to these thresholds. The support of the rule A → B is the number of transactions where A and B are observed jointly. In other words, it is the probability to observe association of occurrences of A and B in a transaction database: sup (A→B) = P(AB). The confidence of A→B is the number of transactions where A and B occur jointly compared to the total number of transactions where only A occurs. In other words, the confidence is the probability to observe occurrences of B when A occurs: conf(A→B) = P(AB)/P(A). A transaction database D is formally defined as a set of transactions T={$t_1,t_2...t_n$} and a set of items I={$i_1, i_2...i_n$}, where $t_1,t_2...t_n \subseteq$ I.

In the other hand, sequential rules mining aims at discovering association rules where the transactions are ordered based on their time of occurrence. Transactions with such sequential nature are referred to as sequences and constitute a sequence database. Formally defined, a sequence database D' is a set of sequences S={$s_1, s_2,...,s_n$} and a set of items I={$i_1, i_2,...,i_n$}, where each sequence s_x is a temporally ordered list of transactions s_x={$X_1, X_2, ..., X_n$} such that $X_1, X_2, ..., X_n \subseteq$ I [2]. A set of items that occur together is called an itemset and is non-empty. A sequence is maximal if it is not contained in any other sequence. The length |s| of a sequence is defined by the number of itemsets that it contains. A sequential rule A⇒B is a relationship between two itemsets A, B such that A, B $\subseteq$ I and A∩B = ∅. A⇒B means that each occurrence of items A in a sequence is followed by an occurrence of items B in the same sequence.

Temporal order is not always sufficient for the extraction of interesting rules. Sometimes, one needs to use additional background knowledge to constrain the mining of patterns or rules with characteristics that are assumed to define or enhance their usefulness and significance. For example in [11], the authors propose a solution to mine sequential patterns from customers' transaction datasets considering the categories to which the customers belong (e.g.: the customer socio-professional profile). Likewise, in [12], the proposition is to mine sequential patterns based on the existence of a relationship between events reported in the sequences.

For our part, we want to keep the temporal order of actions, gestures and perceptions in recorded simulation sequences. However, we are further interested in mining those rules based on the importance of actions, gestures and perceptions they contain within a specific phase of a simulated surgery. In fact, the set of sequences recorded from a simulation session is not homogeneous: traces from some phase of the simulation can be

overrepresented compared to others. These actions would be therefore invisible to classical rules mining algorithms. Hence, our aim is to propose a solution to mine items (actions, perceptions and gestures) that are significant enough within a specific phase even if
they are underrepresented given the whole set of simulation sequences.

3   Recording Multi-source Simulation Traces in TELEOS

In this section, we present the method used to capture actions, perceptual behaviors
and gestures in the learning environment of the simulation-based Intelligent Tutoring
System dedicated to orthopedic surgery, TELEOS. The complementary sensing devices used in TELEOS consist of an eye-tracker that records learners' visual perceptions and a haptic arm that records learners' gestures and haptic perceptions [7]. Other
types of actions executed in a simulated percutaneous surgery are recorded from the
user interface. In this study, we focus on simulation of vertebroplasty, a type of percutaneous surgery performed to treat fractured vertebrae.

The simulation interface of TELEOS is composed of sections that represent the
main artefacts of a percutaneous operating room. Namely, as illustrated in Fig. 1.a, it
includes a 3D model section where the patient's model is displayed; the current and
previous X-rays sections and the settings panel that embeds three settings subsections: the fluoroscope settings panel; the cutaneous marking panel and the trocar
manipulation panel. These sections represent the areas of interest (AOI) of the interface, that is, areas that will be recorded throughout the simulation process when they
are fixed by the user. The AOIs associated to the X-rays embed the points of interest
of the targeted vertebra, that is, specific parts of the vertebra that should be analyzed
on X-rays to support decisions on surgical actions and gestures. Fig 1.b shows the
learners' visual perceptions, including fixed areas and points of interest, as monitored
and recorded by a scanpath analyzer [6]. The points of interest have been determined
by expert surgeons for each modeled clinical case and integrated as annotations to the
patients' models as summarized in Fig. 2.

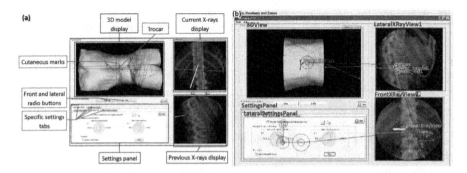

Fig. 1. a) TELEOS simulation interface. b) Visual path traced by the scanpath analyzer

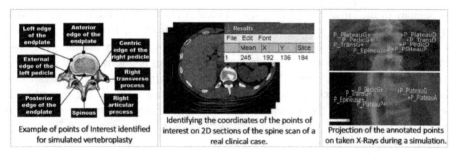

Fig. 2. Identification and annotation process of vertebra with points of interest

Table 1. Conceptual representation of traces from each source

Sequence representation	Parameters
Eye-tracking trace: $S_e: <t; AOI_{i=1,m} \mid POI_{j=0,n}; f_{xy}; r_{mean}; r_{max}; d>$	t: timestamp (Unix format) $AOI_{i=1,m} \mid POI_{j=0,n}$: areas of interest and potential embedded points of interest f_{xy}: coordinates (x, y) of the fixation areas r_{mean}: mean radius of the fixation area (in pixels) r_{max}: maximum radius of the fixation areas (in pixels) d: duration of the fixation (in milliseconds)
Haptic arm trace: $S_h: <t; T_{xyz}; T'_{xyz}; F_{xyz}; S_{xyz}>$	T_{xyz}: coordinates (x,y,z) of the tip of the trocar $T'_{x'y'z'}$: coordinates (x',y',z') of the handle of the trocar F_{xyz}: force applied on the trocar in the plan (x,y,z) S_{xyz}: speed of displacement of the trocar in (x,y,z)
Simulation interface action trace: $S_s: <t; A; R_{xyz}; R'_{x'y'z'}; X_{xy}; X'_{x'y'}; C_{xy}; C'_{xy}; C''_{xy}; T_{xyz}; T'_{xyz}>$	A: punctual action name $R_{xyz}, R'_{x'y'z'}$: coordinates (x,y,z) of the fluoroscope for anteroposterior or (x',y',z') for lateral Xrays $X_{xy}, X'_{x'y'}$: coordinates (x,y) of the current Xray and (x',y') of the prevoisus Xray $CR_{xy}, CR'_{x'y'}$ and $CR''_{x''y''}$: position of the left, right and transversal cutaneous marks. T_{xyz} and $T'_{x'y'z'}$: coordinates (x,y,z) and (x',y',z') of the tip and the handle of the trocar.

The surgical gestures consist of different types of prehension of the trocar, the force applied for its manipulation and the consequent speed of its progression, as well as its incline, orientation and direction of insertion. The data required for modeling these gestures was collected on artificial patients models [7]. The instrumentation used included dynamometers inserted in the models for recording data related to the force and the rate of progression of the trocar at different important insertion stages. The main insertion stages considered for vertebroplasty are skin contact, bone contact, pedicle entry, crossing of the vertebral body until the point of validation of the trocar trajectory. The cognitive interest of training for the positioning of the trocar and adaptation of gestures based on perceived resistance on the trajectory of insertion through the body, are discussed in [7]. The collected data were used to configure a haptic arm that renders the bones and body resistance through the insertion trajectory.

Finally, actions captured from the simulation software are punctual as opposed to the continuity of a visual path or the spatial and temporal dynamism of a gesture. As opposed to traces sent and recorded continuously by the complementary sensing devices, these actions are recorded only at their execution. This is for example the trig- gering of an X-ray or the tracing of a cutaneous mark. An action can be described as a photography of the simulation state at the moment it occurs. It is thus caracterized not only by its name but also by the positions of the tools at the same moment. Traces from the three sources are recorded independently. Their conceptual representation is presented in Table 1. They are heterogeneous in their content types and formats, and their time granularities. In fact, traces from the simulator are alphanumeric as well as traces from the eye-tracker. On the contrary, those from the haptic arm are numeric. Their lengths are also all different. Finally, the eye-tracker and the haptic arm record traces continuously whereas the simulator records traces exclusively when an action is executed from the interface.

4   Generating Perceptual-Gestural Sequences

In this section we describe the treatment performed for generating perceptual-gestural sequences from the heterogeneous multisource simulation traces that we presented in the previous section. The transformation process is realized through a chain of single-function software that we refer to as "operators".

4.1   Traces Merging and Semantization

To produce perceptual-gestural sequences out of TELEOS multisource traces, we first apply the merging operator that links action to the perceptions that support their execution. The result expected is a set of sequences that render the perceptual-gestural aspect of each interaction. Then, the semantization operator is applied for transposing changes in the coordinates of the simulation tools into semantic states. These changes are the consequences of executed actions and gestures. The semantic denominations used for TELEOS are based on the standard anatomical terms of location (e.g. *"the fluoroscope has a caudal incline"; "the trocar is quickly inclined on the sagittal axis"*). The states of the tools are reported from sequence-to-sequence for keeping track of the current simulation state, i.e., the positions of all the tools, in each generated perceptual-gestural sequence. In its actual version, the semantization operator uses a simple mapping method that takes as input the coordinates of the simulation tools as Euclidean vectors and link the changes of these coordinates through the interaction sequences into manually recorded semantic denominations. In other terms, the semantization operator does not currently exploit an ontology but a taxonomy from the standard anatomical terms of location.

4.2   Traces Enrichment

In TELEOS, elements of knowledge put into play by interns during a simulation are diagnosed based on their adequacy with a set of expert controls through a Bayesian network [9]. These controls are elements of knowledge formulated by expert surgeons and integrated into the knowledge model of the simulator. The evaluation items computed on top of these controls are referred to as "situational variables". An annotation operator is used to enrich the sequences with related situational variables. Table 2 shows one example of control and situational variables, the actions they are associated with and steps of the simulation in which these actions can be executed. Fig. 3 gives an overview of the treatment process. Annotations are represented in the sequences like any other action or interaction element in the learning environment. Conceptually, each annotation is an action from the system generated as a consequence of actions, gestures and perceptions from the learner. This representation fosters mining of the annotations as potential frequent patterns associated to learner's interactions in association rules.

Table 2. An example of control and situational variable

Action	Phase	Control	Situational Variable
Check the position of the trocar on a profile radio	Insertion	At the cutaneous entrance spot, the trocar must be tipped towards the pedicle.	Orientation of the trocar at the cutaneous entrance spot.

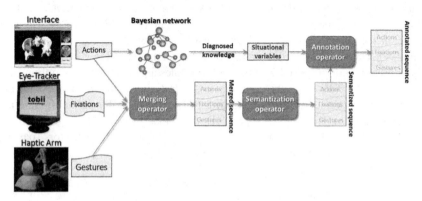

Fig. 3. Schema of the treatment process for generating perceptual-gestural sequences from heterogeneous multisource simulation traces

At this stage of the treatment process, we have a representation of the sequences on top of which we can proceed to knowledge extraction tasks. Table 3 shows the conceptual representation of generated perceptual-gestural sequences and their representation as annotated with situational variables (computed expert evaluations).

Table 3. Conceptual representation of generated perceptual-gestural sequences

Sequence representation	Parameters
Generated perceptual-gestural sequence: S_{pg}: $<t;$ $(\mathsf{F}, f);$ $(\mathsf{T}, \tau);$ $A;$ $AOI_{i=1,m}[\delta_k];$ $POI_{i,j=0,n}[\delta_k]>$	t: timestamp (Unix format) F: semantic denomination of the trocar manipulations f: states of the trocar T: semantic denominations of the fluoroscope manipulation τ: states of the fluoroscope A: punctual action name AOI_i: areas of interest $\quad POI_{j,i}$: points of interest related to AOI_i δ_k: semantic categorization of fixation durations
Annotated perceptual-gestural sequence: Sa: $<(\mathsf{t}_i, S_{i=1,\eta})$; $(\mathsf{V}_{q=1,v}[\upsilon_{r=1,w}])>$	t_i: temporal order tags of sequences V_q: situational variables υ_r: values of the situational variables

5   Mining Sequential Rules

We present in this section the CMRules algorithm that has been proposed for mining sequential rules common to several sequences in sequence databases. Then we present the modified version that we propose such that items can be mined considering their significance in the context of a phase.

CMRULES proceeds by considering first that an input sequence database D has a corresponding transaction database D' when the temporal information of sequences are ignored. For D and D', each sequential rule r: A⇒B of the set of sequential rules S has a corresponding association rule r': A→ B in S'. Since sup(A∎B) is always lower or equal to sup(A∪B), the relationships sup(r') ≥ seqSup(r) and conf(r') ≥ seqConf(r) holds for any sequential rule r and its corresponding association rule r'. An association rule mining algorithm is applied at this stage to extract association rules from the transaction database with *minsup = minSeqSup* and *minconf = minSeqConf*. Then, CMRules calculates the sequential support and sequential confidence of each association rule in the sequence database, and discard all rules below the *minSeqSup* and *minSeqConf*. The remaining rules are the expected sequential rules.

Fig. 4 presents our proposed version, the PhARules algorithm. We not only want to extract sequential rules that are common to several simulation sequences but also consider their importance in the context of a phase. We formally define a phase as a subset of sequences $P_i= \{s_{i1}, ... s_{im}\} \subseteq D$ such that $P_1 \cap ... \cap P_i \cap ... \cap P_n = \emptyset$ and $P_1 \cup ... \cup P_i \cup ... \cup P_n = D$. A phase P_i is characterized by a set of descriptors (parameters) $a_i = \{a_{i1},..., a_{im}\}$ such that $\forall s_{ij} \in D$, $s_{ij} \in Pi$ *iff* $a_i \Rightarrow s_{ij}$.

```
INPUT : a phase descriptors database, a sequence database D, minSeqSup, minSeqConf
OUTPUT : the set of phase-related sequential rules
PROCEDURE:
    1.  Consider the sequence database D as a transaction database D'
    2.  Group sequences by phase based on phase descriptors and generate
        transaction databases D'₁, ... ,D'ₙ (n = number of phases)
    3.  Find all association rules for each database D'ᵢ. Select minsup = minSeqSup
        and minconf = minSeqConf
    4.  Compute seqSup and seqConf of each association rule r D'ᵢ in Dᵢ. Eliminate
        each rule r in Dᵢ such that:
        a.  seqSup(r) < minSeqSup
        b.  seqConf(r) < minSeqConf
    5.  Return the set of phase-related sequential rules
```

Fig. 4. The PhARules algorithm

6   Evaluations and Findings

We present in this section the evaluations conducted on PhARules execution performance and the interestingness of the phase-related sequential rules that it extracts. The traces used for this experiment were recorded from 9 simulation sessions of vertebroplasty performed by 5 interns and 1 expert surgeon from the Orthopedic and Traumatology Department of the University Hospital of Grenoble. The proposed simulation exercises consisted of treating a fracture of the 11th and/or the 12th thoracic vertebra. For the first part of the conducted evaluations, all 9 simulation sessions traces were joined into one dataset. Table 4 summarizes the characteristics of the data. The dataset is available for download here: goo.gl/zS37Ly.

Table 4. Characteristics of the dataset *(#= number; it=items; its= itemset; seq= sequence)*

# Seq				#its	#it	#distinct it	Avg # its/seq	Avg # it/seq	Avg #dis- tinct it/seq
Total	Phase 1	Phase 2	Phase 3						
616	171	89	356	10 618	20 605	47	17.2 (σ=13)	33.45 (σ=22.1)	20.9 (σ=7.9)

6.1   Evaluating the Execution Performance of PhARules

To compare the performance of PhARules and CMRules, we used the joint set of sequences from the 9 simulation sessions of vertebroplasty. We conducted the performance tests on a HP ZBook embedding an Intel® Core™ i7-4800MQ CPU of 2.7 GHz and 16 GB of RAM. We applied the two algorithms for *minSeqConf* = 0.7 fixed on a random selection, for a variation of *minSeqSup* ranging from 1.0 to 0.1. Fig. 5 summarizes the obtained results. The *minSeqSup* for which no rules were found are not presented in the graphics. We can notice that CMRules outperformed PhARules regarding execution time and memory usage especially for *minSeqSup* smaller or equal to 0.15. However, PhARules seemed to keep a more stable level of memory usage through variations of *minSeqSup* greater than or equal to 0.15. PhARules reported also better results regarding rules count for almost all applied *minSeqSup*.

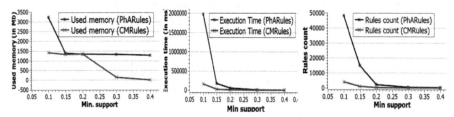

Fig. 5. The comparative performance of PhARules and CMRules on memory usage *(left)*, execution time *(center)* and number of rules count *(right)*

Further, as presented in Fig. 6, PhARules extracted rules from the three different phases of simulation sessions of vertebroplasty for the same variations of *minSeqSup*. Conversely, no significant knowledge patterns related to phases 1 and 2 of the vertebroplasty simulation sessions have been detected by CMRules: all extracted rules were from the third phase.

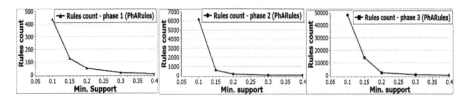

Fig. 6. Rules count obtained by PhARules by phase for a variation of *minSeqSup*

6.2   Evaluating the Interestingness of Phase-Related Sequential Rules

After the evaluation of execution performance of PhARules, we wanted to assess the interestingness of the reported rules with respect to expert surgeons' belief. After the mining process, we used a post processing operator to select rules containing specific characteristics, namely for this experiment, the operator selected rules that contain punctual actions or gestures, perceptions, states of the tools and situational variables in either their *if*-clause or their *then*-clause. We refer to these rules as perceptual-gestural. An example of perceptual-gestural rule is given in Fig. 7.

> **Cutaneous Marking Phase.** (The fluoroscope is positioned for frontal X-rays with a cranial incline); (the learner positions the slider on the patient's body); (the learner takes a frontal X-ray); (the learner visualizes the position of the spinous process of the targeted vertebra on the X-ray)
> ⇒ The transverse cutaneous mark is correct. The left cutaneous mark is correct

Fig. 7. An example of selected perceptual-gestural sequential rule

We applied the PhARules algorithm on each of the 9 simulation sessions sequences separately with a minimum support of 0.3 and a minimum confidence of 0.7. A total of 188 803 general rules have been reported. The rules selector identified 3 895 perceptual-gestural rules out of those. We randomly pulled out 20 perceptual-gestural rules to be evaluated by 5 vertebroplasty experts. Four of these experts are teaching surgeons. They were asked to estimate from their belief the didactic interestingness of each rule in a Likert scale ranging from 1 to 5, 1 being *very low* and 5, *very high*.

The overall average of the scores for the didactic interestingness of the rules is 3.8 out of 5. The weakest average rating is 3.0 for one rule; the average ratings for the 19 other rules range from 3.2 to 4.4, including 12 with an average score greater than or equal to the overall score of 3.8. This reveals that the selected rules are likely of rather high or very high didactic interestingness in average from the experts' point of view. We then computed Jaccard distance upon the experts' ratings to evaluate their agreement. The obtained results denote high level of agreement among them. In fact, the largest distance observed between experts' ratings is of 22% between experts 3 and 5. Fig. 8 shows the histogram for the distribution of the rules on the Likert scale by each expert and the corresponding Jaccard distance matrix among experts' ratings two-by-two.

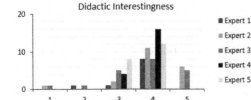

	Expert 1	Expert 2	Expert 3	Expert 4	Expert 5
Expert 1	0				
Expert 2	.19	0			
Expert 3	.20	.15	0		
Expert 4	.13	.10	.15	0	
Expert 5	.15	.20	.22	.14	0

Fig. 8. Histogram of the distribution of the rules scores by each expert and the corresponding Jaccard distance matrix among experts' ratings two-by-two

7   Conclusion and Future Works

We presented in this paper our method to transform multisource heterogeneous traces of vertebroplasty simulations into coherent perceptual-gestural sequences. We also presented our method to mine surgery phase-related sequential rules from the set of represented sequences. Our proposition for sequential rules extraction is the PhARules algorithm (PHase-Aware sequential rules mining algorithm) which is a modified version of the existing algorithm, CMRules. The proposed modifications led to the extraction of sequential rules common to several sequences based on their significance within distinct parts of the dataset and not their significance within the whole dataset. In fact, the dataset is not a homogeneous set of sequences. Namely, the context considered in this study are execution phases of simulated vertebroplasty. We showed that our algorithm applied on traces recorded from the simulation-based Intelligent Tutoring System TELEOS (Technology-Enhanced Learning Environment for Orthopedic Surgery), was able to extract interesting sequential rules related to the distinctive phases of simulated operations of vertebroplasty. However, PhARules needs to be optimized for better performance on execution time and memory usage. Further, in its actual version, the algorithm extract many rules which are difficult to be all exploited in more advanced treatment as their high number increase the risk of redundancy and irrelevancy. Consequently, we envisage to improve the rules selection process in order to lower the amount and increase the relevancy of retained rules based on main characteristics shared by the top-rated ones in this study. Then, we will evaluate the effective gain obtained from the simulator's tutoring services namely, knowledge diagnosis and pedagogical guidance, by enriching its knowledge base with extracted and selected rules by PhARules. We finally plan to test the performance of PhARules on larger datasets as well as its genericity on traces related to other domains involving perceptual-gestural knowledge.

Acknowledgements. This work has been partially supported by the LabEx PERSYVAL-Lab (ANR-11-LABX-0025-01). The authors would like to thank Dr. J. Tonetti, Dr. M. Boudissa, Dr. L. Bouyou-Garnier, Dr. G. Kershbaumer and Dr. S. Ruatti for their kind participation in this study.

References

1. Agrawal, R., Imielminski, T., Swami, A.: Mining Association Rules Between Sets of Items in Large Databases. In: SIGMOD Conference, pp. 207–216 (1993)
2. Agrawal, R., Srikant, R.: Mining Sequential Patterns. In: Proc. Int. Conf. on Data Engineering, pp. 3–14 (1995)
3. Fournier-Viger, P., Nkambou, R., Mephu Nguifo, E.: Building Intelligent Tutoring Systems for Ill-Defined Domains. In: Nkambou, R., Bourdeau, J., Mizoguchi, R. (eds.) Advances in Intelligent Tutoring Systems. SCI, vol. 308, pp. 81–101. Springer, Heidelberg (2010)
4. Fournier-Viger, P., Nkambou, R., Mayers, A., Mephu Nguifo, E., Faghihi, U.: A Hybrid Expertise Model to Support Tutoring Services in Robotic Arm Manipulations. In: Batyrshin, I., Sidorov, G. (eds.) MICAI 2011, Part I. LNCS(LNAI), vol. 7094, pp. 478–489. Springer, Heidelberg (2011)
5. Fournier-Viger, P., Faghihi, U., Nkambou, R., Mephu Nguifo, E.: CMRules: Mining sequential rules common to several sequences. Journal Know.-Based Syst. 25(1), 63–76 (2012)
6. Jambon, F., Luengo, V.: Analyse oculométrique « on-line » avec zones d'intérêt dynamiques: application aux environnements d'apprentissage sur simulateur. In: Actes de la Conférence Ergo'IHM sur les Nouvelles Interactions, Créativité et Usages, Biarritz France (2012)
7. Luengo, V., Larcher, A., Tonetti, J.: Design and implementation of a visual and haptic simulator in a platform for a TEL system in percutaneous orthopedic surgery. In: Westwood, J.D., Vestwood, S.W. (eds.) Medecine Meets Virtual Reality 18, pp. 324–328 (2011)
8. Luengo, V., Vadcard, L., Tonetti, J., Dubois, M.: Diagnostic des connaissances et rétroaction épistémique adaptative en chirurgie. In: Revue d'Intelligence Artificielle, vol. 25(4), pp. 499–524. Lavoisier. Hermes Science Publications (2011)
9. Minh Chieu, V., Luengo, V., Vadcard, L.: Student Modeling in Orthopedic Surgery Training: Exploiting Symbiosis between Temporal Bayesian Networks and Fine-grained Didactical Analysis. In: International Journal of Artificial Intelligence in Education 20, pp. 269–301. IOS Press (2010)
10. Lynch, C., Ashley, K., Aleven, V., Pinkwart, N.: Defining Ill-Defined Domains; A literature survey. In: Proc. Intelligent Tutoring Systems for Ill-Defined Domains Workshop, ITS 2006, pp. 1–10 (2006)
11. Rabatel, J., Bringay, S., Poncelet, P.: Mining Sequential Patterns: A Context-Aware Approach. In: Guillet, F., Pinaud, B., Venturini, G., Zighed, D.A. (eds.) Advances in Knowledge Discovery and Management. SCI, vol. 471, pp. 23–41. Springer, Heidelberg (2013)
12. Stendardo, N., Kalousis, A.: Relationship-aware sequential pattern mining. CoRR 1212, 5389 (2012)

Data Driven Order Set Development Using Metaheuristic Optimization

Yiye Zhang$^{(\boxtimes)}$ and Rema Padman

Carnegie Mellon University, Pittsburgh, PA 15213, USA
yiyez@andrew.cmu.edu

Abstract. An unanticipated negative consequence of using healthcare information technology for clinical care is the cognitive workload imposed on users due to poor usability characteristics. This is a widely recognized challenge in the context of computerized provider order entry (CPOE) technology. In this paper, we investigate cognitive workload in the use of order sets, a core feature of CPOE systems that assists clinicians with medical order placement. We propose an automated, data-driven algorithm for developing order sets such that clinicians' cognitive workload is minimized. Our algorithm incorporates a two-stage optimization model embedded with bisecting K-means clustering and tabu search to optimize the content of order sets, as well as the time intervals where specific order sets are recommended in the CPOE. We evaluate our algorithm using real patient data from a pediatric hospital, and demonstrate that data-driven order sets have the potential to dominate existing, consensus order sets in terms of usability and cognitive workload.

1 Introduction

Information technology (IT) is playing an increasingly critical role in the day-to-day practice of healthcare [1]. However, an unintended consequence of widespread healthcare IT deployment and use is the physical and cognitive workload imposed on users due to poor system usability [2]. A recent report from the US Agency for Healthcare Research and Quality (AHRQ) pointed out that poor usability−−such as poorly designed screens, hard-to-navigate files, conflicting warning messages, and need for excessive keystrokes or mouse clicks−−adversely affects clinical efficiency and data quality [3]. Excessive cognitive workload imposed by technology on healthcare IT users have profound impacts on behavior [4], and lead to insufficient customization of the system to workflow and information overload [1,5]. Therefore, there is a need to re-design healthcare IT systems that take into account the potential cognitive complexity associated with its use such that healthcare software applications can be accepted more readily and lead to safer, more efficient usage.

This paper addresses this challenge in the context of order sets, a core component of computerized provider order entry (CPOE) systems, which are intended to electronically aid clinicians to place orders efficiently and accurately [6]. Figure 1 is a screenshot of an Admission Orders Asthma order set which includes a

© Springer International Publishing Switzerland 2015
J.H. Holmes et al. (Eds.): AIME 2015, LNAI 9105, pp. 47–56, 2015.
DOI: 10.1007/978-3-319-19551-3_6

list of orders administered to Asthma patients upon admission. Some orders are defaulted-ON ('incl?' box is checked), such that they are automatically selected when the order set is selected, while others are relevant but defaulted-OFF('incl?' box is blank), and can be manually selected to add to the automatically selected orders when needed. Defaulted-ON items can be de-selected by clinicians as well. Aside from using order sets, items can be ordered as a la carte orders, which refer to individual orders listed in CPOE without relation to others.

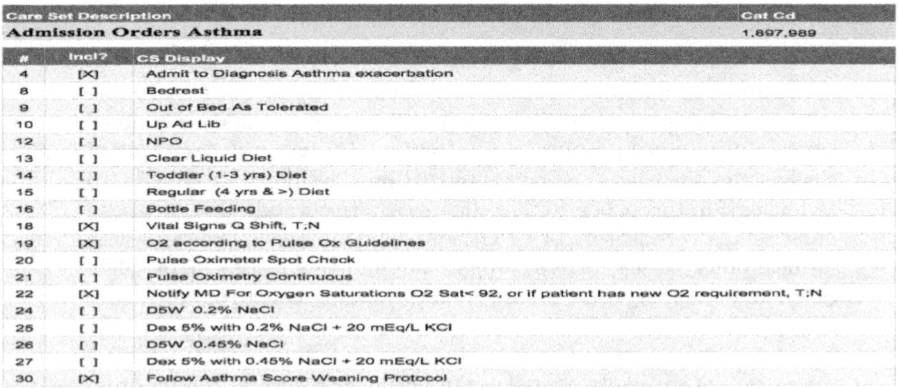

Care Set Description			Cat Cd
Admission Orders Asthma			1,897,989
#	**Incl?**	**CS Display**	
4	[X]	Admit to Diagnosis Asthma exacerbation	
8	[ ]	Bedrest	
9	[ ]	Out of Bed As Tolerated	
10	[ ]	Up Ad Lib	
12	[ ]	NPO	
13	[ ]	Clear Liquid Diet	
14	[ ]	Toddler (1-3 yrs) Diet	
15	[ ]	Regular (4 yrs & >) Diet	
16	[ ]	Bottle Feeding	
18	[X]	Vital Signs Q Shift, T;N	
19	[X]	O2 according to Pulse Ox Guidelines	
20	[ ]	Pulse Oximeter Spot Check	
21	[ ]	Pulse Oximetry Continuous	
22	[X]	Notify MD For Oxygen Saturations O2 Sat< 92, or if patient has new O2 requirement, T;N	
24	[ ]	D5W 0.2% NaCl	
25	[ ]	Dex 5% with 0.2% NaCl + 20 mEq/L KCl	
26	[ ]	D5W 0.45% NaCl	
27	[ ]	Dex 5% with 0.45% NaCl + 20 mEq/L KCl	
30	[X]	Follow Asthma Score Weaning Protocol	

Fig. 1. Screenshot of an order set

Figure 2 illustrates the medical order placement process using order set and a la carte orders. Well-designed order sets allow faster order placement by grouping multiple relevant orders by clinical purpose, such that users can enter multiple system-suggested orders designed for various conditions in one setting, instead of placing a la carte orders one at a time. Yet, historical data indicate tremendous variability and insufficient usage of order sets [7], but more frequent use of a la carte orders, due to the inconsistency of current order set content with the best practices [2]. This potentially results in decreased ordering efficiency and patient safety, while increasing health IT fatigue and resistance to use [8].

Order sets are traditionally developed manually using a consensus approach by clinician experts in the domain of interest [6]. This is a time-, labor- and knowledge-intensive approach that does not scale well with the increasing pace of scientific discovery and the challenges associated with translating the science to the bedside. Alongside, considerable data and information are being gathered on a daily basis as orders are placed in clinical information systems such as CPOE that are deployed widely in healthcare organizations. This usage data reflects both best practice via the available order sets in the system as well as new discoveries that clinicians have incorporated into their daily practice. In this paper, we propose an automated order set development process, taking advantage of the large amount of electronic medical information compiled via CPOE to learn new order sets that are more efficient and up to date with current practice. The development process incorporates a two-stage optimization procedure

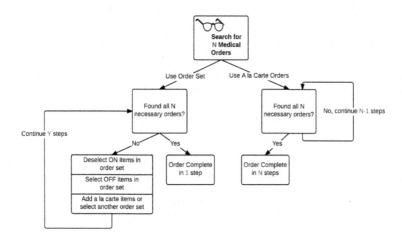

Fig. 2. Medical order placement using order set and a la carte orders

using bisecting K-means clustering and tabu search with the objective of minimizing the amount of cognitive workload incurred during order placement. The resulting order sets from the automated process can then be evaluated by expert clinicians before they are deployed in CPOE.

2 Methods

Several previous studies from real-world EMR implementations have reported the number of order sets built and used, and there have been attempts to create ambulatory order sets or lab corollary orders through data mining and machine learning techniques [9-13]. Zhang et al proposed a two-stage optimization approach embedded with bisecting K-means clustering to create data-driven order sets [7], and this paper aims to improve the performance of this algorithm by incorporating tabu search, a metaheuristic optimization procedure [14].

Tabu search is a metaheuristic search algorithm for complex optimization problems that prevents the search process from being trapped in locally optimal solutions [14,15]. It has been applied in healthcare for supporting prostate cancer diagnosis by identifying signals from a large amount of data [16], and optimization of supply distribution in hospitals [17], among others. Three main components of tabu search are the use of flexible memory structures, control mechanism of the memory structures, and memory functions of different time spans. Specifically, starting with an initial solution i, tabu search generates a subset V of candidate solutions and identifies the best solution j in V for the next move. If the stopping criteria are met, the search is terminated or transferred to initiate a memory function such as intensification or diversification.

If not, tabu search records j as the next solution to move to, and marks it as a tabu move that prevents the move from occurring for a user-defined number of times, unless aspiration criteria are met. Aspiration criteria allow tabu moves when they result in solutions that are better than the current solutions. These features of tabu search approach are particularly suited to the order set optimization problem by allowing the search process to efficiently improve the clusters resulting from the K-means procedure [7].

Table 1. Cognitive click cost (CCC)

		Action	
		Select	De-select
	A la carte	1.2	–
Order	Order set	1.2	–
Type	Default-ON	0.2	1.5
	Default-OFF	0.5	0.1

We develop order sets such that optimal orders are presented to clinicians at the optimal time interval, such that users incur the least amount of cognitive workload while making order placement. This is modeled as a two-stage optimization problem, where we seek to minimize cognitive click cost (CCC), a cognitive measure on order set usage developed by Zhang et al [7]. CCC assigns a cognitive workload coefficient to each order placement task in Figure 2. The default setting for each order is pre-defined. If an order has been used by more than 80% of the patients in the historical data, it is set as ON, and OFF otherwise. Due to space limitations, we refer to Zhang et al [18] for a more detailed formulation of the problem.

Definition 1. *Cognitive Click Cost In an action of order placement where clinician selects multiple orders for a patient,*

$$CCC = 1.2A + 1.2K + 0.2\sum_{k=1}^{K} on_{k,on} + 1.5\sum_{k=1}^{K} on_{k,off}$$
$$+0.5\sum_{k=1}^{K} off_{k,on} + 0.1\sum_{k=1}^{K} off_{k,off} \tag{1}$$

where A is the number of a la carte orders, K is the number of order sets, $on_{k,on}$ and $on_{k,off}$ are defaulted-ON orders from order set k that are kept as ON, or turned OFF, respectively. $off_{k,on}$ and $off_{k,off}$ are defaulted-OFF orders from order set k that are kept as OFF, or turned ON, respectively.

Example 1. As shown in Table 1, choosing an order set or a la carte order requires 1.2 units of CCC, and adding a defaulted-OFF item to the order set orders requires 0.5 unit of CCC. An order set that is perfectly aligned with the workflow will only incur $1.2 + 0.2x$ unit of CCC, where x is an integer number of defaulted-ON items in the order set. There will be no additional clicks to de-select defaulted-ON orders, to select defaulted-OFF orders, or to add a la carte orders. In this case, given x is at least 2, using order set will generate less cognitive workload compared to selecting x a la carte orders, which incur $1.2x$ units of CCC.

A sketch of the algorithm is shown in Algorithm 1. Given a time span from *start* to *endtime* in hours, within each *interval* that is at least 2 hours long, we use bisecting K-means clustering to cluster n orders that were placed in the particular time interval, based on the number of co-occurrence of each order with the rest of the orders in patients' order lists. All clusters with more than 2 orders are considered as order sets, and the rest of the 1-order clusters are considered as a la carte orders. Parameter k^* that produced the lowest $CCC_{k^*,t}$ is saved as the tentative best solution $S_{k^*,t}$ in interval t. Then, in tabu search we perturb $S_{k^*,t}$ by adding or deleting orders from order sets. In the deletion step, the algorithm randomly removes an item from a cluster, and in the addition step the algorithm randomly moves an item from one cluster to another. Recent 7 moves are saved in tabu list, unless the tabu move results in lower CCC than the current best solution. Further, we compare $CCC_{k^*,t}$ post tabu search across all intervals with the same *start*, such that the interval with the lowest $CCC_{k^*,t}$ is saved as the optimal interval t^*, and we have found the best solution S_{t^*} in interval t. The number of hours *run* to run the algorithm before comparing $CCC_{k^*,t}$ is defined by users. The ending time point end_{t^*} in interval t becomes the starting time point *start* of the $t+1$ interval.

Algorithm 1. Two-stage optimization using tabu search

---

    while $start \leq endtime - interval$ **do**
        for $end = start + interval$ to $\min(start + run, endtime + 1)$ **do**
            for $k = 2$ to $n - 1$ **do**
                apply bisecting K-means clustering on order items with $K = k$
                save solution $S_{k,t}$
                calcualate $CCC_{k,t}$ given $S_{k,t}$
            end for
            $CCC_{k^*,t} = \min(CCC_{k,t})$
            save $S_{k,t}$ as S_t
            save end as end_t
            apply Tabu search on S_t
        end for
        $CCC_{k^*,t^*} = \min(CCC_{k^*,t})$
        save S_{t^*} as best solution in time interval
        $end_{t^*} = start$
    end while

In addition to CCC to evaluate the algorithm's performance, we use coverage rate, defined by Zhang et al as the number of items used by a patient from an order set divided by the total number of items in the order set [7].

Definition 2. *Average Coverage Rate The average coverage rate (ACR) across K order sets, M order entries, and P patients is*

$$\frac{1}{K}\sum_{1}^{K}(\frac{1}{M}\sum_{1}^{M}(\frac{1}{P}\sum_{1}^{P}\frac{n_{p,m,k}}{n_k})) \tag{2}$$

where $n_{p,m,k}$ is the number of unique items given to patient p from order set k during order entry m, and n_k is the total number of orders in order set k.

The higher the ACR, the fewer modification needs to be made to order sets during order placement. Hence, ACR is another measure to confirm the usability of data-driven order sets.

3 Experiments

3.1 Data

This dataset comes from a large pediatric hospital where all inpatient orders have been entered directly into the CPOE since 2002. Diagnosis and severity are captured by the drug description and severity of illness using All Patient Refined Diagnosis Related Groups (APR-DRGs). All patient identifying information was removed to create a de-identified dataset for the study. For this study, we use data from 179 pneumonia patients, with moderate severity, who used a total of 462 unique orders from 55 unique order sets in 2011. Table 2 lists the summary statistics on order placement. As the table shows, there are 253 unique order set orders that have never been used, while there are 187 orders that were used by patients, but are not part of any order sets. The summary statistics show that there is a gap between actual workflow and order sets design, which may be improved through data-driven order set development.

The order sets were trained using 96 patients whose final diagnoses were "Pneumonia, Organism unspecified", and we tested their generalizability using a test set, which includes patients whose final diagnoses included "Pneumonia, Organism unspecified" , "Bacterial Pneumonia, Unspecified", "Viral Pneumonia, Unspecified", "Pneumonia due to Mycoplasma Pneumoniae", "Asthma, unspecified with (acute) exacerbation", "Influenza with Pneumonia", and "Acute Chest Syndrome". Whereas the training set included patients with only the most common diagnosis "Pneumonia, Organism unspecified", the test set is used to test the usability of order sets under the real setting, where patients are admitted with diverse backgrounds, multiple conditions and complications. Patients with a final diagnosis of "Pneumonia, Organism unspecified" are randomly divided into the training and test set, and all patients whose final diagnoses were others are put into the test set.

The distribution of order actions for Pneumonia patients with moderate condition is shown in Figure 3. The horizontal axis represents the time of ordering since admission. Negative time entries are the times patients spent in emergency rooms, pre-admission to the inpatient setting. Primary vertical axis is the average

Table 2. Summary Statistics of Patient Population

	Count
Number of patients	179
Number of unique order sets used	55
Number of unique orders used	462
Number of order set orders not used from order sets	253
Number of unique orders used that are not part of any order set	187
Average number of order placement per patient (sd)	37 (17)
Average total number of orders per patient (sd)	74 (32)
Average ratio of a la carte vs. order set items	2
Average number of symptoms exhibited during hospital stay	4.7

count of orders per patient per hour, with red indicating order set items and blue indicating a la carte items. Except for two peaks at hours -10 and 0, orders are largely placed as a la carte.

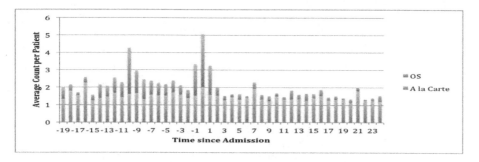

Fig. 3. Distribution of Order Actions in Pneumonia Patients with Moderate Conditions

3.2 Optimization Results

The extended algorithm incorporating tabu search resulted in a reduction of 33% in CCC compared to the current solution. This outperforms the previous algorithm incorporating just bisecting K-means which achieved 19% reduction in CCC compared to the existing solution [7]. Table 3 describes the optimization results from an experimental evaluation. Ten optimal time intervals were found over the duration of interest, between 15 hours prior to admission and 24 hours after admission. Table 3 lists the number of order sets, number of order items, and number of orders that were not placed in an order set (a la carte items) in each time interval. In both training and test sets, average coverage rates of order sets from the optimization are significantly higher than those from the current order sets (p-value < 0.05 using Mann-Whitney test). In addition, the duration of the time intervals are longer than those obtained from previous methods, which tended to be 2-hour intervals, indicating that order sets generated using tabu search are more robust to changes in workflow, hence easier to implement.

Table 4 presents 2 example order sets created using the new metaheuristic optimization procedure. The table lists the time interval when they were created, orders, default setting, and order type. Orders in the 1st order set were

Table 3. Optimization results

	Optimization			Train set			Test set		
time interval	# order set	# order set item	# a-la-carte item	# pati-ents	orig-inal ACR	new ACR	# pati-ents	orig-inal ACR	new ACR
-15, -11	4	8	15	8	.27	.50	6	.19	.50
-11, -7	15	34	11	17	.30	.49	16	.39	.47
-7, -1	24	89	20	86	.25	.27	75	.26	.31
-1, 2	24	49	174	96	.46	.50	80	.47	.49
2, 7	28	81	47	74	.41	.37	68	.31	.37
7, 11	21	56	12	65	.34	.40	52	.38	.42
11, 14	12	28	35	56	.26	.48	50	.26	.46
14, 20	25	55	73	78	.45	.47	62	.26	.49
20, 22	13	28	26	46	.36	.47	30	.25	.46
22, 24	8	19	35	47	.41	.42	23	.25	.40

Table 4. Example order sets

Order set	Time interval	Order	Default	Type
1	-1,2	Glucose	OFF	Pharmacy
		Electrolytes	OFF	Laboratory
2	-11,-7	Admit	ON	Patient Care
		Subsequent Pulse Oximetry Continuous	ON	Respiratory Care
		Acetaminophen	OFF	Pharmacy

originally ordered as a la carte orders in the data, and the optimization process determined that placing them into a single order set would reduce CCC and increase coverage rate during the admission period. In the 2nd order set, 'Admit to' and 'Acetaminophen' are part of a large general admission order set, and 'Subsequent Pulse Oximetry Continuous' is part of a 2-order pulse oximetry order set. Data shows that these two order sets tend to be used together upon patients' admission, and often times just part of the general admission order set is used. Hence, the incomplete use of the general admission order set and its common co-use with the pulse oximetry order set may be reflected in the creation of the 2nd order set. Also, in the pulse oximetry order set, 'Subsequent Pulse Oximetry Continuous' is defaulted-ON, and 'Initial Pulse Oximetry Continuous' is defaulted-OFF. It is possible that only the defaulted-ON item, 'Subsequent Pulse Oximetry Continuous,' was selected into the machine-generated order set to lower the cost.

4   Discussion

In a previous study, we applied a two-stage optimization embedded with just bisecting K-means on order data from asthma, appendectomy and pneumonia patients. We found that the algorithm performs well on asthma and appendectomy data, but significant improvement was challenging for pneumonia data, possibly due to the diverse complications suffered by these patients. Results from this study, incorporating tabu search in the optimization, indicate that the metaheuristic-enhanced optimization approach dominates currently implemented solution and previous data-driven methodology, potentially easing the process of keeping order sets up to date with current best practice by generating a feasible initial solution for expert review.

Future work will require clinicians to perform clinical evaluation of the optimized order sets, such that unrealistic order combinations can be identified and eliminated, and machine-generated order sets can be correctly classified and named. This algorithm also should be tested on other clinical conditions with varying levels of patient diversity to improve generalizability and coverage rates. For example, we can incorporate intensification and diversification on tabu search, such that more consistent increase in coverage rates can be obtained while reducing CCC. In this study we do not differentiate the cognitive workload among clinicians of different experiences and familiarity with IT. Factoring in the individual differences, or altering the objective function from CCC to other meaningful measures, may produce order sets that meet different goals.

5   Conclusion

In this study, we developed order sets based on how the content of order sets or a la carte orders alter the amount of cognitive workload incurred by clinicians upon usage. The optimization sought to minimize cognitive click cost (CCC) by clustering orders that tend be given together to patients, and further, by perturbing the order set assignment using tabu search. We evaluate this approach using data on 179 pneumonia patients with moderately severe condition, who exhibited nearly 5 symptoms, on average, during their hospital stay. A total of 174 order sets comprising 447 order items were created from the optimization process. Evaluation of machine-generated order sets demonstrate the algorithm's potential in creating order sets that meet the workflow and increase usability of health IT components.

Acknowledgement. We are greatly indebted to the vision, contributions and support of the late Dr. James E. Levin that made this study possible.

References

1. HIMSS Analytics: Healthcare IT Data, Research, and Analysis, http://www.himssanalytics.org/hc_providers/emr_adoption.asp.
2. Horsky, J., Kaufman, D.R., Oppenheim, M.L., Patel, V.L.: A framework for analyzing the cognitive complexity of computer-assisted clinical ordering. J. Biomed. Inform. 36(12), 422 (2003)
3. Schumacher, R.M., Lowry, S.Z.: NIST Guide to the Processes Approach for Improving the Usability of Electronic Health Records (November 2010)

4. Ash, J.S., Berg, M., Coiera, E.: Some unintended consequences of information technology in health care: the nature of patient care information system-related errors. J. Am. Med. Inform. Assoc. 11(2), 104–112 (2004)
5. Jung, M., Riedmann, D., Hackl, W.O., Hoerbst, A., Jaspers, M.W., Ferret, L., Lawton, K., Ammenwerth, E.: Physicians' Perceptions on the usefulness of contextual information for prioritizing and presenting alerts in computerized physician order entry systems. BMC Med. Inform. Decis. Mak. 12(1), 111 (2012)
6. Payne, T.H., Hoey, P.J., Nichol, P., Lovis, C.: Preparation and use of preconstructed orders, order sets, and order menus in a computerized provider order entry system. J. Am. Med. Inform. Assoc. 10(4), 322–329 (2003)
7. Zhang, Y., Padman, R., Levin, J.E.: Paving the COWpath: data-driven design of pediatric order sets. Journal of the American Medical Informatics Association: JAMIA 21(e2), e304–e311 (2014)
8. Ash, J.S., Sittig, D.F., Poon, E.G., Guappone, K., Campbell, E., Dykstra, R.H.: The extent and importance of unintended consequences related to computerized provider order entry. J. Am. Med. Inform. Assoc. 14(4), 415–423 (2007)
9. Klann, J., Schadow, G., McCoy, J.M.: A recommendation algorithm for automating corollary order generation. In: AMIA Annu. Symp. Proc., vol. 2009, pp. 333–337 (2009)
10. Ali, N.A., Mekhjian, H.S., Kuehn, P.L., Bentley, T.D., Kumar, R., Ferketich, A.K., Hoffmann, S.: Specificity of computerized physician order entry has a significant effect on the efficiency of workflow for critically ill patients. Crit. Care Med. 33(1), 110–114 (2005)
11. Wright, A., Sittig, D.F.: Automated development of order sets and corollary orders by data mining in an ambulatory computerized physician order entry system. In: AMIA Annu. Symp. Proc., pp. 819–823 (2006)
12. Munasinghe, R.L., Arsene, C., Abraham, T.K., Zidan, M., Siddique, M.: Improving the utilization of admission order sets in a computerized physician order entry system by integrating modular disease specific order subsets in, a general medicine admission order set. J. Am. Med. Inform. Assoc. 18(3), 322–326 (2011)
13. Hulse, N.C., Del Fiol, G., Bradshaw, R.L., Roemer, L.K., Rocha, R.A.: Towards an on-demand peer feedback system for a clinical knowledge base: a case study with order sets. J. Biomed. Inform. 41(1), 152–164 (2008)
14. Glover, F.: Tabu search-part I. ORSA Journal on Computing 1(3), 190–206
15. Glover, F.: Tabu search-part II. ORSA Journal on Computing 2(1), 4–32
16. Bai, X., Padman, R., Ramsey, J., Spirtes, P.: Tabu Search-Enhanced Graphical Models for Classification in High Dimensions. INFORMS Journal on Computing Summer 20, 423–437 (2008)
17. Michelon, P., Dib Cruz, M., Gascon, V.: Using the tabu search method for the distribution of supplies in a hospital. Annal. Op. Res. 50(1), 427–435 (1994)
18. Zhang, Y., Padman, R., Levin, J.E., Mengshoel, O.: Data-driven Order Set Development in the Pediatric Environment: Toward Safer and More Efficient Patient Care. Heinz College Working Paper. Carnegie Mellon University (2015)

Conceptual Modeling of Clinical Pathways: Making Data and Processes Connected

Carlo Combi[1], Barbara Oliboni[1(✉)], and Alberto Gabrieli[2]

[1] Dipartimento di Informatica, Università di Verona, Verona, Italy
{carlo.combi,barbara.oliboni}@univr.it
[2] Dipartimento di Anestesia e Terapia Intensiva, AOUI Verona, Verona, Italy

Abstract. In this paper, we propose a framework for seamless conceptual modeling of both data and processes, and the seamless integration of temporalities for both clinical data and clinical tasks. Moreover, we apply our approach to model the clinical pathway for managing patients with ROSC (Return Of Spontaneous Circulation) in a real ICU clinical setting.

1 Introduction

Clinical pathways are used for managing quality in the standardization of care processes. They refer to clinical guidelines and their main aim is the organized and efficient patient care based on evidence-based practice [4]. Clinical pathways can be considered as an application of process management in the context of patient healthcare. This means that in the conceptual modeling of clinical pathways, we can take advantage of process models proposed in the literature for the conceptual modeling of business processes [3].

A very crucial point to highlight is that information accessed during the execution of clinical tasks are used for both performing activities and supporting medical decisions. Indeed, each activity described in a clinical pathway implies the execution of specific diagnostic/therapeutic (decision-making) actions, often based on patient clinical data. In classical approaches, the process-related information is usually designed separately, and is often conceptually represented by traditional data models. As a matter of fact, BPMN 2.0, the well-known framework for business process modeling, allows one to represent the process-related information as Data Objects, but a true integration between data and processes in conceptual modeling is still a research goal. Moreover, clinical pathways and the related clinical information are characterized by relevant temporal aspects, as both clinical data and processes need to be interpreted according to their temporal context, to possible temporal constraints, and considering their temporal evolution [4].

According to this scenario, in this paper we propose a new framework for the seamless conceptual modeling of both data and processes for clinical pathways, and the seamless integration of temporalities for both clinical data and clinical tasks. A preliminary version of our framework, which did not consider all temporal aspects and adopted a different process model, is discussed in [1]. Moreover,

© Springer International Publishing Switzerland 2015
J.H. Holmes et al. (Eds.): AIME 2015, LNAI 9105, pp. 57–62, 2015.
DOI: 10.1007/978-3-319-19551-3_7

we discuss the application of our framework to the real world clinical pathway for managing patients with ROSC (Return Of Spontaneus Circulation) [5] by considering process requirements collected from the medical team of the Borgo Trento Hospital (Verona - Italy).

2   Seamless Conceptual Modeling of Clinical Pathways and Data

The framework we propose for the seamless conceptual modeling of clinical pathways and related data is based on a process model (notation), on a data model, and on some new concepts, and related diagrams, allowing the designer to link process and data schemata. In particular, we adopt the workflow conceptual model proposed in [3], while for representing the related data, we refer to TIMEER [2], and we describe a possible solution for connecting process and information views. As a matter of fact, we model the connection between the activities of a process and the related key information at a conceptual level. At this aim, we define the notion of *core entitity*. A *core entitity* is part of the TIMEER diagram representing information related to the considered clinical process. The instance of a *core entitity* is named *core instance*. The graphical representation of a *core entitity* is characterized by the presence of a box (containing the label n) under the rectangle representing the TIMEER entity. The label n in the box represents the number of core instances of the core entity. *Core entitities* represent information that are significant for the whole process, i.e., information that are needed to most activities.

In the conceptual modeling of the considered context, a given designed process can be connected to one or more core entities. At instance level, a process case (which is an instance of the considered process) can manage one or more instances of a *core entitity*. In a TIMEER diagram also entities that are not considered and represented as *core entitities* may be present. These *simple* entities may have instances that are involved in a relationship with a *core instance* (CI) or not (NCI). In the former case we define each of them as *core-instance-related* (CIR), while in the latter as *not-core-instance-related* (NCIR). An involved TIMEER relationship can be classified either *direct* or *indirect*. If the relationship relates a core entity and a simple entity, then the relationship is direct, while if a path of relationships between the core and the simple entities exists, then the relationship is indirect. In a similar way, we can classify instances of relationships. If a relationship instance involves a core instance or is indirectly connected to a core instance through a path of relationships, it is a *core-instance-involving* instance (CII). Otherwise, if a relationship instance does not involve a core instance, then it is *not-core-instance-involving* instance (NCII).

A clinical pathway is composed of activities (tasks). Each task may be related to the part of the TIMEER diagram representing the information the physician needs to perform the task itself. A *task view* indicates what is the information a physician has to access to properly execute activity. The *task view* is composed by a set of entities and relationships belonging to the considered TIMEER diagram.

The task is in a *view association* with each entity and relationship included in the *task view*. For each view association, it is possible to specify a set of *view constraints* stating how the key information guides the whole process.

The *view constraints* express the type of access to the considered information, the view cardinality, and the set of instances the agent executing the task has access to. A *view constraint* has the form

$< $ `AccessType` $ >< $ `QualTime` $ > [(< $ `MinC` $ >, < $ `MaxC` $ >)|< $ `InstGroup` $ >|< $ `Path` $ >]$

where `AccessType` $\in \{read, write\}$ defines in which way the physician performing the task can access the related information; `QualTime` $\in \{start, during, end\}$ specifies the qualitative constraint for fixing the moment the physician performing the task has to access to information; (`MinC` $\in \{0, N\}$, `MaxC` $\in \{1, N\}$), $N \in \mathbb{N}$ defines the minimum and maximum number of accessible instances; `InstGroup` $\in \{CI, NCI, CIR, NCIR, CII, NCII\}$ defines the group of instances accessible from the physician performing the task; and `Path` $= relName_1; ...; relName_n, n \in \{1, N\}$ is composed of relationship names and specifies the path to follow for reaching the core entity starting from the entity/relationship involved in the considered constraint.

3   Conceptual Modeling of ROSC Pathway

In this paper, we consider the clinical process for managing patients with ROSC, i.e., patients having had a cardiac arrest, underwent to a resuscitation attempt, and give signs of the return of spontaneus circulation, such as breathing, coughing, movement, palpable pulse or a measurable blood pressure. The clinical pathway related to the management of patients having had a cardiac arrest is based on the clinical guideline about postresuscitation care [5], benefits from success of postcardiac arrest therapeutic hypotermia [6], and implements the care process starting from evidence-based practice of the medical team of the Borgo Trento Hospital.

The immediate treatment of emergency is decisive for having best chance of recovery and survival. In Fig. 1 we report the process describing activities to perform in the immediate postarrest phase. The diagram of Fig. 1 starts with the cardiac arrest treatment (task *T1*), and finishes with the admission of the patient in the Intensive Care Unit (task *T25*). Activities in the diagram are coordinated with respect to their execution flow. As an example, activities (*T5*, *T6*, and *T7*) performed for alerting computed tomography team, medical emergency team and cardiologists must be executed in parallel, and thus they are enclosed between a split and a join total connectors (identified by *+1*). The workflow schema models temporal contraints by defining the execution duration of task, i.e., the allowed time-stamped interval the task must be executed within, the temporal span allowed for executing the connector activity, and the edge duration (delay) representing the time span between the ending instant of the predecessor and the starting instant of the successor. Moreover, the workflow diagram allows the definition of relative constraints, i.e., the definition of the time distance (duration) between the starting/ending instants of two nonconsecutive workflow nodes. The notation for limiting this temporal aspect is

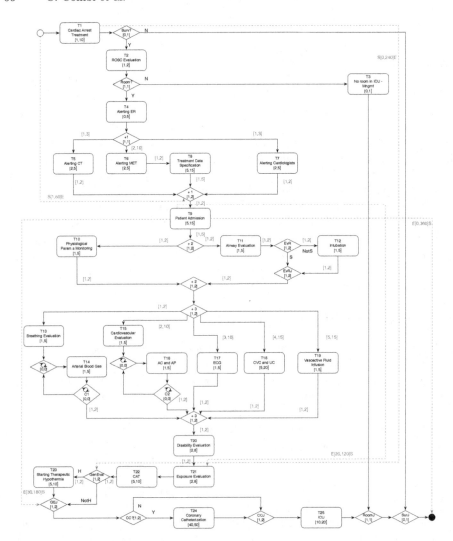

Fig. 1. Workflow diagram describing activities in the immediate postarrest phase

$I_F[MinDurarion, MaxDuration]I_S$, where $I_F \in \{S, E\}$ represents the instant (S for starting and E for ending) of the first node to use, and I_E the same information for the second one. As an example, in the diagram of Fig. 1 the time distance between the start event and the join total connector ($+1$) is expressed as $S[1, 60]E$ and specifies that within 60 minutes the patient must be admitted to the Shock Room.

In Fig. 2 we show the task view related to task *T23* (*Starting Therapeutic Hypothermia*) being part of the workflow diagram of Fig. 1. Involved physicians consider this task a very important step in the clinical process for managing patients with ROSC. This is due to the fact that postarrest patients receiving therapeutic hypothermia seem to have a favourable neurologic recovery. An example of view association connects (by using a line ending with a filled diamond) task *Starting Therapeutic Hypothermia* with the core entity *Admission*, since the physician must be able to read information about the admitted patient, i.e., the core instance. The related view constraint (*read start (1,1) CI*) specifies that the physician reads the unique instance (*CI*) of the entity *Admission* at the beginnig of its performance.

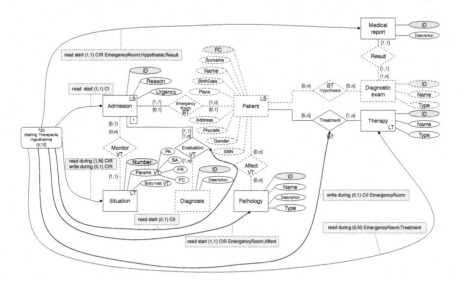

Fig. 2. Graphical representation of a task view (dotted lines represent no visible information)

4   Conclusions

In the medical domain, a very important issue to consider is the fact that process activities intertwined with data. Clinical activities are often characterized by decision-making aspects, and thus need to manage related, decision-supporting information. In this paper, we dealt with this topic and proposed a framework for seamless conceptual modeling of both data and processes, by considering also temporal aspects[1].

References

1. Combi, C., Degani, S.: Seamless (and temporal) conceptual modeling of business process information. In: ADBIS 2011. CEUR Proceedings, vol. 789, pp. 23–32 (2011)
2. Combi, C., Degani, S., Jensen, C.S.: Capturing temporal constraints in temporal ER models. In: Li, Q., Spaccapietra, S., Yu, E., Olivé, A. (eds.) ER 2008. LNCS, vol. 5231, pp. 397–411. Springer, Heidelberg (2008)

---

[1] We wish to thank our former student Alice Pizzolato, for her contribution to the design of ROSC pathway.

3. Combi, C., Gozzi, M., Posenato, R., Pozzi, G.: Conceptual modeling of flexible temporal workflows. ACM Transactions on Autonomous and Adaptive Systems 7(2), 19 (2012)
4. Combi, C., Keravnou-Papailiou, E., Shahar, Y.: Temporal Information Systems in Medicine. Springer-Verlag New York, Inc., New York (2010)
5. Nolan, J.P., et al.: European resuscitation council guidelines for resuscitation 2010 section 1. executive summary. Resuscitation 81(10), 1219–1276 (2010), European Resuscitation Council Guidelines for Resuscitation 2010
6. Perman, S.M., et al.: Timing of neuroprognostication in postcardiac arrest therapeutic hypothermia. Critical Care Medicine 40(3), 719–724 (2012)

Data Mining and Machine Learning

Distributed Learning to Protect Privacy in Multi-centric Clinical Studies

Andrea Damiani[1], Mauro Vallati[2], Roberto Gatta[1(✉)], Nicola Dinapoli[1],
Arthur Jochems[3], Timo Deist[3], Johan van Soest[3], Andre Dekker[3],
and Vincenzo Valentini[1]

[1] Radiotherapy Department, Università Cattolica del Sacro Cuore, Rome, Italy
{ad61965, roberto.gatta.bs,nicola.dinapoli.74,vvalentini}@gmail.com
[2] School of Computing and Engineering, University of Huddersfield, Huddersfield, UK
m.vallati@hud.ac.uk
[3] Department of Radiation Oncology (MAASTRO), GROW School for Oncology and
Developmental Biology, Maastricht University Medical Centre,
Maastricht, Netherlands
{arthur.jochems,timo.deist,johan.vansoest,andre.dekker}@maastro.nl

Abstract. Research in medicine has to deal with the growing amount
of data about patients which are made available by modern technologies. All these data might be used to support statistical studies, and for
identifying causal relations. To use these data, which are spread across
hospitals, efficient merging techniques as well as policies to deal with this
sensitive information are strongly needed. In this paper we introduce
and empirically test a distributed learning approach, to train Support
Vector Machines (SVM), that allows to overcome problems related to
privacy and data being spread around. The introduced technique allows
to train algorithms without sharing any patients-related information, ensuring privacy and avoids the development of merging tools. We tested
this approach on a large dataset and we described results, in terms of
convergence and performance; we also provide considerations about the
features of an IT architecture designed to support distributed learning
computations.

Keywords: Distributed learning · Patient privacy preserving ·
Multi-centric clinical studies

1 Introduction

Modern research in medicine has to deal with a growing number of variables
coming from the world of images, genomics, proteomics, etc. Given this huge
number of variables, medical research requires an extremely large number of
clinical cases to be studied, in order to support statistical inference and avoid
overfitting issues. Considering the fact that each hospital only has a limited
number of patients, cooperation among hospitals is needed to recruit adequately
large cohorts of patients.

© Springer International Publishing Switzerland 2015
J.H. Holmes et al. (Eds.): AIME 2015, LNAI 9105, pp. 65–75, 2015.
DOI: 10.1007/978-3-319-19551-3_8

The most used method to do this type of research is the multi-centric study which requires some specific techniques for collecting and merging data. Traditional approaches are based on sharing Excel files, FileMaker or Access Databases, populated and maintained locally and then sent via e-mail. This approach has been overcome by the web, and the development of *ad hoc* websites and commercial products allowing a more flexible (and reliable) way to collect clinical data (e.g., https://www.openclinica.com/). However the exploitation of the Internet and its technologies raises a number of questions related to the privacy of involved data. Also the use of a central website means hospitals need to query their own information systems and subsequently enter the data in the central study system, which is often a manual, resource intensive process. The issue of guaranteeing patients privacy while performing research in medicine is becoming more and more present in the public debate. In fact, IT infrastructures and Machine Learning techniques encourage the development of multi-centric studies, dealing with increasing numbers of features and patient records, thus meeting the needs expressed by the medical research community [7]. On the other hand this poses serious questions about the need of protecting the privacy of those involved in the studies. The best way to avoiding any privacy-related issue, while still exploiting multi-centric data, is to avoid sharing clinical data among different hospitals, training algorithms by sharing only few aggregate parameters among hospitals and guaranteeing the global convergence (*consensus*) to an acceptable shared mathematical model. The use of cryptography to send clinical data is not an effective solution: in fact, in this approach, a decryption key is used to reconstruct the dataset *far from the institution that collected it* before doing the analysis. We hypothesise in this study that Distributed Learning techniques are a good answer to this pressing issue [9].

It is well known that many Machine Learning algorithms lead to convex optimisation problems; if this is the case, as in our examples, the well-known Method of Lagrange Multipliers offers a solution, for instance, via the *dual ascent* algorithm. Interestingly, when a condition known as *strong duality* holds, together with additivity of the objective function, dual decomposition is possible and a form of parallel, privacy-preserving learning can be achieved, as shown by Dantzig and Wolf [3]. Unfortunately, the dual ascent method is not very robust with respect to convergence and is also quite demanding in terms of assumptions. In order to overcome these limitations, the so called *augmented Lagrangian* was introduced, in which a regularisation term is included, thus improving both the problem's differentiability and its convergence under milder assumptions. As a trade-off, separability is lost, and with it, so is distributed learning. Recently, several authors (e.g., [4][2]) proposed a novel approach for Distributed SVMs, in which DL across nodes is achieved through the exchange of limited information, namely a (subset of) the problem's support vectors. While this approach gives good results by reducing the amount of data being transferred, i.e. the communication overhead, among nodes, it is not the preferred approach in medical environments. In this context, support vectors correspond to patients data, which should not be shared for the aforementioned privacy reasons. Among existing methods addressing the privacy issue, such as [8], [2], we found the approach proposed by Boyd [1] particularly interesting for two reasons.

First, it addresses the problem of Privacy Protection Distributed Learning with a method that leaves all patient data, including both features and outcomes, safely at the institution that collected them; this allows performing multi-centric studies even under the strictest privacy policy, either today or in the future. Second, the method is general: different learning algorithms, all leading to a convex optimisation problem, can be implemented under the same framework: we successfully experimented Support Vector Machines, L1 regularised linear regression (LASSO), and Logistic regression.

In this paper we propose the implementation of a Distributed Learning solution to train predictive models without sharing clinical data by exploiting the well-known Alternating Direction Method of Multipliers (ADMM) algorithm [1], which is a technique used to solve convex optimisation problems in parallel. Although several techniques handling similar problems have been proposed (see, e.g. [14]), ADMM has been selected due to its generality: it can handle logistic regression, L-1 regularised linear regression, or SVM.

2   Background

In this section we present the ADMM algorithm and we introduce the notion of convergence in distributed learning algorithms. We advise the interested reader to refer to [1][13][15] for an in-depth theoretical analysis.

2.1   Summarising Privacy Preserving Data Mining (PPDM) through ADMM

A general convex model fitting problem, like the LASSO (L-1 regularised linear regression), logistic regression or SVM, can be expressed as

$$\text{minimize} \quad l\left(A\xi - b\right) + r(\xi) \tag{1}$$

where $\xi \in \mathbb{R}^n$ is the vector of unknown parameters, $A \in \mathbb{R}^{m \times n}$ is the feature matrix (or a matrix that can be built from it and the label vector through affine transformations), $b \in \mathbb{R}^m$ is the output (sometimes called *labels*) vector, $l : \mathbb{R}^m \to \mathbb{R}^n$ is a convex loss function, and $r : \mathbb{R}^n \to \mathbb{R}$ is a convex regularisation function.

We also add a further hypothesis, that both $l()$ and $r()$ are additive, and it can be proved [13] that SVM's, logistic regression and LASSO loss functions all fall in this category, and that the typical regularisation functions, and namely the norm-1, norm-2 and norm-∞ functions, are all separable in the sense above described. This is crucial: if an objective function is not additive, i.e. *commutative* and *associative*, then this solution cannot be pursued.

Our examples all fall under the category of the *global variable consensus with regularisation* problem:

$$\text{minimize } f(x) = \sum_{i=1}^{N} f_i(x_i) + g(z) \tag{2}$$
$$\text{subject to } x_i - z = 0 \qquad\qquad i = 1, \ldots, N$$

in which $g(z) = \lambda\|z\|$ is the regularisation term with parameter λ and the N constraints enforce consensus among nodes. The ADMM iterations for this problem, with *augmented Lagrangian* parameter ρ, are

$$x_i^{k+1} := \operatorname*{argmin}_{x_i} \left(f_i(x_i) + (\rho/2) \left\| x_i - z^k + u_i^k \right\|_2^2 \right)$$
$$z^{k+1} := \operatorname*{argmin}_{z} \left(g(z) + (N\rho/2) \left\| z - \bar{x}^{k+1} - \bar{u}^k \right\|_2^2 \right) \tag{3}$$
$$u_i^{k+1} := u_i^k + x_i^{k+1} - z^{k+1}$$

The algorithm amounts to a Gauss-Seidel pass for $x-$ and $z-$ updates, followed by a dual $u-$update performed via gradient ascent. The $x-$update can be performed in parallel on all the involved nodes and then the other two updates happen at a Master, i.e. *central* level, for consensus.

By exploiting results from the Proximity Operators theory, the iterations (3) can be further simplified according to the structure of the regularisation term, as in the computation schema for for Support Vector Machines (L_2 regularised):

$$x_i^{k+1} := \operatorname*{argmin}_{\xi} \left(1^T (A_i\xi + 1)_+ + (\rho/2) \left\| \xi - z^k + u_i^k \right\|_2^2 \right)$$
$$z^{k+1} := \frac{N\rho}{(1/\lambda) + N\rho} \left(\bar{x}^{k+1} + \bar{u}^k \right) \tag{4}$$
$$u_i^{k+1} := u_i^k + x_i^{k+1} - z^{k+1}$$

A similar approach can be used for Logistic Regression and LASSO.

2.2 Convergence

When the f and g functions are closed, proper, and convex, and the extended Lagrangian L_0 has a saddle point, we have (proof can be found in [1]):

(a) *Residual Convergence* $r^k = x^k - \bar{x}^k \to 0$ as $k \to \infty$, meaning that consensus is eventually achieved.
(b) *Objective convergence* $f(x^k) + g(z^k) \to p^*$ as $k \to \infty$: the iterations converge toward the unique optimal point.
(c) *Dual variable convergence* $u^k \to u^*$ as $k \to \infty$, where u^* is a (scaled) dual optimal point.

Stopping Criteria. The stopping check is performed at the Master level, as follows:

The $\|r^k\|_2$ and $\|s^k\|_2$ quantities are obtained from

$$\|r^k\|_2^2 = \sum_{i=1}^{N} \|x_i^k - \bar{x}^k\|_2^2 \text{ and } \|s^k\|_2^2 = \|\bar{x}^k - \bar{x}^{k-1}\|_2^2 \qquad (5)$$

and the ϵ^{pri} and ϵ^{dual} are defined as

$$\begin{aligned} \epsilon^{pri} &:= \sqrt{n}\,\epsilon^{abs} + \epsilon^{rel} \max\{\|x^k\|_2, \|-z^k\|_2\} \\ \epsilon^{dual} &:= \sqrt{n}\,\epsilon^{abs} + \epsilon^{rel} \rho\|u^k\|_2 \end{aligned}$$

We stop the iterations when

$$\|r^k\|_2 \le \epsilon^{pri} \qquad \text{and} \qquad \|s^k\|_2 \le \epsilon^{dual} \qquad (6)$$

Reasonable values for ϵ^{rel} are usually in the range $10^{-4} - 10^{-3}$, while the value of ϵ^{abs} is problem-dependent.

From an analysis of the stopping conditions, we see that the first one computes the standard deviation among nodes, thus enforcing consensus; the second one computes the difference between the models obtained by two consecutive iterations. Asking that both quantities are small is equivalent to checking that consensus achievement does not happen at the cost of an excessive suboptimality.

It should also be noted that the method guarantees convergence to the optimal solution, and that this solution is the same that would have been obtained had all the data been consolidated at the same site; alas, convergence is generally not fast. On the other hand, the first ten iterations usually lead close to final solution; depending on the problem at hand, a balance can then be found between accuracy and time complexity.

3   Infrastructure

In the proposed approach, software agents, called Slave Nodes (SN) are sent to each hospital, train on local data and exchange part of the results with an external arbiter, called the Master Node (MN). The MN collects all the results, calculates new coefficients and sends them back to SNs. The computation is performed and after a finite number of cycles, all the Slave Nodes converge to the same result. It should be noted that the exchanged parameters do not allow in any case, from a mathematical point of view, the derivation of any information about any single patient. The general schema of interactions is shown in Figure 1. In a first step (top left) nodes calculate the vector X at time $t+1$ by considering $X(t)$, $z(y)$ and $y(t)$. After computation, $X(t+1)$ is sent to the Master node (top right). Master is now able to calculate $z(t+1)$ and $u(t+1)$ (top right), and returns $z(t+1)$ and $u(t+1)$. Finally, the value of t is incremented, and the process is repeated until the stopping criteria are satisfied.

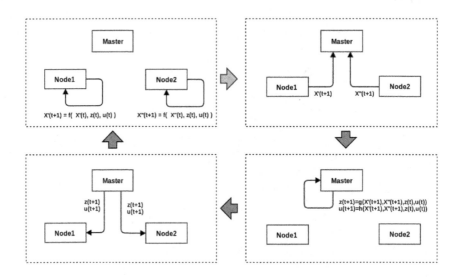

Fig. 1. The general schema of interactions between Master and Nodes

4   Empirical Analysis

Our experimental analysis is aimed at investigating the adaptation proposed by Boyd et al. [1], in terms of convergence and performance, with regards to the number and type of clinical variables included in the model.

In order to evaluate the performance on different optimising engines, we developed three different implementations of the Distributed SVM: namely in R, Mathematica and MATLAB. Implementations were tested on 5,542 simulations, on the R implementation[1]. Each simulated study was different and data was randomly generated [2]. Concerning the statistical distribution of clinical variables, we considered a single clinical outcome with two classes, i.e., survived versus dead. For each centre and for each computation we defined a random number M of clinical cases (called sample points) and an arbitrary number of K independent clinical variables (covariates), defining a $K-$dimensional space. Given a centre, the j_{th} clinical case is a t-uple built as:

$\{Class, V_1, V_2, ..., V_M\}$ where $Class = \{-1, +1\}$ is the clinical outcome (i.e. 1 = survived, -1 = dead) and the generic V_j is the clinical variable (independent variable, or covariate) which has value:

$$O_j^{Class} = N(N(Class, sd2), sd1) \tag{7}$$

---

[1] R implementation can be found at https://github.com/kbolab/pancabbestia.git
[2] Data used for the experimental analysis are available at: http://helios.hud.ac.uk/scommv/storage/csvData.tar.gz

	sd1	sd2	nodes	num.of.cov	rho	lambda	alpha	samples	accuracy	iterations
sd1	1	0.01	0.02	0	0.01	0	-0.01	0.01	0.01	0.03
sd2	0.01	1	0	-0.01	0	0.01	0.02	0	-0.05	0
nodes	0.02	0	1	-0.04	-0.02	0	-0.03	-0.01	-0.02	0.05
num.of.cov	0	-0.01	-0.04	1	-0.01	-0.02	-0.11	-0.01	0.58	0.39
rho	0.01	0	-0.02	-0.01	1	0.02	0.01	-0.01	-0.01	-0.01
lambda	0	0.01	0	-0.02	0.02	1	0.01	0	0.01	0.11
alpha	-0.01	0.02	-0.03	-0.11	-0.11	0.11	1	0.02	-0.04	0.08
samples	0.11	0	-0.01	-0.01	-0.01	0	0.02	1	-0.01	-0.01
accuracy	0.11	-0.05	-0.02	0.58	0.11	0.11	-0.04	-0.01	1	0.11
iterations	0.03	0	0.05	0.39	-0.01	0.11	0.08	-0.01	0.11	1

Fig. 2. Cross Correlation Matrix built using the Pearson correlation method

where $N(\mu, \sigma)$ is a normal distribution with mean and standard deviation μ and σ, respectively. In our analysis, $sd1$ is a factor introduced to have different levels of linear separability of the space, and $sd2$ is used to reproduce the presence of significantly different statistics, for a feature, across sites (i.e., a bias due to different patient population across the nodes). Both $sd1$ and $sd2$ were obtained by a uniform distribution probability: in our case $sd1 = Unif[0.5, 0.9]$ and $sd1 = Unif[0, 0.5]$. This cited model built the clinical variables independently but not identically distributed.

Used optimisers are the optimx package for R [12] (which itself includes a large number of optimisers), CVS for MATLAB [5,6] and the embedded Quasi-Newton Methods in Mathematica. In our experimental analysis we considered, for each computation, the following features:

number of nodes: uniformly distributed between 2 and 10. It represents the number of hospitals involved in computation;
number of features: an integer, taken from a uniform distribution from 2 to 10;
$sd1$, $sd2$: the previously introduced factors for controlling the population of considered hospitals.
ρ, α, λ: uniformly distributed between 1.2 and 1.8. These parameters control the convergence speed of the DL mathematical model;
number of samples per nodes: uniformly distributed from 50 to 500. It represents the simulated number of patients per hospital. Per our experience these cover small to large university hospital for rectal cancer.

The experimental analysis is focused on computations that converge within 2,000 iterations, which means 4882 experiments (660 experiments took more than 2,000 iterations). Results are shown in Figure 2. According to such results, the feature which can play a significant role seems to be the number of covariates, or clinical variables, which affects both accuracy of final model and the number of interactions needed to converge. Also, the number of clinical variables plays an important role, in particular in terms of the number of iterations. This means that a statistical analysis based on a backward elimination for covariates selection seems to be a costly strategy in terms of time. Attention should be thus be paid to feature selection, possibly by applying a forward selection or more advanced techniques, such as [16][10].

5   Discussion

The performed analysis allows us to derive interesting insights:

- policies about Internet connections are very heterogeneous among different hospitals. In most cases, with the exception of a VPN, hospitals do not accept connections from external Internet site, including for research or clinical activities purposes. Moreover, a VPN connection can be slow and unstable. On the other hand, almost all hospitals allow web browser connection, so an HTTP connection can be a good solution both for the accessibility of the channel and the availability of technology to work with. The problem of "one way" data, in a context of web-technologies, can be solved by polling from a client located inside the hospital towards a web server, which manages the messages between nodes. This solution, while apparently solving all issues, is time consuming, because an infrastructure based on a polling strategy in normally slower than an asynchronous one, and generates a lot of redundant network traffic.
- R, Mathematica and MATLAB work well as computation engines, but they show inhomogeneous performances as optimisers. Differences in performance can be significant [15][11]. This can affect convergence in terms of both efficacy and efficiency.
- In a distributed learning scenario, the Data Manager has a different role than his current one. In particular, he is no more in charge of evaluating and manipulating data directly. Although such activities are still important and can not be avoided, in a DL scenario they should be guaranteed in a different way. Distributed Learning can effectively solve the problem of privacy, but it poses new challenges regarding lexical/syntactic/semantic data check, consensus about the ontology, identification of statistical biases among centres, which still have to be solved.

Finally, we investigated the critical issues of a proposed DL architecture, by also testing some simple proofs of concept. A first set of tests was made by running the algorithm developed in Mathematica on a VPN, simulating computation among 4/5 nodes. Then we implemented the same framework in PHP, in

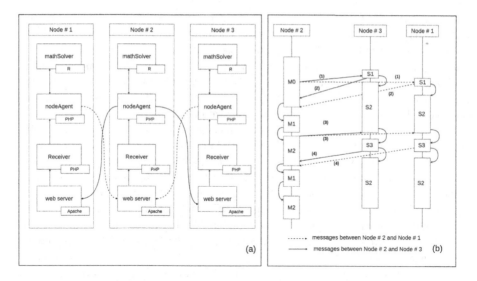

Fig. 3. A general architecture of technologies used (left), and a simplified sequence diagram regarding message exchanging to begin a calculus (right)

order to experiment a web-based implementation and shed some light on weaknesses. Figure 3 shows the implemented nodes structure. Node#2 plays the role of *master*. Despite the different roles in computation, the nodes structure is the same. Differences arise in the web-technologies integrating different scripts written in R. Right part of Figure 3 shows a simplified sequence diagram regarding message exchanging needed to begin a calculus. (1) the *master* asks to Node#3 and Node#1 if they are available for a computation, and waits for a response. Message (1) forces Nodes #3 and #1 to change state to S1; they therefore become *slave* nodes, and prepare the environment for the computation. Finally, they move autonomously to state S2, which means "ready for computation". Once the *master* has received all the "ok" from recruited *slaves* (2), it changes its state to M1, in order to calculate vectors U and Z. Then, the master goes into state M2, sends the calculated vectors (3) and waits for answers. *Slaves* receive (3), move to state S3, in which they calculate their own X vectors, and at the end they send back X to the *master* using the message (4). *Master* gets back all X from *slaves*, and turns again to state M2 to calculate the new vectors, Z and U, for the second iteration.

6 Conclusion

Modern medical technologies are making a large and always increasing amount of information available about patients. On the one hand, this potentially allows us to gain a better understanding of causal relations between observed variables. On the other hand detecting such casual relations needs large patients data in order to perform reliable and meaningful investigations. Since each hospital only treats a limited number of patients, multi-centric studies are more and more common. Multi-centric studies raise a number of issues, mainly related to the way in which patients data are collected, merged and shared. In particular, privacy of patients is an important factor that must be guaranteed. Several countries are currently studying quite restrictive laws to protect patients privacy. Given this context, avoiding privacy-related issues, but still being able to exploit multi-centric data, is possible by using distributed learning techniques.

In this paper, we introduced and empirically tested a distributed learning approach, based on the ADMM algorithm. The proposed technique allows one to train algorithms without sharing any patient-related information, therefore ensuring privacy and avoiding the development of tools to merge patients at a central site. Our experimental analysis, performed on a large set of simulated data, showed the importance of the number of covariates, with regards to number of iterations for convergence and performance. Finally, we discussed the critical parts of the architecture that can support this sort of distributed learning computations.

Future works include the development of the required large IT infrastructure for using the distributed learning approach in real-world multi-centric studies.

References

1. Boyd, S., Parikh, N., Chu, E., Peleato, B., Eckstein, J.: Distributed optimization and statistical learning via the alternating direction method of multipliers. Found. Trends Mach. Learn. 3(1), 1–122 (2011)
2. Caragea, D.: Learning Classifiers from Distributed, Semantically Heterogeneous, Autonomous Data Sources. Ph.D. thesis (2004)
3. Dantzig, G.B., Wolfe, P.: Decomposition principle for linear programs. Operations Research 8, 101–111 (1960)
4. Caragea, D., Reinoso, J., Silvescu, A., Honavar, V.: Statistics gathering for learning from distributed, heterogeneous and autonomous data sources (2003)
5. Grant, M. C., Boyd, S. P.: Graph implementations for nonsmooth convex programs. In: Blondel, V.D., Boyd, S.P., Kimura, H. (eds.) Recent Advances in Learning and Control. LNCIS, vol. 371, pp. 95–110. Springer, Heidelberg (2008)
6. Grant, M., Boyd, S.: Cvx: Matlab software for disciplined convex programming, version 2.1 (March 2014)
7. Gummadi, S., Housri, N., Zimmers, T.A., Koniaris, L.G.: medical record: a balancing act of patient safety, privacy and health care delivery. The American Journal of the Medical Sciences 348(3), 238–243 (2014)
8. Vaidya, J., Yu, H., Jiang, X.: Privacy-preserving SVM classification. Knowledge and Information Systems 14(2), 161–178 (2008)
9. Lindell, Y., Pinkas, B.: Privacy preserving data mining. In: Bellare, M. (ed.) CRYPTO 2000. LNCS, vol. 1880, pp. 36–54. Springer, Heidelberg (2000)
10. Nguyen, M.H., de la Torre, F.: Optimal feature selection for support vector machines. Smart Computing Review 3(43), 584–591 (2010)
11. Mullen, K.M.: Continuous global optimization in r. Journal of Statistical Software 60(6) (2014)
12. Nash, J.C., Varadhan, R.: Unifying optimization algorithms to aid software system users: optimx for r. Journal of Statistical Software 43(9), 1–14 (2011)

13. Parikh, N., Boyd, S.: Proximal algorithms. Foundations and Trends in Optimization 1(3), 123–231 (2014)
14. Que, J., Jiang, X., Ohno-Machado, L.: A collaborative framework for distributed privacy-preserving support vector machine learning. In: AMIA Annual Symposium Proceedings, vol. 2012, pp. 1350–1359 (2012)
15. Koenker, R., Mizera, I.: Convex optimization in r. Journal of Statistical Software 60(5) (2014)
16. Kumar, V., Minz, S.: Feature selection: A literature review. Smart Computing Review 4(3) (2014)

Mining Hierarchical Pathology Data Using Inductive Logic Programming

Tim Op De Beéck[1(✉)], Arjen Hommersom[2], Jan Van Haaren[1],
Maarten van der Heijden[2], Jesse Davis[1], Peter Lucas[2], Lucy Overbeek[3],
and Iris Nagtegaal[4]

[1] Department of Computer Science, KU, Leuven, Belgium
{tim.opdebeeck,jan.vanhaaren,jesse.davis}@cs.kuleuven.be
[2] Institute for Computing and Information Sciences,
Radboud University, Nijmegen, The Netherlands
{arjenh,m.vanderheijden,peterl}@cs.ru.nl
[3] Registry of Histo- and Cytopathology in the Netherlands, Utrecht, The Netherlands
[4] Department of Pathology, Radboud University Medical Centre,
Nijmegen, The Netherlands

Abstract. Considerable amounts of data are continuously generated by pathologists in the form of pathology reports. To date, there has been relatively little work exploring how to apply machine learning and data mining techniques to these data in order to extract novel clinical relationships. From a learning perspective, these pathology data possess a number of challenging properties, in particular, the temporal and hierarchical structure that is present within the data. In this paper, we propose a methodology based on inductive logic programming to extract novel associations from pathology excerpts. We discuss the challenges posed by analyzing these data and discuss how we address them. As a case study, we apply our methodology to Dutch pathology data for discovering possible causes of two rare diseases: cholangitis and breast angiosarcomas.

1 Introduction

The nationwide network and registry of histo- and cytopathology in the Netherlands (PALGA) aims to facilitate communication and information flow within the field of pathology and to provide information to others in health care. PALGA began collecting pathology reports generated in The Netherlands in 1971 and has complete coverage of all pathology laboratories in both academic and non-academic hospitals in The Netherlands since 1991 [3]. Currently, its database contains approximately 63 million excerpts of pathology reports, which are coded using a variant of the SNOMED classification system that was originally developed by the College of American Pathologists [5]. Each year, approximately three million excerpts are added.

The pathology database provides a rich data source for answering medically relevant questions, usually in the form of testing associations between concepts in the data like diagnoses, morphology, etc. This currently leads to roughly 25

J.H. Holmes et al. (Eds.): AIME 2015, LNAI 9105, pp. 76–85, 2015.
DOI: 10.1007/978-3-319-19551-3_9

to 30 publications per year. Typical examples that use the PALGA data include studying incidence of rare diseases (e.g., Brenner tumours of the ovary), as well as mortality of diseases, co-morbidities, and cancer. However, using data mining and machine learning techniques to find completely novel associations, instead of testing predefined hypotheses, is completely unexplored with this data. The sheer size of the data presents significant opportunities to find medically relevant associations by mining the data.

It is well recognized in the literature that medical data is one of the most challenging types of data to analyze [4]. Typical challenges associated with medical databases include their sheer volume and heterogeneity, inconsistencies, selection biases, and significant amounts of missing data. In this paper, we discuss the specific challenge of how to effectively cope with the specific structure (e.g., relationships, time dependencies, hierarchies, etc.) present in pathology data. Structure within data can be beneficial as it may be exploited during learning, however, standard data analysis techniques typically assume the data are flat.

In this paper, we focus on discovering novel associations within pathology data using inductive logic programming (ILP) techniques. Using an inductive logic programming approach provides several benefits compared to both propositional machine learning approaches (e.g., decision trees, rules sets, etc.) and traditional pattern mining approaches (e.g., association rule mining, sequence mining, etc.). Propositional machine learning approaches require that each example is defined by a fixed-length feature vector. For the PALGA data, it is non-trivial to define such a feature set because different patients can have different numbers of entries in the database. The relational nature of ILP allows us to avoid this problem by simply creating one fact for each entry in the database. Furthermore, it is well known that by introducing the appropriate background knowledge, ILP can more naturally capture the hierarchical organization of the codes [14,16] compared to both propositional learners and pattern mining.

2 Description of the Data

In this section, we present two case studies and the structure of the data.

2.1 Case Studies

The goal of this work is to investigate whether it is possible to automatically extract useful relationships between pathologies. In particular, we are interested in finding possible causes of certain pathologies. In collaboration with pathologists, we selected two case studies to evaluate the techniques proposed in the remainder of this paper. The first case study deals with *cholangitis*, which is an inflammation of the bile ducts. The second case study aims to learn associations with *breast angiosarcomas*, which is a tumour in the walls of blood vessels. For both cases studies, we obtained data from patients who were diagnosed with these diseases. As controls, we obtained data from patients with colitis ulcerosa

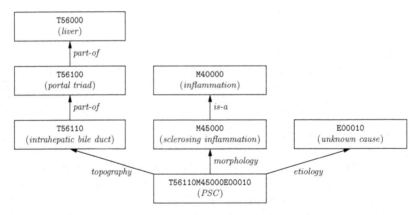

Fig. 1. Hierarchy of the primary sclerosing intrahepatic cholangitis (PSC) code

and Crohn's disease for cholangitis, and patients with angiosarcomas not in the breast and neavus mamma for breast angiosarcomas. We also acquired data representing a general population to avoid a selection bias.

2.2 Hierarchical Coding

The data consist of diagnoses from excerpts of pathological reports that are coded based on the SNOMED classification system. Each diagnosis consists of multiple codes including at least the topography (i.e., location), the procedure for obtaining the material, and a finding (i.e., pathological morphology or diagnosis). For example, a particular instance of colitis ulcerosa may be coded by the following code: `colon,biopsy,colitis ulcerosa`.

The coding poses significant challenges. First, the number of codes per diagnosis varies. For example, there may be multiple topographies such as colon and duodenum as well as multiple morphologies within the same diagnostic rule. Combinations of codes are also relevant. For example, skin (`T01000`) and breast (`TY2100`) should be interpreted as *skin of the breast*. Also, combinations of topographies and morphologies are important. For example, angiosarcoma of the breast may be coded by `TY2100`, `T01000` (skin of breast) and `M91203` (angiosarcoma). Moreover, a code itself can contain a hierarchical structure as is illustrated in Figure 1. Exploiting the structure within a code is a key challenge.

3 Background on Inductive Logic Programming

In this section, we give some background on sequential data mining using ILP.

3.1 First-Order Logic and Logic Programming

First-order logic (FOL) is a formalism to represent objects and their relations in a structured format. Due to its expressiveness, FOL is widely used in machine learning applications. This project only requires a subset of FOL, limiting the alphabet to three types of symbols. *Constants* (e.g., a diagnosis d_i), referring to specific objects in the domain, start with a lower-case letter. *Variables* (e.g., `Patient`), ranging over objects in the domain, are denoted by upper-case letters. *Predicates* $p\backslash n$, where n is the arity (i.e., number of arguments) of the predicate, represent relations between objects.

Given these symbols, several constructs can be defined: *atoms* $p(t_1, ..., t_n)$, where each t_i is either a constant or a variable; *literals*, i.e., an atom or its negation; *clauses*, a disjunction over a finite set of literals; and *definite clauses*, i.e., clauses that contain exactly one positive literal. Definite clauses can be written as an implication $B \Rightarrow H$. The body B consists of a conjunction of literals, whereas the head H is a single literal. Variables in definite clauses are presumed to be universally quantified. For example, the rule diagnosed(Patient, carcinoma) $\Rightarrow$ diagnosed(Patient, angiosarcoma) states that if a `Patient` has been diagnosed with a `carcinoma`, he or she has also been diagnosed with an `angiosarcoma`.

In the following, clauses are given a logic programming semantics. In brief, a logic programming engine first replaces each variable by an object of the variable's domain. Then, the engine checks whether the resulting instantiation of the head of the rule is true if the instantiation of the body is true. In this case the rule is said to *cover* an example (i.e., a set of variable instantiations). The *coverage* of the rule is the number of examples covered.

3.2 Inductive Logic Programming

Inductive logic programming (ILP, [9]) aims to learn hypotheses for a given concept. More formally, we define ILP as follows:

Given: A concept C, a background knowledge K, a language specification L, an optional set of constraints I, a non-empty set of *positive* examples E+ of C (i.e., examples of C), and a set of *negative* examples E− of C (i.e., examples of not C).

Learn: A set of clauses S, in the form of a logic program, that respects the constraints I and covers all of the positive examples in E+ and none of the negative examples in E−.

ILP is well-suited to be used in this medical setting as it yields interpretable rules and allows a user to iteratively narrow down the search space by defining background knowledge K and constraints I on acceptable hypotheses.

3.3 Aleph

We use the Aleph ILP system to learn the hypotheses [12]. The system iteratively learns first-order definite clauses from positive and negative examples.

To learn a clause, Aleph proceeds as follows. First, it randomly picks a positive example, which is called the seed example, and searches the background knowledge for facts known to be true about the seed (saturation step). The system combines these facts to construct the most-specific clause that covers

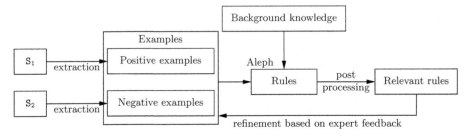

Fig. 2. Overview of our method for extracting knowledge from PALGA data using ILP

the seed (i.e., the bottom clause). Second, Aleph generalizes these facts as the generalizations of facts explaining the seed might also explain other examples (search step). Typically, Aleph employs a breadth-first search that considers the shortest clauses first. From these clauses, the system works its way through the search space in a general-to-specific manner towards the bottom clause. The search process can be further constrained by bounding the clause length and the number of clauses that should be tested.

Several metrics exist to evaluate each generated clause. Usually, these metrics try to capture how well the clause discriminates between positive and negative examples. A commonly used metric for this purpose is the m-estimate [8], which is a smoothed ratio between the number of positive examples covered and the total number of examples covered (i.e., the precision of the clause).

Aleph's global search strategy affects how it proceeds from one iteration to another. One commonly used strategy is the "cover-removal" approach which removes all positive examples that are covered by a previously learned clause from the set of positive examples. Hence, successive iterations focus on learning rules that apply to currently uncovered examples (i.e., none of the learned rules covers them). Another approach is to use every positive example as a seed once such that more rules are learned.

4   Empirical Evaluation

4.1   Methodology

More formally, we address the following learning task in this paper:

Given: A disease of interest d_t, SNOMED-structured patient records, and hierarchical domain knowledge.
Learn: Novel associations in the data that provide clinical experts with new insights about disease d_t.

In the following, we discuss the steps taken to address this task. Figure 2 provides a schematic overview.

Sampling the Medical Database. Our approach requires two samples of the database. We extract positive examples from a sample S_p, which are patients

Table 1. The records of a patient X

Patient ID	Date	Diagnosis
X	06/06/2011	T67000—P11400—T67000M40030
X	22/06/2011	T56000—P11400—P30700—T56110M45000E00010—M55800

who suffer from the target disease d_t, and negative examples from a sample S_n, which are patients who have **not** been diagnosed with d_t. While S_p mainly consists of patients who have been diagnosed with d_t or a strongly related disease, S_n represents the general population. This approach avoids a selection bias that could make it harder to discriminate between positive and negative examples.

Extracting Examples. An example corresponds to a patient p_i's records. If a patient p_i was diagnosed with d_t at a time t_i, we label the example as *positive* and add a ground fact $d_t(p_i, t_i)$ to the set of positive examples. We add all diagnoses d_i of p_i at time $t_j < t_i$ (i.e., before the first diagnosis of the target disease) as background knowledge as ground facts $\texttt{diagnosis}(p_i, \texttt{normD}_i, t_j)$.

While each diagnosis d_i is a highly-structured sequence of codes, we need to normalize the sequence to $\texttt{normD}_i$. Our normalization procedure sorts the codes alphabetically and ensures they were entered consistently. While not essential, this procedure allows to more easily detect duplicate diagnoses, which avoids learning hypotheses consisting of multiple atoms describing the same diagnosis.

We construct the *negative* examples in a similar way. We search S_n for patients p_j who have never been diagnosed with the target disease d_t and add a ground fact for each such patient to the set of negative examples.

We now illustrate this process for the records of a patient X, which are shown in Table 1, to learn rules about cholangitis. We search X's records chronologically for codes corresponding to cholangitis. The second record, which dates from 22 June 2011, mentions the code T56110M45000E00010 referring to primary sclerosing cholangitis. Hence, we label X as a positive example and add the following fact to the set of positive examples: $\texttt{cholangitis}(\texttt{x}, 22/06/2011)$. In addition, we add all X's records that were recorded before 22 June 2011 as background knowledge. For this example, we generate the following three ground facts: $\texttt{diagnosis}(\texttt{x}, \texttt{M40030T67000}, 06/06/2011)$, $\texttt{procedure}(\texttt{x}, \texttt{P11400}, 06/06/2011)$, and $\texttt{topography}(\texttt{x}, \texttt{T67000}, 06/06/2011)$.

Adding Background Knowledge. To exploit the structure of the data during learning, we add a hierarchy of codes as background knowledge, which we provide as a set of clauses (see Figure 1). For example, the clause $\texttt{diagnosis}(\texttt{P}, \texttt{normD}_j, \texttt{T})$ $\Rightarrow \texttt{diagnosis}(\texttt{P}, \texttt{normD}_i, \texttt{T})$ specifies that diagnosis d_i is more general than diagnosis d_j. This approach allows us to learn more generally applicable rules.

Configuring and Running Aleph. Aleph has many parameters that influence the number of learned clauses. If configured too strictly, it learns no clauses at all. If configured too loosely, it learns many uninteresting clauses which makes manually inspecting the learned clauses a slow and tedious process.

Table 2. The top-five rules for cholangitis with their coverage of positive and negative examples, and m-estimate. The abbreviated notation is explained in the text.

Rule	|E+|	|E−|	m-est.
brush ∧ colon ∧ no tumour ⇒ cholangitis	55	0	0.90
extra hepatic bile duct ∧ liver ∧ no abnormalities ⇒ cholangitis	51	0	0.90
brush ∧ liver ∧ no tumour ⇒ cholangitis	50	0	0.89
ductus choledochus ∧ colon ∧ no tumour ⇒ cholangitis	50	0	0.89
ductus choledochus ∧ colon ∧ no abnormalities ⇒ cholangitis	45	0	0.89

The following parameters highly influence the number of generated clauses: `minpos` denotes the minimum number of positive examples that a clause *must* cover, `noise` denotes the maximum number of negative examples that a clause *can* cover, and `minacc` denotes the minimum precision (i.e., the percentage of covered examples that should be positive).

As a global search strategy, the `induce_max` setting is a good choice when performing knowledge discovery as it picks each positive example as the seed once. Hence, it generates more clauses and ensures that the order in which the seeds are picked does not influence the clauses that are learned. The `explore` parameter forces Aleph to continue the search until all remaining elements in the search space are definitely worse than the current best element [12].

Scoring the Learned Clauses. We sort the clauses according to their coverage of positive examples. In case of a tie, we sort the clauses according to their m-estimate. This approach allows us to easily discover and inspect the top clauses.

4.2   Experimental Results

We applied the above methods to both case studies. For cholangitis, we constructed 1,292 positive examples from S_{p1} containing 402,939 records of 78,911 patients. For angiosarcoma of the breast, we constructed 303 positive examples from S_{p2} containing 28,557 records of 14,424 patients. We constructed 7,958 negative examples for cholangitis and 7,963 negative examples for angiosarcoma of the breast from S_n containing 53,439 records of 7,963 patients.

Running Aleph with a `minpos` of 10, a `minacc` of 0.5, and `noise` values of 10, 50, and 100 resulted in a total of 6,775 rules for cholangitis, and 945 rules for angiosarcoma of the breast. Among the best-scoring rules, there are several examples where the background knowledge capturing the hierarchical structure was used to construct rules. For example, a high-scoring rule for cholangitis is:

$$\texttt{diagnosis}(P, \texttt{auto-immune disease}, T_1) \land \texttt{topography}(P, \texttt{liver}, T_2) \land$$
$$\texttt{morphology}(P, \texttt{fibrosis}, T_3) \Rightarrow \texttt{cholangitis}(P, T)$$

where $T_1, T_2, T_3 < T$. While "auto-immune disease" does not explicitly appear in the data, Aleph used the background knowledge to derive it as a generalization of the more specific code "auto-immune hepatitis".

Table 3. The top-five rules for cholangitis after feedback from the pathologist with their coverage of positive and negative examples, and m-estimate

Rule	E+	E−	m-est.
liver ∧ colitis ulcerosa ⇒ cholangitis	91	6	0.87
cholestasis ∧ colon ⇒ cholangitis	30	0	0.87
cirrhosis ∧ external revision ⇒ cholangitis	25	0	0.86
auto-immune hepatitis ⇒ cholangitis	49	3	0.85
cirrhosis ∧ fibrosis ⇒ cholangitis	31	1	0.85

We presented the 50 top-scoring rules containing at least one morphology or diagnosis to a gastro-intestinal specialist of the Radboud University Medical Centre in The Netherlands. Table 2 presents the top-five rules for cholangitis using a shorthand notation. For example, the first rule corresponds to:

$$\texttt{procedure}(P, \texttt{brush}, T_1) \wedge \texttt{topography}(P, \texttt{colon}, T_2) \wedge$$
$$\texttt{diagnosis}(P, \texttt{no tumour}, T_3) \Rightarrow \texttt{cholangitis}(P, T)$$

where $T_1, T_2, T_3 < T$.

The specialist confirmed that the high-scoring rules are in accordance with existing medical knowledge. In particular, as expected, rules for cholangitis are related to inflammatory bowel diseases and rules for angiosarcoma of the breast are related to breast cancer. Yet, for finding novel disease associations, we identified three limitations. First, there is a large number of rules that can be found within the data, which makes medical validation challenging. Second, some of the high-scoring rules are irrelevant because they are, for example, an artifact of *diagnosis by exclusion* (e.g., no tumour, no abnormalities). For example, the method of obtaining the sample (e.g., brush) is predictive but medically irrelevant. Third, for exploratory data analysis, it is only of interest which other morphologies occur before the diagnosis of interest. Repetition of the same morphology or diagnosis leads to a large number of rules, which may only differ in, for example, location.

The interpretability of ILP-learned rules facilitates the interaction with and feedback from domain experts. Inspired by the above limitations, we added a post-processing step by removing rules containing particular codes (e.g., no tumour) and rules for which there are higher-scoring rules that contain the same morphology or diagnosis. For the cholangitis case study, this results in a list of only 30 rules that cover at least 10 positive examples. Table 3 presents a few of the best-scoring rules using the same shorthand notation as in Table 2. Some of the associations, such as the strength of the association between Crohn's disease and cholangitis (with 16 positive and no negative examples), were considered surprising and warrant further investigation.

4.3   Comparison with Sequential Pattern Mining

Sequential pattern mining is an alternative to the proposed ILP approach. We applied several sequential pattern mining variants to the cholangitis case study (i.e., CMRules, RuleGrowth, ERMiner, TNS, and TopSeqRules), using the data mining framework SPMF [6]. To do so, we used sample S_{p1} to construct sequences of diagnoses of patients who have been diagnosed with cholangitis. Each patient corresponds to one sequence, while each record corresponds to an itemset in the sequence. We only consider the records up until the first diagnosis of cholangitis.

Running the rule mining algorithms yields 389 distinct rules. However, the post-processing procedure from the previous section retains none of these rules. Inspecting the rules before post-processing, allows us to identify three limitations of propositional mining algorithms: (*i*) no abstractions are found using these algorithms, which makes the rules less interpretable, (*ii*) many of the rules found are irrelevant for a specific disease of interest (e.g., the rule `liver => biopt`), and (*iii*) no specific rules for cholangitis are discovered.

5 Conclusions

In recent years, there has been considerable interest in extracting knowledge from the data collected in electronic health records (EHRs), though it is recognized that there are considerable challenges involved [7,10]. Nonetheless, several attempts have been made to mine the EHR, typically used for predictive modelling, e.g., in order to support clinical decisions or for the identification of risk factors [1,2,13,15]. However, exploratory data mining to find novel relationships between diseases is something which has not been studied as far as we are aware.

This paper presented a case study of applying inductive logic programming (ILP) to extract interesting rules from a pathology data set. This paper posited that ILP is particularly suited to this task for three reasons. First, is its ability to handle structure such as the hierarchical organization of diagnosis codes and time. This not only allows improving the learning process, as in [11], but also to abstract from specific codes to more abstract ones. Second, ILP returns interpretable rules which facilitate an iterative mining process with domain experts. Third, ILP is a discriminative approach so it can focus its discovery efforts on target variables of interest. In the case studies, we found that ILP was able to exploit the structure in the data and that it produced more meaningful patterns than sequential pattern mining. Furthermore, we illustrated how we were able to revise the mining process based on the feedback of a domain expert. In the future, we will continue to explore adding additional domain knowledge to further guide the search process. Finally, rules considered interesting by the medical experts will be verified using traditional statistical methods to make them acceptable to the medical literature.

Acknowledgments. AH and MVDH are supported by the ITEA2 MoSHCA project (ITEA2-ip11027). JVH is supported by the Agency for Innovation by Science and Technology in Flanders (IWT). JD is partially supported by the Research Fund KU Leuven (CREA/11/015), EU FP7 MC-CIG (#294068) and FWO (G.0356.12).

References

1. Bellazzi, R., Zupan, B.: Predictive data mining in clinical medicine: current issues and guidelines. International Journal of Medical Informatics 77(2), 81–97 (2008)
2. Bennett, C., Doub, T.: Data mining and electronic health records: Selecting optimal clinical treatments in practice. In: Proc. of DMIN 2010, pp. 313–318 (2010)
3. Casparie, M., Tiebosch, A., Burger, G., Blauwgeers, H., Van de Pol, A., van Krieken, J., Meijer, G.: Pathology databanking and biobanking in the netherlands, a central role for PALGA, the nationwide histopathology and cytopathology data network and archive. Analytical Cellular Pathology 29(1), 19–24 (2007)
4. Cios, K., Moore, W.: Uniqueness of medical data mining. Artificial Intelligence in Medicine 26(1), 1–24 (2002)
5. Cote, R., Robboy, S.: Progress in medical information management: Systematized nomenclature of medicine (SNOMED). JAMA 243(8), 756–762 (1980)
6. Fournier-Viger, P.: Spmf: A sequential pattern mining framework (2011), http://www.philippe-fournier-viger.com/spmf
7. Jensen, P., Jensen, L., Brunak, S.: Mining electronic health records: towards better research applications and clinical care. Nature Reviews Genetics 13(6), 395–405 (2012)
8. Lavrač, N., Dzeroski, S., Bratko, I.: Handling imperfect data in inductive logic programming. Advances in Inductive Logic Programming 32, 48–64 (1996)
9. Muggleton, S., De Raedt, L.: Inductive logic programming: Theory and methods. The Journal of Logic Programming 19, 629–679 (1994)
10. Ramakrishnan, N., Hanauer, D., Keller, B.: Mining electronic health records. Computer 43(10), 77–81 (2010)
11. Singh, A., Nadkarni, G., Guttag, J., Bottinger, E.: Leveraging hierarchy in medical codes for predictive modeling. In: Proc. of ACM Conference on Bioinformatics, Computational Biology, and Health Informatics, pp. 96–103. ACM (2014)
12. Srinivasan, A.: The Aleph manual. Machine Learning at the Computing Laboratory. Oxford University (2001)
13. Sun, J., Hu, J., Luo, D., Markatou, M., Wang, F., Edabollahi, S., Steinhubl, S., Daar, Z., Stewart, W.: Combining knowledge and data driven insights for identifying risk factors using electronic health records. In: Proc. of AMIA Annual Symposium., vol. 2012, p. 901. American Medical Informatics Association (2012)
14. Vavpetič, A., Lavrač, N.: Semantic subgroup discovery systems and workflows in the sdm-toolkit. The Computer Journal 56(3), 304–320 (2013)
15. Wang, F., Lee, N., Hu, J., Sun, J., Ebadollahi, S.: Towards heterogeneous temporal clinical event pattern discovery: a convolutional approach. In: Proc. of the 18th ACM SIGKDD, pp. 453–461. ACM (2012)
16. Žáková, M., Železný, F.: Exploiting term, predicate, and feature taxonomies in propositionalization and propositional rule learning. In: Kok, J.N., Koronacki, J., Lopez de Mantaras, R., Matwin, S., Mladenič, D., Skowron, A. (eds.) ECML 2007. LNCS (LNAI), vol. 4701, pp. 798–805. Springer, Heidelberg (2007)

What if Your Floor Could Tell Someone You Fell? A Device Free Fall Detection Method

Roberto Luis Shinmoto Torres$^{(\boxtimes)}$, Asanga Wickramasinghe, Viet Ninh Pham, and Damith Chinthana Ranasinghe

Auto-ID Lab, The University of Adelaide, Adelaide, SA 5005, Australia
roberto.shinmototorres@adelaide.edu.au

Abstract. Falls in the home environment are a serious cause of injury in older people leading to loss of independence and increased health related financial costs. In this study we investigate a device free method to detect falls by using simple batteryless radio frequency identification (RFID) tags in a smart RFID enabled carpet. Our method extracts information from the tags and the environment of the carpeted floor and applies machine learning techniques to make an autonomous decision regarding the posture of a person on the floor. This information can be used to automatically seek assistance to help the subject and decrease the negative effects of 'long-lie' after a fall. Our approach does not require video monitoring or body worn kinematic sensors; hence preserves the privacy of the dwellers, reduces costs and eliminates the need to remember to wear a device. Our results indicate a good performance for fall detection with an overall F-score of 94%.

Keywords: Falls detection · Passive RFID · Ambient assisted living · Dense sensing

1 Introduction

Falls among older population is a very significant healthcare issue. Falls are major cause of injuries and can severely reduce life expectancy if the person is lying on the ground for more than an hour (long lie) after falling [19,18]. Moreover, the cost associated with falls for medical expenses in 2012 was US $30 billion and this annual cost is expected to reach US $67 billion by 2020 [6]. In a recent extensive study conducted in two Canadian long-term care facilities over three years, Robinovitch et al. [21] recorded 227 falls from 130 subjects and identified the most frequent causes of falls as incorrect weight shifting (41%), tripping or stumbling (21%), hit and bump (11%) and loss of support (11%).

Several approaches have been developed for detecting falls, these can be divided into body worn sensors [3,17,2], environmental sensors [16,20,4,15,22] and hybrid approaches [10]. The problem with most worn sensor approaches is the size of the sensors and body straps for attachment that can be inconvenient for the user. In the case of environmental approaches some studies are based on video monitoring which has raised privacy concerns [8].

© Springer International Publishing Switzerland 2015
J.H. Holmes et al. (Eds.): AIME 2015, LNAI 9105, pp. 86–95, 2015.
DOI: 10.1007/978-3-319-19551-3_10

Alternative approaches using floor based sensing technologies have been developed such as that of Klack et al. [15] where multiple sensors and micro-controllers are embedded into the solid floor; however, this study is yet to report falls detection performance results. The study of Braun et al. [4] presented an arrangement of capacitive proximity sensors able to detect a person lying on the floor; nonetheless, similar to the previous method, no results on performance have been reported. The study of Werner et al. [22] used accelerometers mounted on the floor in order to detect possible falls using floor vibrations, this method was tested only with mannequins and has a processing delay of 30 s to issue an alarm; this demands large storage of data prior to processing which is not practical for a memory and power constrained stand-alone deployment such as using an RFID reader as falls detector.

In contrast, we propose and evaluate an approach to instrument the floor that does not utilize battery powered kinematic sensors but uses the capabilities and reported data from batteryless radio frequency identification (RFID) tags integrated into floor carpeting to detect a fall. We employ machine learning techniques in order to obtain predictions of falls from the observed RFID tag signals. These batteryless RFID tags are paper thin and can emit signals, potentially indefinitely, without maintenance. We also use the extensive study of Robinovith et al. [21] and the detailed video data on actual falls of older people to design our experimental study to ensure the validity of our results. The main contributions of this study are: i) design, develop and test a smart RFID tag integrated carpet (*smart carpet*) that is capable of detecting falls with minimum delay; ii) construct a machine learning based method that requires no more post-processing than sorting and averaging tag signals and therefore fast and efficient to implement on simple embedded systems; and iii) evaluate the approach with simulated falls following specific falling instances from older people as captured in the detailed recent study conducted over three years by Robinovith et al. [21].

The rest of the paper is organized as follow, Section 2 describes our technological approach, Section 3 refers to our experimental methodologies used in the trial, Section 4 shows our results and discussion and future work are presented in section 5.

2   Device Free Approach

2.1   Technology

The objective of our instrumented carpet approach is to obtain human motion patterns which are reflected in data variations using RFID technology. We use RFID, a wireless technology capable of precisely identifying objects and people autonomously; basic components of modern RFID platforms are RFID tags, readers and antennas and backend systems [13]. Passive RFID tags are batteryless and use the radio frequency (RF) energy radiated from the reader antennas to power its circuitry and return a signal encoded with a digital identification code. In our proposed application RFID tags are integrated into a floor carpet.

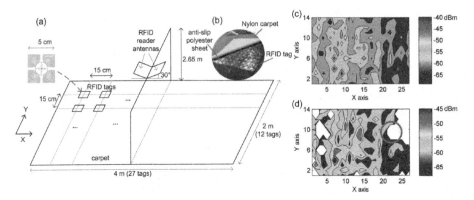

Fig. 1. Overall experimental setting. (a) RFID tag. (b) Smart carpet with embedded RFID tags. (c) Temperature map of average RSSI readings per tag for a 4 hour trial in an empty room showing the different levels of power received from the smart carpet tags. (d) Temperature map over a 0.5 s duration indicating the location (red circle) of a person walking where the large white space are tags occluded by the person while other white spaces are unread tags.

The smart carpet has a three layered structure (see Figure 1(b)). The top layer is a commercially available 3 mm nylon carpet. The middle layer consists of RFID tags placed within two sheets of 0.5 mm plastic to hold the tags in position, and for convenience, the bottom layer is a 3 mm anti-slip polyester sheet. The nylon carpet and the polyester sheet are selected based on their dielectric characteristics and experimental evaluation of the structure to ensure that the tags can be read at least 2 m from the antenna. This design not only cloaks the tags but also mimics a real-world deployment as RFID tags are not directly exposed but integrated into the carpet.

The RFID tags are the most important part of our smart carpet. The design of the RFID tag antenna and the RFID chip used determine the read range and supported capabilities of the tag, including compliance for RFID communication protocols such as ISO-18000-6C [11]. We selected the Smartrack FROG 3D[1] tag (see Figure 1(a)) from commercially available RFID tags not only due to its operational range (> 6 m when covered by 3 mm plastic) but also due to its orientation insensitivity with respect to the RFID reader antenna.

The tag layout is important as it determines: i) the amount of information available for identifying falls; and ii) time taken to inventory all the tags in a given area and subsequently determine the latency of the fall detection approach. We placed tags at 15 cm intervals between tag centers in both horizontal and vertical directions to form a grid as shown in Figure 1(b). This layout is selected as the average width of a human (chest depth) is around 24 cm [9]; thus we ensure that at least one tag will be completely occluded by the human body even when a person is lying on their side. Furthermore, this tag layout requires 378 (14×27) tags to monitor an 8 m² (2 m×4 m) area. The cost of each tag is less

---

[1] https://www.smartrac-group.com/frog-3d.html

than US $0.50 making this deployment inexpensive to implement (although the cost of the present RFID infrastructure, i.e. 2 antennas and a reader is about US $1600.00, this cost is not recurrent and is also reducing over time [1]).

As shown in Figure 1, we utilized two RFID reader antennas placed 2.65 m above the ground in opposing directions, angled approximately 30° to the horizontal plane and pointed towards the ground and an Impinj Speedway R-420 (Firmware version: 5.2.1) RFID reader. From every observed RFID tag we obtain its identification code, the antenna that read the tag and the received signal power indicator (RSSI) of the tag signal. This value of reported RSSI from each tag is of interest as it represents the strength of the signal reflected from the tag captured by the reader antenna [13]; this value is dependent on the distance (inversely proportional to its fourth power) and given that tags and antennas are fixed, variations of RSSI can provide information related to physical activity in the vicinity of the tag and reader antennas.

2.2 Classifiers

Given that we are only interested in identifying if a person has fallen, we focus on a simplified binary class casting of our classification problem. Hence we build a predictive model to determine if a set of RFID tag observations is a Fall or a No-fall. In addition, less complex models are simpler and faster and can be eventually integrated into an RFID reader itself.

For this study, we focus on a pair of distinctly different classifiers that are easy to deploy and embed in the limited resource hardware of an RFID reader. In particular, we consider the linear SVM, a method that finds the optimal separating hyperplane that maximises the margin between two convex sets of classes [7], and decision trees (DT), a method that predicts a label based on learnt decision rules from the input features. Although methods such as conditional random fields (CRF) can model temporal/sequential relationships between stages, they require more processing power and memory during inference; hence not suited for embedded deployments. We used the tool Liblinear [12] and the CART (classification and regression tree) [5] algorithm in Matlab[2] to evaluate the linear SVM and DT respectively.

In order to learn movements and postures of people in the monitored region, we used two information sources: i) the set of tags in the smart carpet observed by the RFID reader over a duration, T, of 0.5 s; and ii) RSSI information of each tag during T. The observation interval was determined through extensive experiments to select the minimum time to inventory over 95% of the RFID tags in our smart carpet to ensure the availability of an adequate amount of information for monitoring human movements. A modern RFID reader can be configured to deliver reports of tags observed every $T = 0.5$ s and thus the tag data stream can be explicitly partitioned at the reader level.

Given a set of RFID tag observations, we can represent the status of observed and un-observed tags in the smart carpet as a matrix, R, such that $r_{(i,j)} =$

---

[2] MATLAB, The MathWorks Inc., Natick, MA, 2013

$\sum_{\tau=0}^{T}(\mathbb{1}_{(i,j)})$ where $\mathbb{1} = \{1,0\}$ denotes the presence or observation of a tag and (i,j) is the coordinate of the tag in the RFID tag grid. Similarly, RSSI information can also be represented as a matrix, S, such that $s_{(i,j)} = \overline{\text{RSSI}}_{(i,j)} \in \mathbb{R}$; RSSI values of un-observed tags were assigned -100 dBm as a value much lower than the minimum of -70 dBm (see Figure 1(c)). In order to reduce the processing cost of operating on several hundreds of features per set of observations, we also consider the possible reduction of the granularity of tag level data necessary to detect a fall. Therefore we investigated two formulations:

1. Use information from all tag positions, in our case 378 tags in a 14×27 tags array arrangement (All tags case).
2. Use information from tags divided in quadrants, in our case 2×3 tags per quadrant, providing in total, information for 63 (7×9) quadrants (Quadrants case).

For the first case we vectorized R and S, and concatenated them to formulate a feature vector $f \in \mathbb{R}^{756}$ for the classification task. In the second case features were calculated based on the quadrants containing 6 tags. We considered this quadrant size (i.e. 2×3) as these number of tags are the minimum divisors greater than one for each smart carpet dimension (in number of tags). Given a set of tags in a quadrant, $Q_{(m,n)}$, we obtained number of tags $r^{q}_{(m,n)} = \sum_{t \in Q_{(m,n)}} r_t$ and the mean RSSI of tags $s^{q}_{(m,n)} = \sum_{t \in Q_{(m,n)}} s_t / r^{q}_{(m,n)}$ in the quadrant as features. Here, (m,n) represents the coordinate of the quadrant, and r_t and s_t represents the presence and RSSI for tag t respectively. Similar to the first case, we arrange these features to form a feature vector $f \in \mathbb{R}^{126}$.

We consider averaging the RSSI values in each quadrant as RSSI values can be regarded regular in a small local vicinity; we confirmed our proposition by measuring the RSSI readings from the smart carpet as shown in Figure 1(c) where we can see that RSSI values are regular in stripes along the Y axis of the smart carpet, as expected, due to the static location of the antennas and tags. We also note the distribution of RSSI is not similar on both sides of the smart carpet as the antennas are dividing the X axis in two; the most probable cause is the location of a wall, parallel to the Y axis about 1 m from the start of the X axis, that can generate a different multipath environment and reflection of RF (radio frequency) waves. We show in Figure 1(d) an RSSI map for a time duration T when a subject (red circle) is walking across the smart carpet where the large white space are blocked tags by the subject while other white spaces are unread tags; this information can also be regarded as regular in a small area.

3   Experimental Procedure

3.1   Study Description

Eight participants (average age of 33.9±8.5 years) and male to female ratio of 3:1 were trialled in this study. Each participant performed a series of activities on the smart carpet that included: i) walking across the area, ii) walking into the area,

(a)

(b)

(c)

(d)

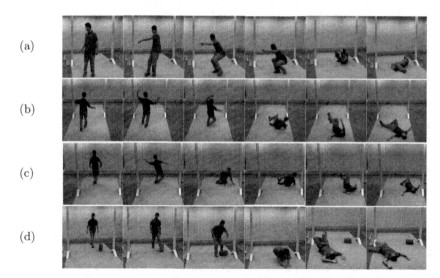

Fig. 2. Four types of falls performed by volunteers following those recorded in Robinovith et al. [21], (a) *Fall 1*: fall backwards rotating body, (b) *Fall 2*: fall sideways by narrowing support base and incorrectly shifting weight, (c) *Fall 3*: fall sideways by tripping on the other leg, (d) *Fall 4*: fall forwards by tripping over an obstacle

squatting down to pick an object and leaving, and iii) falling backwards, sideways and forward; in total 72 falls and 16 object pick ups were performed. Each participant fell into the smart carpet following the motion of falls as captured by Robinovitch et al. [21] where the biomechanic of falls are clearly shown. Using this information each participant fell in the following ways:

1. *Fall 1*: fell backwards by rotating the body shown in Figure 2(a) and performed weight shifting as in Figure (A) in [21],
2. *Fall 2*: fell sideways by narrowing the support base and incorrectly shifting weight as shown in Figure 2(b) and performed as in Figure (B) in [21],
3. *Fall 3*: fell sideways by tripping with one's leg shown in Figure 2(c) and performed as in Figure (C) in [21] and
4. *Fall 4*: fell forwards by tripping with an obstacle shown in Figure 2(d) and performed as in Figure (D) [21].

Each participant fell two to four times per type of fall, as previously described, over the smart carpet shown in Figure 1(b). The data was labelled in real time by a researcher observing the trials for training of the classifiers and comparison with predictions.

For recognizing falls, a fall is detected (or has started) if the classifier predicts two consecutive Fall class labels after a No-fall label. We consider this heuristic to avoid any possible error that may cause preventable false alarms as it is realistically impossible for a fall to last just 1 s. This consideration also means that any fall signal can have a maximum delay of 1 s (note we make a prediction every 0.5 s). We also consider a detected fall as valid if predicted no more than

1 s before an actual fall as stated in the ground truth. This approach overcomes possible ground truth label misalignments with actual fall events (label noise).

3.2   Statistical Analysis

In this study, true positives (TP) were correctly recognized labels (Fall or no-Fall). False positives (FP) are predicted labels that are not in correspondence with the ground truth (i.e. incorrectly identified as target activity). False negatives (FN) are labels that were missed (not predicted). True negatives (TN) are those labels of no-interest correctly predicted. In the case of falls detection, these metrics follow the same considerations except for TN; given that the only event of interest is the detected fall, we do not report TN values.

The performance of the classifiers in predicting Fall or No fall was evaluated using the metrics: i) accuracy = (TP+TN)/(TP+TN+FN+FP) and ii) F-score = 2×TP/(2×TP+FN+FP); whereas for falls detection, we evaluate the performance of our approach using the metrics: i) recall (sensitivity) = TP/(TP+FN); ii) precision = TP/(TP+FP); and iii) F-score. We give importance to F-score, as it represents the harmonic mean of precision and recall as opposed to metrics such as accuracy that only reports the general error of the classifier and can mis-represent the performance especially in cases of imbalanced data [14]. Thus, for classifier performance we present accuracy for completeness.

Evaluation of these metrics was performed using a leave one out cross validation procedure because we need to evaluate each participant independently; hence we train the model without the data of the test participant. For each fold, we used the data of six participants for training, one for validation and one for testing. We used the data from the validation subset for model parameter selection with the goal of selecting the model that presented the highest overall F-score. Finally we report results from the testing subset using the best model parameter. Results are presented as mean ± standard deviation. To compare the results of our classifiers, we evaluate the significance of their performance using a two-tailed independent t-test where a p-value (p) <.05 was considered statistically significant.

4   Results

We evaluated the performance of each classifier using a leave-one-out cross validation (see Section 3.2). The results presented in Table 1 show that SVM-All tags achieve better performance than all other methods. In particular, SVM-All tags achieves significant difference for the class Fall when compared with the other methods ($p < .031$) and a significant difference with DT-Quadrant ($p = .022$) for class No-fall class. All other results were not significant when compared with each other. As shown in Table 1, using information from all tags has better impact on the classification performance for SVM than compressing the information to quadrants. However, that is not the case with DT, where there is no significant difference between DT-All tags and DT-Quadrants.

Table 1. Overall performance metrics for label classification

Classifier	F-score (%)	Accuracy (%)
SVM-All tags	89.40 ± 6.12	90.76 ± 5.51
SVM-Quadrants	80.37 ± 8.07	83.54 ± 6.91
DT-All tags	80.57 ± 10.00	83.87 ± 7.08
DT-Quadrants	81.51 ± 5.42	84.00 ± 4.19

Table 2. Overall performance metrics for fall detection

Classifier	Recall (%)	Precision (%)	F-score (%)
SVM-All tags	95.22 ± 8.85	93.84 ± 8.87	94.21 ± 7.01
SVM-Quadrants	84.01 ± 13.42	76.75 ± 17.79	78.23 ± 9.84
DT-All tags	85.97 ± 13.53	72.97 ± 18.43	78.27 ± 15.68
DT-Quadrants	96.36 ± 5.02	65.68 ± 10.96	77.57 ± 7.77

Table 3. Number of falls detected for each type of fall

Subject	1			2			3			4			5			6			7			8		
	TP	FN	FP	TP	FN	FP	TP	FN	FP	TP	FN	FP	TP	FN	FP	TP	FN	FP	TP	FN	FP	TP	FN	FP
Walk	0	0	0	0	0	0	0	0	0	0	0	0	0	0	0	0	0	0	0	0	0	0	0	0
Fall 1	2	0	0	3	0	0	2	1	0	2	0	0	2	0	0	2	0	0	2	0	0	2	0	0
Fall 2	2	0	0	2	0	0	2	1	0	2	0	0	2	0	0	2	0	0	2	1	0	2	0	0
Fall 3	2	0	0	2	0	0	2	0	0	2	0	0	2	0	0	2	0	0	2	1	0	2	0	0
Fall 4	2	0	0	2	0	0	3	0	0	4	0	0	2	0	0	2	0	0	2	0	0	2	0	0
Pick up	0	0	0	0	0	0	0	0	2	0	0	0	0	0	0	0	0	2	0	0	0	0	0	1

The results for falls detection in Table 2 indicate that SVM-All tags with 94.2% F-score and statistical significance of $p < .02$ deliver better performance than all other methods which achieve an F-score performance of approximately 78%. Table 3 shows the output of the falls detection process for all participants. The worst performer is subject 3 (Table 3) with two FN and FP. We can see that most FPs are caused by the action of picking up an object where the squatting motion has covered enough tags to confuse the predictive model. In total, 5 out of 16 picking up activities were erroneously recognized as falls however, none of the walking was erroneously predicted as falls.

5   Discussion

Our method demonstrates the feasibility of detecting falls using batteryless RFID technology integrated into floor carpeting. Our approach can be easily realized in halls, walkways or open spaces as falls have been observed to occur while ambulating in such areas [21].

In addition, our approach takes advantage of readily available information such as RSSI from an RFID reader to provide all features for classification with little post-processing; therefore our approach based on simple classification models can conveniently be included in a RFID reader's firmware to directly implement the falls detection algorithm and subsequently seek help (via paging or SMS messages to the care givers). The ability to develop a self contained system will greatly simplify deployments in practice.

We have tested our approach with eight young participants, as it is impractical to trial our approach with older subjects for obvious reasons, and our pilot study demonstrates the feasibility of our innovative device free falls detection approach. Moreover, the RFID tag based approach considers body shape and height variations between participants as they occlude the observation of tags on the floor, thus the age of the faller has no other effect on our approach since we have considered the manners in which older people fall. Withal, our approach is blind to variations in gait and body posture characteristics of older people.

In terms of room characteristics, we tested our approach in an empty $8\,\mathrm{m}^2$ area. In a larger room, multiple RFID readers are required where each reader be configured to read only the tags in their area of interest using tag ID filtering, hence issuing an alarm for events in their given area. Future studies must consider current limitations such as trialling a larger cohort and, in terms of deployment, placing objects in the room (e.g. fixed and movable furniture). We must also study the behaviour of multipath in furnished environments and rooms of different sizes to validate our approach with real life scenarios.

In conclusion, the presented approach provides good performance for the detection of falls. This method is capable of producing a response after each 0.5 s with an expected maximum delay of 1 s. Further studies must also work on reducing FP and FN by enhancing our classification algorithm and further improving our features to provide more details to the classifier without increasing complexity.

Acknowledgment. This research was supported by a grant from the Department of State Development (DSD) under the Collaboration Pathways Program.

References

1. Bhuptani, M., Moradpour, S.: RFID Field Guide: Deploying Radio Frequency Identification Systems. Prentice Hall (2005)
2. Bianchi, F., Redmond, S., Narayanan, M., Cerutti, S., Lovell, N.: Barometric pressure and triaxial accelerometry-based falls event detection. IEEE Transactions on Neural Systems and Rehabilitation Engineering 18(6), 619–627 (2010)
3. Bourke, A., van de Ven, P., Gamble, M., OConnor, R., Murphy, K., Bogan, E., McQuade, E., Finucane, P., Laighin, G., Nelson, J.: Evaluation of waist-mounted tri-axial accelerometer based fall-detection algorithms during scripted and continuous unscripted activities. Journal of Biomechanics 43(15), 3051–3057 (2010)
4. Braun, A., Heggen, H., Wichert, R.: Capfloor - a flexible capacitive indoor localization system. In: Chessa, S., Knauth, S. (eds.) EvAAL 2011. CCIS, vol. 309, pp. 26–35. Springer, Heidelberg (2012)
5. Breiman, L., Friedman, J., Stone, C.J., Olshen, R.A.: Classification and regression trees. Wadsworth International Group, Belmont (1984)
6. Centers for Disease Control and Prevention: Cost of falls among older adults (2014), http://www.cdc.gov/homeandrecreationalsafety/falls/fallcost.html
7. Cortes, C., Vapnik, V.: Support-vector networks. Machine Learning 20(3), 273–297 (1995)
8. Demiris, G., Hensel, B.K., Skubic, M., Rantz, M.: Senior residents' perceived need of and preferences for "smart home" sensor technologies. International Journal of Technology Assessment in Health Care 24, 120–124 (2008)
9. Donelson, S.M., Gordon, C.C.: 1995 Matched anthropometric database of US Marine Corps personnel: Summary statistics. Tech. rep., GEO Centers INC (1995), http://www.humanics-es.com/ADA316646.pdf

10. Doukas, C., Maglogiannis, I.: Emergency fall incidents detection in assisted living environments utilizing motion, sound, and visual perceptual components. IEEE Transactions on Information Technology in Biomedicine 15(2), 277–289 (2011)

11. EPCglobal Inc: EPC radio-frequency identity protocols, class-1 generation-2 UHF RFID (2008), http://www.gs1.org/gsmp/kc/epcglobal/

12. Fan, R.E., Chang, K.W., Hsieh, C.J., Wang, X.R., Lin, C.J.: LIBLINEAR: A library for large linear classification. Journal of Machine Learning Research 9, 1871–1874 (2008)

13. Finkenzeller, K.: RFID handbook: fundamentals and applications in contactless smart cards, radio frequency identification and near-field communication. Wiley (2010)

14. He, H., Garcia, E.: Learning from imbalanced data. IEEE Transactions on Knowledge and Data Engineering 21(9), 1263–1284 (2009)

15. Klack, L., Möllering, C., Ziefle, M., Schmitz-Rode, T.: Future care floor: A sensitive floor for movement monitoring and fall detection in home environments. In: Lin, J., Nikita, K.S. (eds.) MobiHealth 2010. LNICST, vol. 55, pp. 211–218. Springer, Heidelberg (2011)

16. Lan, M., Nahapetian, A., Vahdatpour, A., Au, L., Kaiser, W., Sarrafzadeh, M.: Smartfall: an automatic fall detection system based on subsequence matching for the smartcane. In: Proceedings of the Fourth International Conference on Body Area Networks, BodyNets 2009, ICST, Brussels, Belgium, pp. 8:1–8:8 (2009)

17. Li, Q., Stankovic, J., Hanson, M., Barth, A., Lach, J., Zhou, G.: Accurate, fast fall detection using gyroscopes and accelerometer-derived posture information. In: 6th International Workshop on Wearable and Implantable Body Sensor Networks, BSN 2009, pp. 138–143. IEEE (2009)

18. Lord, S.R., Sherrington, C., Menz, H.B., Close, J.C.: Falls in older people: risk factors and strategies for prevention. Cambridge University Press (2007)

19. Oliver, D., Healey, F., Haines, T.P.: Preventing falls and fall-related injuries in hospitals. Clinics in Geriatric Medicine 26(4), 645–692 (2010)

20. Qian, H., Mao, Y., Xiang, W., Wang, Z.: Home environment fall detection system based on a cascaded multi-SVM classifier. In: 10th International Conference on Control, Automation, Robotics and Vision, ICARCV 2008, pp. 1567–1572 (2008)

21. Robinovitch, S.N., Feldman, F., Yang, Y., Schonnop, R., Lueng, P.M., Sarraf, T., Sims-Gould, J., Loughin, M.: Video capture of the circumstances of falls in elderly people residing in long-term care: an observational study. The Lancet 381(9860), 47–54 (2012)

22. Werner, F., Diermaier, J., Schmid, S., Panek, P.: Fall detection with distributed floor-mounted accelerometers: An overview of the development and evaluation of a fall detection system within the project eHome. In: 5th International Conference on Pervasive Computing Technologies for Healthcare, pp. 354–361 (2011)

Domain knowledge Based Hierarchical Feature Selection for 30-Day Hospital Readmission Prediction

Sandro Radovanovic[1], Milan Vukicevic[1,2(✉)], Ana Kovacevic[1,2], Gregor Stiglic[3], and Zoran Obradovic[2]

[1] University of Belgrade, Faculty of Organizational Sciences, Jove Ilića, 154, Belgrade, Serbia
{sandro.radovanovic,milan.vukicevic}@fon.bg.ac.rs
[2] Temple University, Philadelphia, PA, USA
{ana.kovacevic,zoran.obradovic}@temple.edu
[3] University of Maribor, Maribor, Slovenia
gregor.stiglic@um.si

Abstract. Many studies fail to provide models for 30-day hospital re-admission prediction with satisfactory performance due to high dimensionality and sparsity. Efficient feature selection techniques allow better generalization of predictive models and improved interpretability, which is a very important property for applications in health care. We propose feature selection method that exploits hierarchical domain knowledge together with data. The new method is evaluated on predicting 30-day hospital readmission for pediatric patients from California and provides evidence that a knowledge-based approach outperforms traditional methods and that the newly proposed method is competitive with state-of-the-art methods.

Keywords: Re-admission · Feature selection · Domain knowledge

1   Introduction

Hospital re-admissions, one of the major costs of hospital care, often result from preventable errors associated with discharging patients, such as hospital acquired infections, poor planning for follow up care, inadequate communication of discharge instructions, and failure to reconcile and coordinate medications. Timely identification of potential readmissions can have high impact on improvement of healthcare services for patients, by reducing the need for unnecessary interventions and hospital visits, as well as for hospitals, by reducing costs and improving hospital status. Algorithms for prediction of hospital re-admission often fail to produce well performing models because of high dimensionality of data (over 14,000 possible diagnoses in ICD-9 coding) and high level of data sparsity. Additionally, high dimensionality reduces the interpretability of predictive models. This is why it is utterly important to develop efficient feature selection methods that will lead to parsimonious predictive models: ones that will select a low number of features without loss in predictive performance. Even though there is a large number of current state-of the art feature selection techniques [1], only a few [4, 5] exploit domain knowledge represented in hierarchical features.

© Springer International Publishing Switzerland 2015
J.H. Holmes et al. (Eds.): AIME 2015, LNAI 9105, pp. 96–100, 2015.
DOI: 10.1007/978-3-319-19551-3_11

We address this problem by proposing a method that utilizes domain knowledge in the form of ICD-9 hierarchy together with data driven classification techniques. The effectiveness of the proposed approach on predicting readmission on pediatric data from California is evaluated. Additionally, we demonstrate synergetic effects of our method with Lasso logistic regression and show that it outperforms alternative methods.

2   GHFCS – Group Hierarchical Feature Compression and Selection Method

We propose a GHFCS method that exploits domain knowledge in the form of ICD-9 hierarchy of diseases, where one disease can be categorized at most in four levels, from concrete diagnosis (i.e. mononucleosis) to high level concept (i.e. infectious or parasitic disease). The main intuition behind GHFCS is that the most of the specific concepts (features) in hierarchy do not bring good quality information about observed phenomena (in our case, readmission risk). This intuition applies on EHR because of high dimensionality and sparsity of hierarchy (only a small number of examples have the same diagnosis on the most specific level), and this often leads to poor predictive performance of the algorithms. Based on this, GHFCS tends to identify features with high information potential on the highest levels of the hierarchy without losing predictive power. Instead of selecting highly specific diagnoses, we can aggregate those diagnoses to a category from a higher level of the hierarchy. If the higher level category is equally or more informative, it will be used instead of specific categories.

The GHFCS method is based on a bottom up greedy strategy and utilizes all ICD-9 hierarchical levels. First, the dataset is aggregated and fused on each level of hierarchy, creating an augmented feature space where every node in the hierarchy is represented as a feature. Further, greedy filter selection is applied starting from leaves of the hierarchy and comparing them with their parent node based on information theoretic measures (note that any information theoretic measure [1] can be used for assessment of information potential). If the average information potential of child nodes is lower than that of the parent node, then all of the child nodes are removed from hierarchy (only the parent stays as a higher concept). If opposite, the parent node is removed from hierarchy and all of the child nodes are connected to the upper level node (parent of their original parent). This allows preservation of high information potential of low level features and examination of their synergetic influence with features of higher levels. Thus, the greedy assumption is reduced.

In order to evaluate GHFCS we developed a benchmark method: **SHFCS** (Single Hierarchical Feature Compression and Selection). Unlike GHFCS, this strategy tends to keep many more features by comparison of information potential of each child node with its parent (single comparison). We also evaluate current state-of-the art methods with similar strategies. **GTD** (Greedy Top Down) [4] uses a greedy top-down approach and the most informative feature from each hierarchy path. This approach selects features in a vertical manner, and in contrast to GHFCS does not utilize the whole hierarchy (it is ignoring the fact that one feature can be present in more than one hierarchy path). **SHSEL** (Simple Hierarchical Selection) [5] identifies and filters out the ranges of nodes with similar relevance in each branch of the hierarchy, (difference in information potential between a child and parent feature). Further, it selects only features that have greater information than the average of the tree path. Complete hierarchy is utilized, but in contrast to GHFCS, it restricts comparison to children and parent features (does not allow comparison between nodes from different hierarchy paths).

3   Experimental Evaluation

Data: Evaluation is performed on pediatric patient data (HCUP, [2]) from California about 30-day hospital re-admission containing 851 features on the lowest level of hierarchy. Data from January 2009 through December 2010 were used for training (46,682 examples), and 2011 data were used for testing (20,312 examples). Data had 14,000 binary valued features (diagnoses) and high class imbalance (11,884 positive and 55,810 negative cases). Detailed information about the dataset can be found in [6].

Comparison Between Knowledge Based and Traditional FS Methods: In the first experiment we compared the performance of knowledge-based against not-knowledge-based state-of-the-art feature selection techniques (Gini, Relief, ReliefF and MRMR) by means of Area Under Curve (AUC), Feature Space Compression (FSC) and Harmonic Mean (HM) of previous measures (where larger values are better). Figure 1 (left) shows that knowledge based feature selection methods, including our proposed Group method, are better in terms of AUC than methods that do not use domain knowledge.

On Figure 1 (middle) it can be seen that Gini has the lowest FSC by far and that not-knowledge-based methods do not follow the parsimony principle: by increasing FSC, AUC is drastically reduced. On the other side, knowledge based methods give parsimonious solutions which can clearly be seen by inspecting HM on Figure 1 (right). It is important to note that Gini was used as a measure of information potential in knowledge-based methods, which clearly shows the value of utilizing domain knowledge.

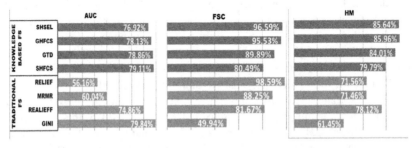

Fig. 1. Comparison of knowledge-based versus not-knowledge based FS methods

Based on results summarized at Figure 1 and for the sake of clarity of presentation in further experiments, we exclude not-knowledge-based methods from further analyses.

Comparison Between Knowledge Based Methods and Integration with Lasso:
Since regularization techniques showed good performance on high dimensional sparse
and imbalanced problems [3] we investigated the potential of combining Lasso regularized feature selection with knowledge based techniques. Figure 1 (left) shows the
levels of AUC and FSC levels obtained from Lasso regression on subsets of features
selected by knowledge based methods, as well as on the complete set of features
(Complete) It can be observed that there are no significant differences in AUC. This is
confirmed by significance testing between all methods (based on 100 times repeated
holdout evaluation of Lasso regression on every). This result points out that GHFCS
and SHSEL lead to the most interpretable solutions without loss of predictive accuracy. In order to better characterize methods, we simulated situations where AUC is
more important than feature compression rate. The results are measured by HM as
suggested in [5]. In our Lasso LR based experiments (summarized at Figure 2), importance of accuracy vs. interpretability (X-axis) is varied from 1 when AUC and
FSC are equally important up to 5 where AUC is drastically more important. GHFCS
shows the best performance in each situation (when AUC is up to 5 times more important). SHSEL showed reduced performance when AUC was more important and
significantly lower performance (on 95% level) compared to GHFCS over all settings.

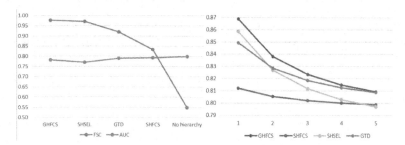

Fig. 2. Comparison between knowledge based methods

4   Conclusion and Future Research

It is shown that in contrast to traditional methods, knowledge-based feature selection
preserves AUC performance and highly reduces feature space. In combination with
Lasso Logistic Regression, GHFCS resulted in the most interpretable result, leaving
20 features (from the initial 851). Two categories (neoplasms and symptoms and
signs) are selected as 1st level features. From the 2nd level, 14 categories are selected,
mostly from the respiratory system,   genitourinary system, skin tissue, sense organs
diseases and injuries. On the 3rd level only food/vomit pneumonitis (ICD 5070) and
exam-clinical trial (ICD V707) are selected. There were no selected features at the
most specific 4th level. High level of aggregation without loss of predictive performance means that whole sub-trees of diseases are not important for predicting pediatric patient readmission. In our future work we will extend GHFCS in order to use
other forms of domain knowledge (ontologies) and apply the method to different prediction tasks.

Acknowledgement. This research was supported by DARPA Grant FA9550-12-1-0406 negotiated by AFOSR, National Science Foundation through major research instrumentation, grant number CNS-09-58854, and by SNSF Joint Research project (SCOPES), ID: IZ73Z0_152415.

References

1. Chandrashekar, G., Sahin, F.: A survey on feature selection methods. Computers & Electrical Engineering 40(1), 16–28 (2014)
2. HCUP State Inpatient Databases (SID), Healthcare Cost and Utiliza-tion Project (HCUP)
3. Jiang, B., Ding, C., Luo, B.: Covariate-Correlated Lasso for Feature Selection. In: Calders, T., Esposito, F., Hüllermeier, E., Meo, R. (eds.) ECML PKDD 2014, Part I. LNCS, vol. 8724, pp. 595–606. Springer, Heidelberg (2014)
4. Lu, S., Ye, Y., Tsui, R., Su, H., Rexit, R., Wesaratchakit, S., Liu, X., Hwa, R.: Domain ontology-based feature reduction for high dimensional drug data and its application to 30-day heart failure readmission prediction. In: International IEEE Conference Conference on Collaborative Computing (2013)
5. Ristoski, P., Paulheim, H.: Feature selection in hierarchical feature spaces. In: Džeroski, S., Panov, P., Kocev, D., Todorovski, L. (eds.) DS 2014. LNCS(LNAI), vol. 8777, pp. 288–300. Springer, Heidelberg (2014)
6. Stiglic, G., Wang, F., Davey, A., Obradovic, Z.: Readmission Classification Using Stacked Regularized Logistic Regression Models. In: Proc. AMIA 2014 Annual Symposium, Washington, DC (November 2014)

A Genomic Data Fusion Framework to Exploit Rare and Common Variants for Association Discovery

Simone Marini[1], Ivan Limongelli[2], Ettore Rizzo[1,2], Tan Da[1],
and Riccardo Bellazzi[1(✉)]

[1] Department of Electrical, Computer and Biomedical Engineering,
University of Pavia, Via Ferrata 1, 27100 Pavia, Italy
{simone.marini,ivan.limongelli,ettore.rizzo,riccardo.bellazzi}@unipv.it
[2] IRCCS Policlinico S. Matteo, Pzz.le Volontari del Sangue 2, 27100 Pavia, Italy
da.tan01@universitadipavia.it

Abstract. Collapsing methods are used in association studies to exploit the effect of genetic rare variants in diseases. In this work we model an enriched collapsing approach by including genes, protein domains, pathways and protein-protein interactions data. We applied the collapsing technique to a data set of epileptic (85 cases) and healthy (61 controls) subjects. The method retrieved 4 genes, 5 domains, 33 gene interactions and 14 pathways showing a significant association with the disease. Collapsed data have been also used as features for prediction models. We found that the use of protein-protein interactions as model features increases the area under ROC curve (+1.5%) if compared to the solely gene-based approach.

Keywords: Collapsing method · Associations study · Rare genetic variants · Epilepsy · Protein-protein interaction · Genetic pathway · Protein domain · Machine learning

1 Introduction

Next generation sequencing technologies have enabled to collect a huge amount of genomic data at increasingly lower costs. In the coming years we expect available sequencing data to explode, allowing the exploitation of both common and rare variants for the characterization of complex diseases. While traditional techniques used in GWAS can test association of common variants in complex diseases, collapsing (or burden) methods aim to combine rare variants within a region of interest (ROI) by collapsing them into a single genetic variable, which is tested for association with the phenotypes of interest. Typically, ROIs correspond to genomic regions that codify proteins, i.e. genes. Several collapsing methods have been proposed [1,2,3,4,5]. Collapsing methods are traditionally aimed to association discovery [2,3,4,5], but collapsed genetic data can be also utilized as features for a classification model [6].

© Springer International Publishing Switzerland 2015
J.H. Holmes et al. (Eds.): AIME 2015, LNAI 9105, pp. 101–105, 2015.
DOI: 10.1007/978-3-319-19551-3_12

We have extended the collapsing approach to include not only gene information, but also protein domains, pathways and protein-protein interactions (PPIs) as ROIs. This framework is a strategy to select and score ROIs that are further used as a genetic signature for complex diseases (or subtypes) of interest, enriching the traditional collapsing method approach by the fusion of multiple biological data sources. Furthermore, we show that by including additional ROIs it is possible to increase the classification performances. Given a set of genomic variants, they are collapsed under four main ROI-categories: NCBI RefSeq genes, KEGG pathways, BioGRID protein-protein interactions and InterPro domains. Each ROI is then scored according to its mutational load within the sample, calculated under an additive variant model based on the work by Tatonetti et al. [6].

2 Methods

Data Set. We analyzed sequencing data of 146 samples corresponding to 85 individuals characterized by different types of either isolated or syndromic epileptic disorders and 61 healthy individuals as controls. Epilepsy cases have been sequenced by a custom gene panel. Note that this panel is an extension of the one utilized by Della Mina et al. [7], and includes 46 more genes, for a total of 109 genes. Controls are divided between 15 healthy individuals sequenced by using the aforementioned gene panel and 61 unrelated whole-exome (Agilent SureSelect v5) sequenced individuals. Genomic variants for each individual have been obtained according to analysis procedures previously described by Della Mina et al.

ROI Score and Feature Encoding. Herby we define a variant as the difference in nucleotide bases between the reference genome (hg19) and the resulting assembled genome for a sample. Human genome is diploid and we expect two alleles for each genomic locus, therefore, when a variant occurs it can be observed in an "heterozygous" or "homozygous" state, i.e. on one or both human genome alleles respectively. Variant frequency typically refers to the frequency of the non-reference allele. Genomic variants have been annotated by using ANNOVAR. NCBI RefSeq and 1000 Genome Project (1TGP, v. april 2012) have been used as gene track and variant frequency sources respectively. Starting from ANNOVAR output, our framework integrates, for each gene variant, (1) protein domains (from InterPro database) overlapping the variant; (2) gene-related pathways from KEGG database; (3) genes resulting from protein-protein interactions (PPIs) recorded into the BioGrid database.

Annotated genes, domains, pathways and PPI-genes constitute our regions of interest (ROIs). Consequently, to each ROI j, for each individual i, a ROI score is assigned by using an additive model similar to the one described by Tatonetti et al. [6]:

$$ROI_{score} = \sum_{k=1}^{N_j} -v_{i,j,k} \tag{1}$$

$$v_{i,j,k} = \sigma_{i,j,k} \log f_{i,j,k} \tag{2}$$

Where N_j is the number of variants overlapping ROI j, $f_{(i,j,k)}$ is the frequency of the genomic variant k of the individual i in 1TGP and $\sigma_{(i,j,k)}$ can be equal to 0, 1 or 2 depending on the number of variant alleles, i.e. non-reference (no variant, heterozygous or homozygous respectively). Each variant therefore contributes to each ROI score per individual. Furthermore, a single variant can contribute to the score of different ROIs. For example, a variant v overlaps the domain D of the gene A; gene A belongs to pathways P_1 and P_2 and also it interacts with gene B and gene C. Therefore, variant v contributes to 6 ROIs: 1 gene (gene A), 1 domain (D) , 2 pathways (P_1 and P_2) and 2 genes given by $PPIs$ (gene B and gene C). Figure 1 shows how gene variants contribute to ROI scores by propagating mutational load to interacting genes at protein level (PPIs).

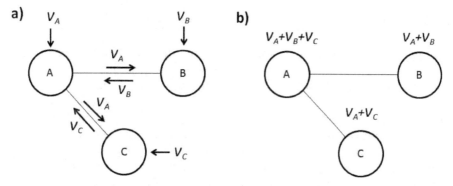

Fig. 1. Protein encoded by gene A interacts with proteins encoded by gene B and gene C. (a) Variant on gene $A_{(vA)}$ contributes to its own score and the score of both gene B and C due to their interaction. In the same way, variants on gene $B_{(vB)}$ and on gene $C_{(vC)}$ both contribute to their own score and the score of gene A. (b) Resulting variant contributions on final PPIs scores.

Each of the four feature groups (genes, domains, pathways and PPIs) has been utilized to generate data sets for patient classification in cases and controls. Data set properties are summarized in Table 1.

Prediction Models. To assess the different feature encoding methods, we trained both Logistic Regression (LoR) and Random Forest (RF) models. These models are designed with Weka framewor to predict if patients belong to case or control group. LoR is a ridge regression (ridge 10^{-8}), while RF exploits 99 trees, with 2 randomly considered features per node. For both models we randomly split each data set into a training set (70%) and a test set (30%). We then trained LoR

Table 1. The resulting list comprises 1080 ROI scores per individual, divided among genes (129), domains (252), pathways (130) and PPIs (569)

ROIs	# features	Description
Genes	129	RefSeq annotated genes. Gene number is greater respect to the gene panel due to gene isoforms
Domains	252	InterPro domains overlapping gene coding regions
Pathways	130	KEGG pathways
PPIs	569	Genes given by PPIs

and RF models on each training set, and measured their area under ROC curve (AUC) on their test sets. We repeated training/test sampling, model learning and AUC measure 100 times, and averaged the measured AUCs for LoR and RF models. Note that during each repetition the patient attribution to training and test sets was consistent among the four feature encodings.

3   Results

Our approach grants both association (knowledge discovery) and prediction (collapsed data as features for a classifier) results. In future studies, we aim to both merge the different data sources and perform feature selection.

Association Study. We measured the statistical significance of ROI scores between cases and controls. T-test statistic or Wilcoxon-test were applied in case of Gaussian or non Gaussian distribution respectively. Bonferroni correction has been used to correct for multiple testing. In this way we retrieved 56 ROIs, divided among genes (4), domains (5), pathways (14) and PPIs (33). It is not surprising that the positive associations found are epilepsy-related, since the sequencing data come from an epilepsy gene panel. For example, the score of CACNA1A gene, encoding for a voltage-gated calcium channel protein, has been found significantly higher in cases respect to controls. CACNA1A has been associated to idiopathic generalized epilepsy and related phenotypes such as episodic ataxia [9,10]. Interestingly, other collapsing methods have been applied on gene panel sequencing data sets of epileptic individuals [7],[10], without leading to significant associations.

Cases/Controls Prediction. Classification results are shown in Table 2. LoR models do not benefit from domains, pathways or PPI enriching; on the other hand, RFs trained on PPIs seem to leverage on interaction information and, on average, they perform better than the other models. Domain and pathway enrichment in general fail to improve classification. We suppose that domains are too much stringent and tend to exclude important disease-related variants (e.g. those in

Table 2. Classification results

	LoR (AUC)	RF (AUC)
Genes	*0.804*	0.872
Domains	0.573	0.777
Pathways	0.725	0.849
PPI	0.788	*0.887*

non-coding regions) while pathways seem to collapse variants belonging to distant genes (even if in the same pathway), adding noise. On the contrary, PPI enrichment accounts only for direct (or close) interacting genes, and its higher performances suggest that disease-related variants tend to gather on proximal interaction network of the considered epilepsy-related genes. Feature selection may further increase the predicted AUCs, and we will surely explore this option in forthcoming studies. We also expect that our framework would take advantage of more exhaustive sequencing data sets (e.g. whole exome or whole genome), although the tradeoff between the benefit due to their completeness and the consequently increased number of features remains to be examined.

References

1. Luo, L., Boerwinkle, E., Xiong, M.: Association studies for next-generation sequencing. Genome Research 21(7), 1099–1108 (2011)
2. Bansal, V., Libiger, O., Torkamani, A., Schork, N.J.: Statistical analysis strategies for association studies involving rare variants. Nat. Rev. Genet. 11(11), 773–785 (2010)
3. Li, Y., Byrnes, A.E., Li, M.: To Identify Associations with Rare Variants, Just WHaIT: Weighted Haplotype and Imputation-Based Tests. American Journal of Human Genetics 87(5), 728–773 (2010)
4. Dering, C., Hemmelmann, C., Pugh, E., Ziegler, A.: Statistical analysis of rare sequence variants: an overview of collapsing methods. Genetic Epidemiology 35(S1), S12–S17 (2011)
5. Price, A.L., et al.: Pooled association tests for rare variants in exon-resequencing studies. Am. J. Hum. Genet. 86(6), 832–838 (2010)
6. Tatonetti, N.P., Dudley, J.T., Sagreiya, H., Butte, A.J., Altman, R.B.: An integrative method for scoring candidate genes from association studies: application to warfarin dosing. BMC Bioinformatics 28(11), S9 (2010)
7. Della Mina, E., et al.: Improving molecular diagnosis in epilepsy by a dedicated high-throughput sequencing platform. Eur. J. Hum. Genet. (2014) (Epub ahead of print)
8. Riant, F., et al.: Identification of CACNA1A large deletions in four patients with episodic ataxia. Neurogenetics 11, 101–106 (2010)
9. Chioza, B., et al.: Association between the alpha-1A calcium channel gene CACNA1A and idiopathic generalized epilepsy. Neurology 56, 1245–1246 (2001)
10. Klassen, T., et al.: Exome sequencing of ion channel genes reveals complex profiles confounding personal risk assessment in epilepsy. Cell 145(7), 1036–1048 (2011)

Collaborative Filtering for Estimating Health Related Utilities in Decision Support Systems

Enea Parimbelli[1(✉)], Silvana Quaglini[1], Riccardo Bellazzi[1,2], and John H. Holmes[3]

[1.]Department of Electrical, Computer and Biomedical Engineering,
University of Pavia, Pavia, Italy
enea.parimbelli@gmail.com
[2] IRCCS Fondazione Salvatore Maugeri, Pavia, Italy
[3] University of Pennsylvania CCEB, Philadelphia, PA, USA

Abstract. A distinctive feature of most advanced clinical decision support systems is the ability to adapt to habits and preferences of patients. However effective preferences elicitation is still among the most challenging tasks to achieve fully personalized guidance. On the other hand availability of data related to patients' lives and habits is steadily increasing, making its exploitation an interesting opportunity for such purposes. In the MobiGuide project decision trees are used to implement shared-decision making using utility coefficients to incorporate patient preferences in the model. The main focus of this paper is the effort devoted to enhance traditional elicitation techniques proposing a methodology to predict patients' health-related utility coefficients. In particular we describe a recommender system, based on collaborative filtering, capable of estimating utilities by means of integrating different data sources such as medical surveys, questionnaires and utility elicitation tools along with patient self-reported experiences in the form of natural language.

Keywords: Collaborative filtering · Health related utility · DSS personalization

1 Introduction

The role of patient preferences in modern clinical decision support systems (CDSS) is assuming a steadily increasing importance. In some cases clinical variables alone cannot drive the decision process to a clear cut optimal solution. Different individuals can value the consequences of decisions in a significantly different way, affecting the final decision. For these reasons individual attitudes, patient's perception of their health status, personal context, job-related requirements and economic conditions should be taken into consideration also in formal decision analysis. This is true even in strictly computer interpretable guideline (CIG) based DSS systems where, according to a recent CDSS review study [1], patient-centric guidance is nowadays regarded as one of the most relevant future research directions. Moreover, in these patient-centric systems, patients are transitioning from their traditional role of passive actors to the one of actual decision makers through shared-decision processes. For these reasons in the context of the MobiGuide project we propose decision theory as a

© Springer International Publishing Switzerland 2015
J.H. Holmes et al. (Eds.): AIME 2015, LNAI 9105, pp. 106–110, 2015.
DOI: 10.1007/978-3-319-19551-3_13

methodological framework for a tool that, during face to face encounters, is used to tailor pre-defined, generic decision models to the individual patient, by involving the patient himself in the customization of the model parameters [2]. These parameters mainly consist in (i) utility coefficients (UCs) used to quantify the desirability of a health state and (ii) out-of-pocket costs for patients. Given the fact that effectively eliciting UCs has a number of challenges that are still unresolved in this paper we will focus on an alternative approach to preferences elicitation based on collaborative filtering and patients' self-reported experiences.

2   Methods

The core of the MobiGuide approach to shared decisions is to use decision trees (DTs) as a probabilistic, decision-theoretic formalism for representing and executing decision tasks. A list of possible decision options branch from the initial node of the DT. When the model is run the number of years spent in a certain health state is "weighted" by a multiplicative UC, which values the quality of that health state. UCs range from 0 (death) to 1 (perfect health), and they are, in principle, very subjective values, since they reflect a patient's feeling about a health state. Including personalized UCs into the model allows to incorporate into a single outcome measure (namely Quality Adjusted Life Years, QALYs) both mortality and morbidity combining a patient's expected length of life with the quality of those life years. It is possible to directly obtain UCs from each specific patient to guarantee the best degree of personalization of the decision problem. For this purpose we developed a web-based software tool named UceWeb which supports three of the main elicitation methods described in the literature [3]. Direct elicitation however can still be affected by some limitations like bias and anchoring effects or intrinsic difficulty of methods like Standard Gamble or Time Trade-Off. This might result in extreme albeit not so rare cases, in the impossibility to perform UCs elicitation. Traditionally in these cases doctors take over the whole responsibility of the clinical decision even if some involvement of the patient would have been appropriate. Some approaches have been proposed to estimate utility functions with limited available data [4]. In a recent work we described a high level architecture of a recommender system capable of predicting UCs for a patient capitalizing on the preferences of similar individuals [5]. In the following we focus on two of the main components of this architecture (NLP and collaborative filtering modules) and present them in more detail along with some advances in our methodological approach.

2.1   Extracting Utilities From Patient Generated Data

Figure 1 shows the functional processing steps we designed to extract UCs data starting from patients' experiences in the form of natural language text. Although several different data sources can potentially be mined to collect data about patients' experiences and quality of life (QoL) in this work we will focus on disease specific discussion boards. The first step of the pipeline shown in Figure 1 is devoted to the creation of a corpus which consists of a collection of discussion threads which have been properly anonymized to comply with patients' privacy requirements. Each thread then undergoes two processing steps: (i) QoL dimension identification and (ii) Degree of negativity assessment. The former is intended to identify those threads where at least one of the 5 QoL dimensions considered in the EuroQol questionnaire (mobility, self-care, usual activities, pain/discomfort, anxiety/depression) is addressed. The latter is intended to assess, by the means of sentiment analysis techniques [6], the degree of negativity associated to each of the identified QoL dimensions. These two information together would allow to virtually score the corresponding EuroQol questionnaire and finally perform the conversion to a proper UC using the standard EuroQol index value calculation algorithm. It is unlikely that we will be able to score all the dimensions of the EuroQol questionnaire for each single patient only looking at what he reported on social media. However, scoring the questionnaire even partially will allow us to derive the boundaries of the interval where the actual UC is contained. These observations, although less precise than UCs directly elicited from a patient, will still be   a valuable resource for training the predictive model.

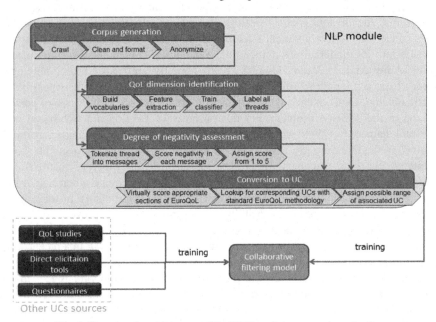

Fig. 1. Functional architecture of the NLP module processing pipeline

2.2   Collaborative Filtering Model

UCs coming from the NLP module presented in the previous section, together with other UCs sources in Fig.1, are then used to train a collaborative filtering model able to predict utilities for those patients who encounter difficulties with traditional elicitation methods. Other data sources are also merged into the training set to improve its quality. This step is important in order not to leave out relevant prior knowledge coming from QoL related studies published in medical literature or UCs elicited for specific subsets of patients (e.g. with disease specific tools). Once properly trained the model would be able to predict UCs for new patients based on the observations of similar individuals in the training set. The similarity measure between patients currently includes some patients' features like age, sex and working status as well as environmental factors like geographic location known to affect perceived QoL. More advanced techniques to define a proper similarity score which include also clinical features like main disorder and comorbidities need to be further investigated and could beneficially impact overall system performance [7].

3   Results

The methodology presented in this article is still work in progress. Nevertheless in this section we present a tentative implementation to demonstrate the technical feasibility of the system. Our scenario is based on one of the shared decisions implemented in MobiGuide where patients[1] have to decide whether to undergo an ablation procedure or stick to antiarrhythmic drug (AAD) therapy. Ablation is a hot topic on atrial fibrillation (AF) discussion forums being a procedure with good success rate but that often needs to be reiterated after some AF episodes recurrences. We used the Medpie framework [8] to collect an initial de-identified corpus of 3757 AF related threads for a total of ~30000 messages. A custom Python information extraction module based on nltk (Natural Language Toolkit) has been developed to mine the corpus and identify threads related to QoL after ablation or during AAD therapy. A mixed approach based on text classification algorithms and regular expression has been used to cope with the very low signal-to-noise ratio present in the corpus trying to achieve maximum recall. For the sentiment analysis of messages we rely on Sentistrength [9] for its ability assess positivity/negativity on a 1 to 5 intensity scale and to effectively cope with the particular lexicon used in web based conversation. The Sentistrength tool also features a machine learning based procedure that makes it easy to customize it to different vocabularies and sentiment lexicons which is very important for the medical domain we are considering. An example taken from the corpus regarding ablation and QoL is reported in the following along with its negativity score and associated UC: "*I was on cumadin, and beta blockers. My episodes were severe in the beginning, I went to the ER half a dozen times...I usually just go about my routine, with less energy of course. Afib seems to take so much away from quality of life...I figure I'll need to get an ablation someday, but I'm in no hurry to take the chance of worsening my condition. I for one am done being treated like a statistic. I want personal attention, not Dr. by numbers.*" (negativity score: 3; QoL dimensions: usual activities and pain/discomfort; UC Upper bound: 0,760[2]) Apart from data mined from social platforms we also plan to include data gathered during the Euro Heart Survey

---

[1]   The eligibility criteria for ablation shared decision consist in: diagnosis of paroxysmal atrial fibrillation and inability to maintain sinus rhythm after one or more antiarrhythmic drug therapy.

[2]   UC calculated using the EQ-5D-5L Crosswalk Index Value Calculator using UK population index values. No further assumptions were done on the score of the missing QoL dimensions.

study which assessed QoL of over 5000 AF patients with EuroQol [10]. Other data sources include UCs collected during the pilot phase of MobiGuide[3] where patients will be periodically filling out questionnaires and performing direct utility elicitation with UceWeb.

4   Conclusion and Future Developments

We presented a methodology based on a collaborative filtering model, NLP and sentiment analysis to cope with those situation where traditional elicitation methods might fail. Applying our proposal to those cases some degree of personalization of CDSS would still be possible and patients could benefit also from experiences reported by others. However not all patients are suitable for our approach and for shared decision in general. Adding to our methodology an additional preliminary step to assess a psychometric measure like locus of control [11] can help to target the most appropriate patients. Other future developments include working to improve the implementation of the single components, run integration testing of the whole pipeline and perform proper evaluation of the system.

References

1. Peleg, M.: Computer-interpretable clinical guidelines: A methodological review. J. Biomed. Inform. 46, 744–763 (2013)
2. Sacchi, L., Rubrichi, S., et al.: From decision to shared-decision: Introducing patients' preferences into clinical decision analysis. Artif. Intell. Med. (2014)
3. Parimbelli, E., Sacchi, L., et al.: UceWeb: a Web-based Collaborative Tool for Collecting and Sharing Quality of Life Data. Met. Inf. Med. (2014)
4. Chajewska, U., Getoor, L., Norman, J., Shahar, Y.: Utility Elicitation As a Classification Problem. In: 14th Conference on Uncertainty in Artificial Intelligence (1998)
5. Parimbelli, E., Quaglini, S., et al.: Use of Patient Generated Data from Social Media and Collaborative Filtering for Preferences Elicitation in Shared Decision Making. AAAI Fall Symposium Series (2014)
6. Greaves, F., Ramirez-Cano, D., et al.: Use of Sentiment Analysis for Capturing Patient Experience From Free-Text Comments Posted Online. J. Med. Internet Res. 15 (2013)
7. Gan, M.: Walking on a user similarity network towards personalized recommendations. PloS One 9, e114662 (2014)
8. Benton, A., Holmes, J.H., Hill, S., Chung, A., Ungar, L.: medpie: an information extraction package for medical message board posts. Bioinforma. Oxf. Engl. 28, 743–744 (2012)
9. Thelwall, M., Buckley, K., Paltoglou, G.: Sentiment strength detection for the social web. J. Am. Soc. Inf. Sci. Technol. 63, 163–173 (2012)
10. Berg, J., Lindgren, P., Nieuwlaat, R., Bouin, O., Crijns, H.: Factors determining utility measured with the EQ-5D in patients with atrial fibrillation. Qual. Life Res. 19 (2010)
11. Craig, A.R., Franklin, J.A., Andrews, G.: A scale to measure locus of control of behaviour. Br. J. Med. Psychol. 57(Pt 2), 173–180 (1984)

---

[3] Planned to start in mid February 2015.

Temporal Data Mining

Updating Stochastic Networks to Integrate Cross-Sectional and Longitudinal Studies

Allan Tucker$^{(\boxtimes)}$ and Yuanxi Li

Department of Computer Science, Brunel University, UK
allan.tucker@brunel.ac.uk

Abstract. Clinical trials are typically conducted over a population within a defined time period in order to illuminate certain characteristics of a health issue or disease process. These cross-sectional studies provide a snapshot of these disease processes over a large number of people but do not allow us to model the temporal nature of disease, which is essential for modelling detailed prognostic predictions. Longitudinal studies on the other hand, are used to explore how these processes develop over time in a number of people but can be expensive and time-consuming, and many studies only cover a relatively small window within the disease process. This paper explores the application of intelligent data analysis techniques for building reliable models of disease progression from both cross-sectional and longitudinal studies. The aim is to learn disease 'trajectories' from cross-sectional data by building realistic trajectories from healthy patients to those with advanced disease. We focus on exploring whether we can 'calibrate' models learnt from these trajectories with real longitudinal data using Baum-Welch re-estimation.

Keywords: Disease progression · Cross-sectional studies · Stochastic networks

1 Introduction

Degenerative diseases such as cancer, Parkinson's disease, and glaucoma are characterised by a continuing deterioration to organs or tissues over time. This monotonic increase in severity of symptoms is not always straightforward however. The rate can vary in a single patient during the course of their disease so that sometimes rapid deterioration is observed and other times the symptoms of the sufferer may stabilise (or even improve - for example when medication is used). Interventions such as medication or surgery can make a huge difference to quality of life and slow the process of disease progression but they rarely change the long term prognosis. The characteristics of many degenerative diseases is therefore a general transition from healthy to early onset to advanced stages. Longitudinal studies [1] measure clinical variables from a number of people over time. Often, the results of multiple tests are recorded, generating Multivariate Time-Series (MTS) data. This is common for patients who have high risk indicators of disease where they are monitored regularly prior to diagnosis.

© Springer International Publishing Switzerland 2015
J.H. Holmes et al. (Eds.): AIME 2015, LNAI 9105, pp. 113–122, 2015.
DOI: 10.1007/978-3-319-19551-3_14

For example, patients with high intra-ocular pressure are brought in to clinic for visual field tests every six months as they are at high risk of developing glaucoma. The advantages of longitudinal data is that the temporal details of the disease progression can be determined. However, the data is often limited in terms of the cohort size, due to the expensive nature of the studies. Cross-sectional studies record attributes (such as clinical test results and demographics) across a sample of the population, thus providing a snapshot of a particular process but without any measurement of progression of the process over time [2]. An advantage of cross sectional studies is that they capture the diversity of a sample of the population and therefore the degree of variation in the symptoms. The main disadvantage of such studies is that the progression of disease are inherently temporal in nature and the time dimension is not captured. For longitudinal analysis, the patients are usually already identified as being at risk and therefore, controls are usually not available and the early stages of the disease may have been missed as is explored in [3]. Previously, a resampling approach known as the Temporal BootStrap (TBS) [6] has been developed that aims to build multiple trajectories through cross sectional data in order to approximate genuine longitudinal data. These 'Pseudo Time-Series' (PTS) can then be used to build approximate temporal models for prediction. This approach has been extended in order to cluster important stages in disease progression using Hidden Markov Models (HMMs) [7]. However, the use of cross-sectional data alone will mean that no genuine timestamps have been used to infer the models and so they only capture an ordering without real temporal information.

In this paper, we explore how to minimise the expensive process of longitudinal data collection by taking models that are learnt from cross-sectional studies using pseudo temporal methods and updating with limited longitudinal data. We do this by using the Baum-Welch algorithm to update stochastic models learnt from pseudo time-series. Essentially, we are integrating cross-sectional and longitudinal data to increase the temporal information and the diversity of data from a large population. Many data integration techniques address representation heterogeneity where similar data is stored in different forms, as is common in bioinformatics data [8].

2   Methods

2.1   Generating Pseudo Time-Series

Let a dataset D be defined as a real valued matrix where m (rows) is the number of samples - here patients - and n (columns) is the number of variables - clinical test data. We define $D(i)$ as the ith row of matrix D. The vector $C = [c_1, c_2, \ldots, cm]$ represents defined classes, where each $c_i \in \{0, 1\}$ corresponds to the sample i, $c_i = 0$ represents that sample i is a healthy case, and $c_i = 1$ represents that sample i is a diseased case. These classifications are based upon the diagnoses made by experts. We define a time-series as a real valued T (row) by n (column) matrix where each row corresponds to an observation measured over T time points. We say that if $T(i)$ was observed before $T(j)$ then

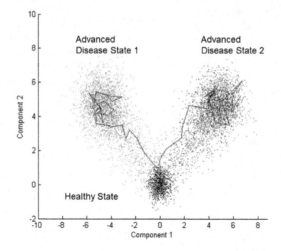

Fig. 1. Example PTS generated from TBS on Simulated Data

$i < j$. We define a set of pseudo time-series indices as $P = \{p1, p2, ...pk\}$ where each pi is a T length vector where $T > 0$. We define p_{ij} as the jth element of p_i and each $p_{ij} \in \{1, ..., m\}$. We define the function $F(p_i) = [p_{i1}, ..., p_{iT}]$ as creating a T by n matrix where each row of $F(p_i) = D(p_{ij})$. A pseudo time-series can be constructed from each pi using this operator. For example, if a pseudo time-series index vector $p_1 = [3, 7, 2]$ then $F(p_1)$ is a matrix where the first row is $D(3)$, the second row is $D(7)$ and the third row is $D(2)$. The corresponding class vector of each pseudo time-series generated by $F(p_i)$ is given by $G(pi) = [C(p_{i1}), ..., C(P_{iT})]$.

To summarise we have defined a set of k pseudo time-series with their associated class labels, sampled from the cross sectional data D indexed by the elements of pi. Building pseudo time-series involves plotting trajectories through cross-sectional data based upon distances between each point using prior knowledge of healthy and disease states. These trajectories can then be used to build temporal models such as Dynamic Bayesian Networks (DBNs) [10] and Hidden Markov Models (HMMs) to make forecasts [11]. The temporal bootstrap involves resampling data from a cross-sectional study and repeatedly building trajectories through the samples in order to build more robust time-series models. Each trajectory begins at a randomly selected datum from a healthy individual and ends at a random datum classified as diseased. The trajectory is determined by the shortest path of Euclidean distances between these two points. The data is first standardised to a mean μ of zero and a standard deviation σ of one as we found that this led to better HMM models. We use the Floyd-Warshall algorithm [12], a well established algorithm used to find the shortest path in a weighted graph. A full description of the algorithm to generate pseudo time-series appears

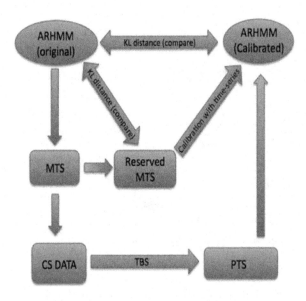

Fig. 2. Simulated Data Experimental Framework

in [6] and an example of pseudo time-series that have been generated from cross-sectional data are shown in Figure 2. Again, this was plotted on the first two components generated using multidimensional scaling.

2.2 The Experiments

We explore two set of experiments that both try to identify whether adding a small number of longitudinal data samples to models learnt from cross-sectional data (via the PTS approach) improves them: i) One on simulated data whereby discovered models are compared to some original time-series model from where the data has been sampled. ii) Another on real data from visual field tests where patients who are at high-risk of developing glaucoma undertake a psychophysical test to identify damage to sectors of their vision. Apart from the clinical test data itself and the clinical diagnosis (glaucomatous or not), no demographic data is included. Here no true original time-series model is known but a comparison can be made to models learnt on the time-series and on sampled cross-sections of the time-series. Firstly, we explore the effect of *updating* models of cross-sectional data, built using PTS, with relatively small numbers of real time series to see if the resulting models are improved. This involves the use of the Baum-Welch re-estimation algorithm applied to a prior HMM. Essentially we want to see if the limitations of pseudo time-series can be overcome (due to there being no time-element) by calibrating them with real time-series. We generate time-series of length 30 from an AutoRegressive HMM (ARHMM) to mimic typical biomedical longitudinal data (MTS in Figure 3). We then randomly sample a single point from these series (CS DATA) to mimic the cross-sectional sampling

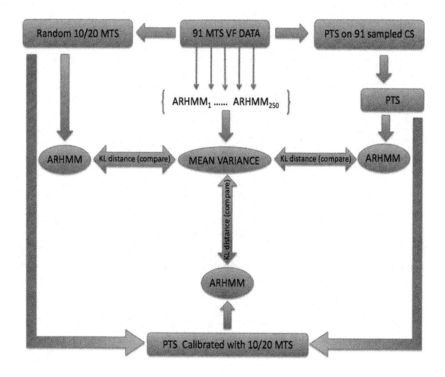

Fig. 3. VF Data Experimental Framework

of a population but reserve 50 for the calibration (Reserved MTS). We start with 500 cross-sectional samples as this was found to be a suitably large size to generate good pseudo time-series and models in [6] and increment by 100 up to 1500 (the size of some increasingly large biomedical cross-sectional studies). We use the Kulbaeck-Leibler distance [13] to explore how close a model learnt from the cross-sectional data using the temporal bootstrap (TBS) is to the original generating model. Experiments involve bootstrapping the data [14] We then add a number of the reserved original time-series generated by the same ARHMM to the pseudo time-series and explore how close new calibrated models are to the original. Increments of 10 time-series were used as these seem to differentiate between the KL distances significantly. We also include how good the model is when learnt solely from the time-series used to calibrate the models. We then apply a similar set of experiments with real VF longitudinal with 91 patient time-series (91 MTS VF DATA in Figure 4). We sample one VF test from each patient's time-series to generate a cross-sectional sample and generate PTS data for learning models from (PTS). We then compare this model as well as ones learnt from a combination of PTS and real time-series (Random 10/20 MTS) to see how quickly we can learn models that are close to the original. This is achieved by comparing these KL distances to the mean KL distance between 200 different ARHMMs learnt from the same original time-series (MEAN VARIANCE). In other words, if we can learn models from the sampled CS data that have similar

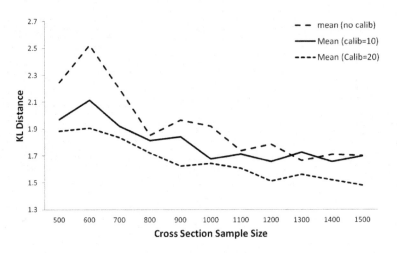

Fig. 4. KL distance for varying cross-sectional study sample sizes with increasing number of longitudinal data for calibration.

KL distances to the general variation in learning a model from the full time-series, then we assume that the models are as close to one learnt from a full time-series.

3   Results

3.1   Simulated Data Results

Figure 5 shows the results for all experiments, learning PTS from cross-sectional samples of varying sizes and either not calibrating, calibrating with 10 time-series, or calibrating with 20 time-series. The first obvious characteristic of these graphs is that calibrating does indeed improve the quality of the models with KL distances that are closer to the original generating ARHMM. This is not surprising seeing that there is no genuine "time" in the PTS generated from the cross-sectional data. What is surprising, is that only a relatively small number of time-series are needed to improve these models, especially when there are lots of samples used from the cross-sectional data. This supports the results from previous studies that the PTS does find good-but-not-perfect models (limited by the lack of real time-series) and that a small number of genuine time-series can calibrate these models. This offers hope that expensive longitudinal studies can be relatively small in size if combined with larger cross-sectional studies that capture the general trajectories and the variability of disease progression within a population. With calibration from 10 time-series, there is a steady decrease in KL distance as cross-sectional sample size increases where more and more reliable PTS are constructed. When the sample size is 1500 we see a KL distance mean of 1.70 ± 0.16. Note that when 10 time-series alone are used to learn the model we get a mean KL distance of 2.08 ± 0.26. This shows that the PTS generated from the cross-sectional data improves on models learnt from the time-series only by incorporating the variability within a larger population captured in the cross-sectional data. With calibration from 20 time-series we see a similar story, where increasing the cross-sectional sample size, build better PTS and results in models that are closer to the original. For 1500 in the cross-sectional sample we see a KL distance of 1.48 ± 0.12. Note that when 20 time-series alone are used to learn the model we get a mean KL distance of 1.78 ± 0.15. Again, it can be seen that the PTS improves on time-series alone but that the integration of both seems to generate the models that best reflect the underlying model. We now explore

Wilcoxon Rank	cs500calib10	cs500calib20	cs1500nocalib	cs1500calib10	cs1500calib20	csfull30	csfull50
cs500nocalib	0.196	0.047	**0.001***	**0.001***	**0.001***	**0.001***	**0.001***
cs500calib10	-	0.455	0.062	0.036	**0.001***	**0.010***	**0.001***
cs500calib20	-	-	0.077	0.130	**0.001***	0.023	**0.001***
cs1500nocalib	-	-	-	0.947	0.119	0.395	0.064
cs1500calib10	-	-	-	-	0.052	0.277	0.047
cs1500calib20	-	-	-	-	-	0.395	0.728
csfull30	-	-	-	-	-	-	0.291
csfull50	-	-	-	-	-	-	-

Fig. 5. Wilcoxon rank comparison between KL distances to original MTS model (significant p values marked with an asterisk P<0.01)

the statistical significance of the differences between these KL distances using the Wilcoxon Rank comparison [15]. Table 1 shows the Wilcoxon Rank statistic comparing the KL distance between different models learnt using the different approaches. An asterisk is used denote significant p values. First of all notice that there are many significant values - indicating that the difference between models learnt using the different approaches are significant. The most important statistics are those that show the models learnt with no calibration and only 500 cross-sectional data points is significantly different to most other models (row 1), but when 1500 cross-sectional data points are used the resulting model is much closer, being most different (though not quite significantly) to the model learnt from 50 full time-series (row 4). By calibrating these models we see a little improvement for 500 CS data points. However, for 1500 datapoints calibrated with 20 time-series, there is no significant difference between the models learnt from the full time-series with much higher p-values.

3.2   Visual Field Data Results

We now explore the effect of calibrating PTS using the real Visual Field time-series data described earlier (Figure 6). As we have no knowledge of the true underlying model, we firstly compare the KL distance between models that are repeatedly learnt from the original 91 patient time-series in order to get an idea of general variance between models and to use this as a base-line. Essentially, if we can generate models using PTS approaches with a KL distance that is not significantly greater than the general variance between different builds of the model on the full data, then we can be confident that the PTS models are of a suitably

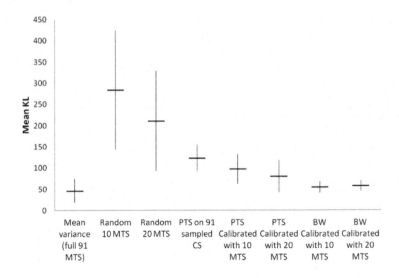

Fig. 6. KL results for VF data with confidence intervals

Wilcoxon Rank	Rand 10	Rand 20	PTS	PTS Cal (10)	PTS Cal(20)	Bayes Cal(10)	Bayes Cal (20)
Mean variance (full 91 MTS)	0.001*	0.001*	0.001*	0.005*	0.011	0.255	0.500
Random 10 MTS	-	0.975	0.023	0.002*	0.001*	0.001*	0.001*
Random 20 MTS	-	-	0.042	0.014	0.010	0.001*	0.001*
PTS on 91 sampled CS	-	-	-	0.452	0.327	0.001*	0.001*
PTS Calibrated with 10 MTS	-	-	-	-	0.773	0.001*	0.002*
PTS Calibrated with 20 MTS	-	-	-	-	-	0.002*	0.006*
Bayes Calibrated with 10 MTS	-	-	-	-	-	-	0.881
Bayes Calibrated with 20 MTS	-	-	-	-	-	-	-

Fig. 7. Wilcoxon rank for VF data (significant p values marked with an asterisk $P<0.01$)

similar quality to those learnt from the full time-series. We then calculate the KL distance between a model learnt from the sampled cross-section using the PTS approach and models learnt from the original 91 time-series. We then incrementally add a number of randomly selected real time-series to calibrate the PTS model to see if this improves the KL distance. We do this in two ways: simply concatenating the data (PTS calibrated), and also using the PTS as a prior which is updated with real time-series - Baum Welch (BW) calibrated Bayes. Finally we calculate the KL distance between learning models using only the calibrating time-series to confirm that the PTS are indeed improving the resulting models. The experiments are repeated 100 times to derive confidence intervals on the KL distances. Figure 7 shows the results of these experiments. Notice firstly that the KL distance between models that have been learnt on the full 91 time-series are in the region of 80-90 with a small confidence interval denoting a relatively small variance from one model learning to the next. The models that are learnt from the sampled cross-section using the PTS approach are impressively close to the time-series models but distinctly higher in KL distance (likely to be because we are lacking real temporal information). When 10 and 20 real time-series are used to calibrate the model, however, we see further improvement in the KL distance resulting in models that are demonstrably closer to the models learnt from all 91 time-series. The updated models that go beyond simply concatenating data appear to perform the best with the lowest KL scores. Finally, models that are learnt from using the relatively small number of calibrating time-series only are clearly worse with much higher distance and large confidence intervals. Looking at the Wilcoxon Rank for significance as before, the important thing to notice in Table 2 is that nearly all of the models are indeed significantly worse than the variation between models learnt on the full longitudinal dataset (significant differences are marked with an asterisk) except for the PTS model calibrated us-ing the updating approach or concatenating with 20 real time-series. This shows that we can learn models that are as good as the natural variation between model building on the full longitudinal dataset by building PTS and calibrating with only 10 real longitudinal samples if we correctly balance the weighting of the cross-sectional PTS and real time-series. We can also see that many of the inferior models are similar in terms of their distances except for the very worst models (learnt from only 10 time-series) which are different from the superior models which are both PTS models that have been calibrated. To summarise, whilst the PTS approach alone does indeed learn very good models, by updat-ing these models with a small number of real time-series we get models that are considerably closer to the models learnt using all the time-series data that is available. What is more, the Baum-Welch approach to updating improves upon a simply concatenation of data. Note that almost all models are significantly different from the general variance form learning the model from the full 91 time-series. The only models that are not significantly different at the 1% level are the PTS models updated with data using the Baum-Welch approach and the PTS model that is updated with 20 time-series by concatenation.

4   Conclusions

In this paper we have explored to what degree pseudo time-series, learnt from building trajectories through a cross-sectional study, can be 'calibrated' by a rel-atively small number of real time-series data form a clinical longitudinal study. The aim is to gain the advantage of both types of study - the population di-versity of symptoms at all stages of a disease process from cross-sectional data; and the inherently temporal information of a disease process from longitudinal data. We have demonstrated that a relatively small number of disease time-series can dramatically improve the quality of disease model if the pseudo time-series has been constructed from a large enough cross-sectional sample. This has been shown to be the case for simulated data based upon a probabilistic model and real-world clinical data where the resultant models are not significantly differ-ent to models learnt from large longitudinal studies. Future work will involve exploring the Baum-Welch updating approach to integrating the longitudinal and cross-sectional data on more datasets. Pseudo time-series naturally model multiple endpoint analysis which is an important topic in modelling disease progression [16]. Future work will explore the explicit understanding of these in terms of identifying subcategories of disease which we have already started to explore [7].

References

1. Albert, P.S.: Longitudinal data analysis (repeated measures) in clinical trials. Statistics in Medicine 18(13), 1707–1732 (1999)
2. Mann, C.J.: Observational research methods. research design ii: cohort, cross sectional, and case-control studies. Emergency Medicine Journal 20(1), 54–60 (2003)
3. Siddiqui, Z.F., et al.: Predicting the post-treatment recovery of patients suffering from traumatic brain injury (TBI). Brain Informatics 2, 33–44 (2015)
4. Frank, A., Asuncion, A.: UCI machine learning repository. Irvine: University of California, school of information and computer science (2010), http://archive.ics.uci.edu/ml (last accessed December 17, 2013)
5. Seber, G.A.F.: In Multivariate Observations. John Wiley and Sons, Hoboken (1984)
6. Tucker, A., Garway-Heath, D.: The pseudo temporal bootstrap for predicting glaucoma from cross-sectional visual field data. IEEE Trans. IT Biomed. 14(1), 79–85 (2010)
7. Li, Y., Swift, S., Tucker, A.: Modelling and analysing the dynamics of disease progression from cross-sectional studies. Journal of Biomedical Informatics 46(2), 266–274 (2013)
8. Shen, R., et al.: Integrative Subtype Discovery in Glioblastoma Using iCluster. Plos One 7(4), e35236 (2012)
9. Inmon, W.H.: Building the Data Warehouse, 2nd edn. John Wiley and Sons (1996)
10. Murphy, K.: Dynamic Bayesian Networks: Representation, Inference and Learning, PhD Thesis, University of Califronia, Berkeley (2002)
11. Rabiner, L.R.: A tutorial on hidden Markov models and selected applications in speech recognition. Proceedings of the IEEE, 257–286 (1989)
12. Floyd, R.W.: Algorithm 97: shortest path. Communications of the ACM 5(6), 345 (1962)
13. Kasza, J., Solomon, P.J.: A comparison of score-based methods for estimating Bayesian networks using the Kullback Leibler divergence. Communications in Statistics: Theory and Methods (2013), arXiv:1009.1463v2 (stat.ME)(in press)
14. Efron, B., Tibshirani, R.: An introduction to the bootstrap (monographs on statistics and applied probability). CRC Press, Boca Raton (1993)
15. Bauer, D.F.: Constructing confidence sets using rank statistics. Journal of the American Statistical Association 67, 687–690 (1972)
16. Pocock, J., Stuart, L., Geller, N., Anastasios, A.T.: The Analysis of Multiple Endpoints in clinical trials. Biometrics 43, 487–498 (1987)

Optimal Sub-Sequence Matching for the Automatic Prediction of Surgical Tasks

Germain Forestier[1]([✉]), François Petitjean[2], Laurent Riffaud[3,4],
and Pierre Jannin[3]

[1] MIPS, University of Haute-Alsace, Mulhouse, France
germain.forestier@uha.fr
[2] Faculty of Information Technology, Monash University, Melbourne, Australia
[3] INSERM MediCIS, Unit U1099 LTSI, University of Rennes 1, Rennes, France
[4] Department of Neurosurgery, Pontchaillou University Hospital, Rennes, France

Abstract. Surgery is one of the riskiest and most important medical acts that is performed today. The desires to improve patient outcomes, surgeon training, and also to reduce the costs of surgery, have motivated surgeons to equip their Operating Rooms with sensors that describe the surgical intervention. The richness and complexity of the data that is collected calls for new machine learning methods to support pre-, peri- and post-surgery (before, during and after).

This paper introduces a new method for the prediction of the next task that the surgeon is going to perform during the surgery (*peri*). Our method bases its prediction on the optimal matching of the current surgery to a set of pre-recorded surgeries.

We assess our method on a set of neurosurgeries (lumbar disc herniation removal) and show that our method outperforms the state of the art by providing a prediction (of the next task that is going to be performed by the surgeon) more than 85% of the time with a 95% accuracy.

1 Introduction

More than half a million surgeries are performed every day worldwide [1], which makes surgery one of the most important component of global health care.

This has motivated the growing interest in Computer Assisted Surgery (CAS) tools. More and more Operating Rooms (ORs) are getting equipped systems with sensing devices that can capture the surgeon's activities and environment. For example, using cameras in pituitary surgery, both the phases of the surgery [2] and the low-level surgical tasks [3] can be detected and recorded automatically. The task performed by the surgeon can also be automatically inferred by combining RFID chips on instruments (for identification) with accelerometers [4]. The collected information is very precise and rich, because it corresponds to the low-level actions and tools that are performed and used by the surgeon. Because it is so precise, the data is however extremely challenging to analyze. For example, two surgeons performing the same surgery on the same patient might exhibit a very different course of specific actions, while being surgically very

© Springer International Publishing Switzerland 2015
J.H. Holmes et al. (Eds.): AIME 2015, LNAI 9105, pp. 123–132, 2015.
DOI: 10.1007/978-3-319-19551-3_15

similar: they might use the same technique, have the same patient outcome, etc. However, from the low-level point of view (the sequence of low-level tasks like *cut, suture,* etc.), these surgeries will look very different from each other.

Extracting useful high-level knowledge from this low-level data has been one of the research themes targeted by the field of Surgical Process Modeling (SPM) [5,6], which aims at understanding surgeries to improve the quality of care. The above-mentioned sensors capture the surgical tasks performed in real-time, which opens the door to using artificial intelligence methods to provide real-time information to the surgical team.

This paper seeks the prediction of the surgeon's subsequent actions, using low-level information only. Such a prediction system is critical for OR management: it will provide useful real-time information to the surgical team (nurses, anesthetist, junior surgeon), while allowing the surgeon to focus on more demanding tasks. Because predicting the next surgical task is central, such a prediction system will also be a keystone to the development of many other systems. Learning to predict the future from past observations is one of the key components that make it possible to bring value to the massive data stores that have been collected in medicine [7].

In this paper, we focus on predicting the next surgical actions from the low-level information that can be captured during the surgery (*e.g.,* [3,8,9]). We use the series of surgical activities performed by the surgeon to represent the course of the surgery. We capture the activity of both hands for three different elements: *used instrument, performed action* and *targeted anatomical structure* [10]. Learning to predict the next activity of the surgeon from such low-level information is extremely challenging, because the next surgical action depends upon high-level information (phase of the surgery, technique used, patient-specific information, so-far reaction of the patient to the surgery, etc.), while a surgery is represented by a series of actions like "*cut,scalpel,skin*".

Intuitively, our approach matches the on-going surgery to every surgery of a reference set of surgeries, and use the next actions that have been performed in the reference set of surgeries to draw a prediction about the next action that will be performed in the current surgery. Our approach includes the three following features:

1. **Optimal registration of a partial surgery:** We propose a method to optimally register the on-going surgery (partial surgery) to any complete pre-recorded surgery. Our approach is based on the Dynamic Time Warping similarity measure [11], which is consistent with surgical processes [12].
2. **Voting for high-confidence prediction:** Using the optimally registered reference set of surgeries, we use voting to draw a high-confidence prediction about the next action that going to be performed by the surgeon.
3. **Detecting when to predict with high-confidence:** Using the agreement rate among multiple predictors, we are able to detect when to perform a prediction and when it is not possible to draw an accurate prediction.

Our framework is assessed using clinical data of lumbar disc herniation surgeries. Dr. L. Riffaud recorded 24 surgeries performed by multiple surgeons as part of a stay at the Neurosurgery Department of the Leipzig University Hospital, Germany. We show that our method outperforms the state of the art by providing a prediction more than 85% of the times with a 95% accuracy.

This paper is organized as follows. In Section 2, we present our solution for high-confidence prediction of the next surgical activity that is going to be performed. In Section 3, we conduct experiments that demonstrate the quality and performance of our approach compared to the state of the art. Finally, we conclude this work and describe future research in Section 4.

2 High-Confidence Prediction of the Next Surgical Activity

We present our proposed approach in this section. We start by presenting our method for optimal sub-sequence matching in Section 2.1. We then present how we use this method to draw high-confidence predictions about the next surgical action in Section 2.2.

2.1 Optimal Sub-Sequence Matching

Let $\mathbb{S} = \{S_1, \cdots, S_N\}$ be the reference set of N sequences (surgeries), $S = \langle s_1, \cdots, s_l \rangle$ be one sequence of this set (a complete surgery), and $S^\star = \langle s_1^\star, \cdots, s_k^\star \rangle$ be a partial sequence (the ongoing surgery). Let us denote $S_{1,l'}$ a sub sequence $\langle s_1, \cdots, s_{l'} \rangle$ of S. Our objective is to find the sub-sequence $S' = S_{1,l'}$ so that the cost of optimally registering the partial sequence $S^\star$ onto the subsequence S' of the reference sequence S is minimal.

Finding the cost of an optimal registration of one sequence onto another has been studied by the literature. The Dynamic Time Warping (DTW) similarity measure [11] makes it possible to find the optimal alignment of two sequences (and thus register them) in $\Theta(l_1 \cdot l_2)$ operations (with l_1 and l_2 the respective lengths of the realigned sequences). The consistency of this measure has been demonstrated for surgical processes in [12,13].

In this section, we 1) introduce a new objective function for finding the sub-sequence S' that best matches $S^\star$, and 2) introduce a new algorithm, based on DTW, that can find S' in $\Theta(k \cdot l)$ operations only.

Objective Function. Our goal is to find the matching point l' in S that minimizes the optimal alignment between $S^\star$ and the sub-sequence $S_{1,l'}$:

$$match(S^\star, S) = \underset{1 \leqslant l' \leqslant l}{\arg\min} \ \mathrm{DTW}(S^\star, S_{1,l'}) \tag{1}$$

Figure 1 presents the intuition about our objective function, compared to DTW's one. Figure 2 presents the trend of this objective function versus the value taken by l' on an example.

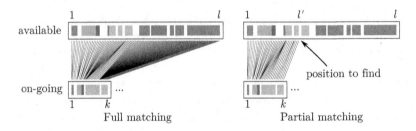

Fig. 1. Illustration of the difference between a full (left) and partial (right) matching

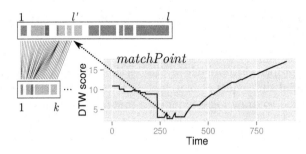

Fig. 2. Illustration of the *matchPoint* resulting of the partial matching

Efficient Algorithm. An exhaustive search among all the possible matching points for l' will take $\Theta(\frac{l \cdot (l+1)}{2} \cdot k) = \Theta(l^2 \cdot k)$ operations. Such a cubic complexity with the length of the matched sequences is incompatible with real-time matching, because a typical surgery will often have more than 10,000 elements long.

We now show how to modify the Dynamic Time Warping (DTW) algorithm to obtain an exact solution in $\Theta(l \cdot k)$ operations without sacrificing the soundness of the process. Note that with 10,000 elements, the difference in the complexity corresponds to an algorithm running 4 orders of magnitude faster than the naive solution. Our solution is presented in Algorithm 1, where we adapted the original DTW algorithm to identify the optimal *matchPoint* (l') during sequences registration. In this algorithm, we kept the core of DTW and we added a condition (*i.e.*, the *if* statement) allowing to store the optimal *matchPoint* during the computation of the matrix storing the partial costs.

Note that although this algorithm can be further optimized depending on δ (*i.e.*, the distance function between elements of the sequences), we chose here to give the algorithm for the general case. Furthermore, this adaptation of the algorithm did no alter the properties of optimality of DTW.

2.2   A Voting Approach to Draw High-Confidence Predictions

Our method uses the proposed optimal sub-sequence matching to draw predictions about the next surgical activity that will be performed. We will use the

---

Algorithm 1. Optimal sub-sequence matching

Require: $S^* = \langle s_1^*, \cdots, s_k^* \rangle$
Require: $S = \langle s_1, \cdots, s_l \rangle$
Let δ be a similarity between the elements of the sequences
Let $m[k, l]$ be a matrix storing partial costs
Let $l' \leftarrow 1$ be the matching point to find
  $m[1, 1] \leftarrow \delta(s_1^*, s_1)$
  for $i \leftarrow 2$ to k **do** $\{m[i, 1] \leftarrow m[i-1, 1] + \delta(s_i^*, s_1)\}$
  for $j \leftarrow 2$ to l **do** $\{m[1, j] \leftarrow m[1, j-1] + \delta(s_1^*, s_j)\}$
  for $j \leftarrow 2$ to l **do**
    for $i \leftarrow 2$ to k **do** $\{m[i, j] \leftarrow \delta(s_i^*, s_j) + \min(m[i-1, j], m[i, j-1], m[i-1, j-1])\}$

    if $m[k, j] < m[k, l']$ **then** $l' \leftarrow j$
  end for
  return l'

---

optimal sub-sequence matching from the on-going surgery S^* to every sequence S_i of $\mathbb{S}$. We can then use this information to draw a probability distribution $\hat{p}_{next}$ over the next possible state of the current surgery. More formally, the maximum likelihood estimate $\hat{p}_{next}$ for the next activity to be s given the previous activities S^* is:

$$\hat{p}_{next}(s|S^*) = \frac{|\{S(match(S^*, S) + 1) = s\}_{S \in \mathbb{S}}|}{|\mathbb{S}|} \quad (2)$$

Finally, we draw a prediction from the maximum a posteriori estimate of $\hat{p}_{next}$ using a majority vote [14], *i.e.*, select s for which $\hat{p}_{next}(s|S^*) \geqslant 0.5$. In order to ensure and confer high-confidence to the system, we do not draw a prediction if no s obtains a majority or in case of ties. Note that $\hat{p}_{next}(s|S^*)$ can be seen as an agreement rate on the prediction: a high value indicates an important agreement amongst the recorded surgeries about the next action that is going to be performed and conversely. The threshold on the agreement rate (0.5 in this paper) can be tuned according to need for a system performing very accurate predictions but in limited number or a large number of predictions with an increased probability of errors. We have developed a web application [1] to allow the reader to try this prediction system easily. An open-source standalone implementation of the method is accessible at the same URL.

3   Experiments

3.1   Clinical Data

Figure 3 presents the dataset. The framework is evaluated using clinical data composed of 24 lumbar disc herniation surgeries recorded at the Neurosurgery Department of the Leipzig University Hospital, Germany. Surgeries contain on average 680 actions. The surgeries involved 10 male and 14 female patients, with

---

[1] http://germain-forestier.info/src/aime2015/ (Accessed: 30 March 2015)

a median age of 52 years. These lumbar disc surgeries are divided into three main steps: (1) approach of the disc, (2) discectomy and (3) closure. The herniated disc is approached via a posterior intermyolamar route. The patients were operated on by five junior and five senior surgeons. Senior surgeons have performed at least a hundred removals of lumbar disc herniation. All the junior surgeons have passed more than two years of their residency program but have only performed a few removals of lumbar disc herniation. In this paper, we focused on the closure phase, because it allows us to ensure that the main surgeon is the one operating (for a junior surgery, his or her senior sometimes takes over the surgery).

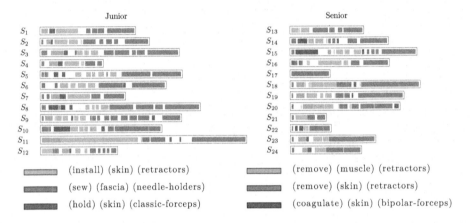

Fig. 3. The dataset of 24 surgeries used for the experiments and the legend for the six most frequent actions

3.2 Methodology

We compare three configurations: using only the senior surgeries, using only the junior surgeries and using all surgeries. Our aim is to observe the influence of the available surgeries (training data) on the quality of the predictions that are drawn. A leave-one-out cross-validation approach was used for each configuration: we select one surgery out of the set of surgeries, and use it as the on-going intervention (this surgery is then removed from the set of reference surgeries). The left-out surgery is used to test our predictions, as if it was progressively discovered. Predictions are made every 5% of the progression of the intervention. We can then compare every prediction with the *actual* activity of the surgery. Every surgery is in turn considered as the on-going intervention.

We evaluate our system using the precision $\mathcal{P}$ (*i.e.*, number of good predictions / total number of predictions), the recall $\mathcal{R}$ (*i.e.*, number of predictions / total number of expected predictions). We also use the F-measure $\mathcal{F}$ (harmonic mean between prediction and recall) to provide an overall evaluation. We compare the results of our method to the one of the Euclidean state-of-the-art method. We use the exact same process, but replace the optimal sub-sequence matching with uniform scaling [15]. Uniform scaling performs a linear transformation that increases or decreases sequences by a scale factor so that they have the same length.

3.3   Results

Figure 4 presents the general results of the F-measure comparing the two methods and the three configurations. We can see that our approach outperforms the

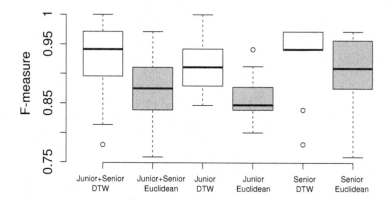

Fig. 4. Results on the three configurations (Junior+Senior, Junior, Senior) for the two methods (DTW in white, Euclidean in gray)

state-of-the-art Euclidean approach, regardless of the considered configuration. The compact dispersion of the results for the senior case (compared the junior case) suggests that seniors have a more homogeneous behavior than junior surgeons, which is consistent with previous studies comparing junior and senior practices [12]. This result also illustrates the influence of the set of available recordings in the quality of the prediction. Even though mixing all the surgeries together provides very good results, the best results are obtained for senior surgeons, whose surgical practice is usually more standardized and homogeneous. This supports our intuition that the more dedicated the training data is to the operating surgeon, the more accurate the predictions will be.

Table 1 details the prediction results for every one of the 24 surgeries (using the 23 remaining surgeries as the training set). A sparkline (*e.g.,*) presents, for each sequence, the evolution of the agreement rate among the predictions over the course of the surgery. The gray rectangle represents the interval (0.5, 1] for which a majority is obtained. The blue dots represent the cases where our system did not provide a prediction (because no majority was obtained), while the red dots represent the inaccurate predictions. The precision of our system is very high: no mistakes are committed for more than half. Overall, our systems exhibits an average precision of 95%: our predictions do not eventuate only 5% of the times.

Table 1. Detailed results for every surgery; results with $\mathcal{F} \geqslant .9$ are shown in boldface

		Junior					Senior		
Surg.	$\mathcal{P}$	$\mathcal{R}$	$\mathcal{F}$	Agreement	Surg.	$\mathcal{P}$	$\mathcal{R}$	$\mathcal{F}$	Agreement
S_1	1.00	0.94	**0.97**		S_{13}	1.00	0.89	**0.94**	
S_2	0.94	0.89	**0.91**		S_{14}	0.94	0.94	**0.94**	
S_3	0.85	0.72	0.78		S_{15}	1.00	0.83	**0.91**	
S_4	1.00	0.94	**0.97**		S_{16}	1.00	0.72	0.84	
S_5	0.94	0.94	**0.94**		S_{17}	1.00	0.83	**0.91**	
S_6	1.00	0.94	**0.97**		S_{18}	1.00	0.89	**0.94**	
S_7	0.88	0.94	**0.91**		S_{19}	1.00	0.94	**0.97**	
S_8	0.94	0.94	**0.94**		S_{20}	0.93	0.83	0.88	
S_9	0.88	0.89	0.88		S_{21}	1.00	0.94	**0.97**	
S_{10}	1.00	0.83	**0.91**		S_{22}	0.94	0.94	**0.94**	
S_{11}	1.00	1.00	**1.00**		S_{23}	1.00	1.00	**1.00**	
S_{12}	0.93	0.78	0.85		S_{24}	0.75	0.89	0.81	

Moreover, our system provides a prediction 89% of the times (recall). This means that for the vast majority of cases, an agreement can be reached and a decision made. Furthermore, the consistency of our voting procedure is confirmed: for all the cases where the MAP (maximum a posteriori) estimate was below the majority threshold, and for which we thus did not provide a prediction (*i.e.*, blue dots in Table 1 – *Agreement* column), the MAP estimate was actually wrong. This confirms the relevance of our approach, by showing that we actually do not provide a prediction when no reliable choice can be made from the training set. This corresponds to the case where not enough similarity can be found between the on-going surgery and the reference set, which can be the case if specific activities are required during the surgery. The highest number of errors are committed in S_{24} with a sequence of four wrong predictions in a row. This corresponds to the green activity in Figure 3, where the surgeon installs the retractors on the skin without stopping, while all the other surgeries exhibit several pauses. Finally, every prediction is made in less than 200 ms, which is compatible with real-time prediction in the OR.

Note that the current system is dependent of the heterogeneity of the sequences inside the reference database. If the reference sequences are highly heterogeneous, the system could have difficulties to perform the partial matching. As the size of the available reference set is limited, we are currently matching all the sequences of the reference database with the target sequence. However, a threshold on DTW score could be used to select only the most similar sequences to perform the prediction.

4   Conclusion

We have presented a method for the prediction of the next surgical task that is going to be performed during the surgery. Our contributions include:

1. definition of the objective function for the registration of a partial sequence to a complete reference sequence.

2. an efficient algorithm, based on DTW, to optimally minimize the above-mentioned objective function.
3. a prediction system that combines our optimal sub-sequence matching with MAP estimation and filtering.

The experiments have shown that our method outperforms the state of the art and provides a prediction more than 85% of the times with a 95% accuracy.

Because the prediction of surgical tasks is central to computer assisted surgery, this work naturally opens up a number of clinical applications. We have mentioned in the introduction how this information can help ensuring a smooth running of the surgery. Another application concerns the training of junior surgeons, where our system could be integrated in a simulation environment in order to provide help and feedback to the junior surgeon [16]. Our system could, on demand, provide a warning to the surgeon about his or her deviation from the standard practice of his or her colleagues. The agreement rate would then inform about the importance of the deviation. In future work, we want to validate this method on a more important dataset (> 300 surgeries) and use our recent work on Dynamic Time Warping [17] to improve the predictions.

Supplementary Materials

Prediction package: Java package containing the source code for the proposed method. (Java ARchive file) – http://germain-forestier.info/src/aime2015/source-code-aime-2015.jar (Accessed: 30 March 2015)

Acknowledgments. This research has been supported by the Australian Research Council under grant DP120100553. The authors would like to thanks all the surgeons involved in this work as well as Professor Ann Nicholson having reviewed the paper.

References

1. Haynes, A.B., Weiser, T.G., Berry, W.R., Lipsitz, S.R., Breizat, A.H.S., Dellinger, E.P., Herbosa, T., Joseph, S., Kibatala, P.L., Lapitan, M.C.M., et al.: A surgical safety checklist to reduce morbidity and mortality in a global population. New England Journal of Medicine 360(5), 491–499 (2009)
2. Lalys, F., Riffaud, L., Morandi, X., Jannin, P.: Automatic phases recognition in pituitary surgeries by microscope images classification. In: Navab, N., Jannin, P. (eds.) IPCAI 2010. LNCS, vol. 6135, pp. 34–44. Springer, Heidelberg (2010)
3. Lalys, F., Riffaud, L., Bouget, D., Jannin, P.: An application-dependent framework for the recognition of high-level surgical tasks in the OR. In: Fichtinger, G., Martel, A., Peters, T. (eds.) MICCAI 2011, Part I. LNCS, vol. 6891, pp. 331–338. Springer, Heidelberg (2011)
4. Meißner, C., Meixensberger, J., Pretschner, A., Neumuth, T.: Sensor-based surgical activity recognition in unconstrained environments. Minimally Invasive Therapy & Allied Technologies, 1–8 (2014)
5. Lalys, F., Jannin, P.: Surgical process modelling: a review. International Journal of Computer Assisted Radiology and Surgery 8(5), 1–17 (2013)

6. Forestier, G., Petitjean, F., Riffaud, L., Jannin, P.: Non-linear temporal scaling of surgical processes. Artificial Intelligence in Medicine 62(3), 143–152 (2014)

7. Liu, Z., Hauskrecht, M.: Clinical time series prediction with a hierarchical dynamical system. In: Peek, N., Marín Morales, R., Peleg, M. (eds.) AIME 2013. LNCS(LNAI), vol. 7885, pp. 227–237. Springer, Heidelberg (2013)

8. Ruda, K., Beekman, D., White, L.W., Lendvay, T.S., Kowalewski, T.M.: Surgtrak – a universal platform for quantitative surgical data capture. Journal of Medical Devices 7(3), 030923 (2013)

9. Ahmidi, N., Gao, Y., Béjar, B., Vedula, S.S., Khudanpur, S., Vidal, R., Hager, G.D.: String motif-based description of tool motion for detecting skill and gestures in robotic surgery. In: Mori, K., Sakuma, I., Sato, Y., Barillot, C., Navab, N. (eds.) MICCAI 2013, Part I. LNCS, vol. 8149, pp. 26–33. Springer, Heidelberg (2013)

10. Mehta, N., Haluck, R., Frecker, M., Snyder, A.: Sequence and task analysis of instrument use in common laparoscopic procedures. Surgical Endoscopy 16(2), 280–285 (2002)

11. Sakoe, H., Chiba, S.: Dynamic programming algorithm optimization for spoken word recognition. IEEE Transactions on Acoustics, Speech and Signal Processing 26(1), 43–49 (1978)

12. Forestier, G., Lalys, F., Riffaud, L., Collins, D.L., Meixensberger, J., Wassef, S.N., Neumuth, T., Goulet, B., Jannin, P.: Multi-site study of surgical practice in neurosurgery based on surgical process models. Journal of Biomedical Informatics 46(5), 822–829 (2013)

13. Forestier, G., Lalys, F., Riffaud, L., Trelhu, B., Jannin, P.: Classification of surgical processes using Dynamic Time Warping. Journal of Biomedical Informatics 45(2), 255–264 (2012)

14. Kittler, J., Hatef, M., Duin, R.P., Matas, J.: On combining classifiers. IEEE Transactions on Pattern Analysis and Machine Intelligence 20(3), 226–239 (1998)

15. Yankov, D., Keogh, E., Medina, J., Chiu, B., Zordan, V.: Detecting time series motifs under uniform scaling. In: International Conference on Knowledge Discovery and Data Mining, pp. 844–853. ACM (2007)

16. Zhou, Y., Bailey, J., Ioannou, I., Wijewickrema, S., O'Leary, S., Kennedy, G.: Pattern-based real-time feedback for a temporal bone simulator. In: Symposium on Virtual Reality Software and Technology, pp. 7–16. ACM (2013)

17. Petitjean, F., Forestier, G., Webb, G., Nicholson, A., Chen, Y., Keogh, E.: Dynamic Time Warping averaging of time series allows faster and more accurate classification. In: IEEE International Conference on Data Mining (2014)

On the Advantage of Using Dedicated Data Mining Techniques to Predict Colorectal Cancer

Reinier Kop[1(✉)], Mark Hoogendoorn[1], Leon M.G. Moons[2],
Mattijs E. Numans[3], and Annette ten Teije[1]

[1] Department of Computer Science, VU University Amsterdam, De Boelelaan 1081,
1081 HV, Amsterdam, The Netherlands,
{r.kop,m.hoogendoorn,annette.ten.teije}@vu.nl
[2] Department of Gastroenterology and Hepatology,
Utrecht University Medical Center, Heidelberglaan 100,
3584CX Utrecht, The Netherlands
l.m.g.moons@umcutrecht.nl
[3] Department of Public Health and Primary Care, Leiden University Medical Center,
Hippocratespad 21, 2333 ZD Leiden, The Netherlands
m.e.numans@lumc.nl

Abstract. Electronic Medical Records (EMRs) provide a wealth of data that can be used to generate predictive models for diseases. Quite some studies have been performed that use EMRs to generate such models for specific diseases, but most of them are based on more traditional techniques used in medical domain, such as logistic regression. This paper studies the benefit of using advanced data mining techniques for Colorectal Cancer (CRC). CRC is the second most common cancer in the EU and is known to be a disease with very a-specific predictors, making it difficult to generate good predictive models. In addition, the EMR data itself has its own challenges, including the sparsity, the differences in which physicians code the data, the temporal nature of the data, and the imbalance in the data. Results show that state-of-the-art data mining techniques, including temporal data mining, are able to generate better predictive models than currently available in the literature.

Keywords: Colorectal cancer · Data mining · Machine learning

1 Introduction

It is well known that more and more data about the medical state and history of patients is stored in electronic medical records (EMRs). In a variety of countries (such as the Netherlands, in which the present study is performed), the general practitioner (GP) acts as a proxy to secondary care and receives and oversees all information about a patient from relevant sources. A variety of studies have been performed using this type of GP EMRs, e.g. [7,11]. Analysis of this data may contribute to an early detection of diseases and more effective treatments. Conventional methods used in the medical domain are however unable to take full advantage of this data as they are directed in a top-down manner. Conversely, machine learning (ML) methods may allow for more data exploitation (e.g. [10]).

© Springer International Publishing Switzerland 2015
J.H. Holmes et al. (Eds.): AIME 2015, LNAI 9105, pp. 133–142, 2015.
DOI: 10.1007/978-3-319-19551-3_16

In this paper, we try to explore whether advanced ML approaches can be used for the prediction of colorectal cancer (CRC). CRC is a disease for which early diagnosis has shown to be difficult due to its a-specific symptoms but also of crucial importance as the life expectancy greatly reduces if diagnosis takes place in a late stage of the disease [5]. Several predictive models have been generated in this domain using EMR data whereby the models by Hippisley-Cox & Coupland [7] and Marshall et al. [11] are the most well-known. However, they (in part) make use of datasets enriched with specific data regarding known predictors for CRC. We have access to an anonymized GP dataset of over 200.000 patients, in which no data enrichment has taken place. Using this dataset we generate predictive models using random forests [3] (RF), SVM [15] and the simpler CART algorithm [4]. In addition, we use a sophisticated approach (based on [2]) to generate and exploit temporal patterns to see whether this benefits the accuracy of the predictions. Given the variety in the quality of the datasets across studies (which makes it difficult to directly compare results), we compare the outcome with an application of the previously generated models on our dataset. Finally, we investigate whether new predictors are identified.

This paper is organised as follows: In Section 2, we discuss the data and how it is pre-processed. We treat our methodology in Section 3. The results are presented in Section 4. We conclude with a discussion in Section 5.

2   Dataset Description and Preparation

For this study, anonymized EMRs from two GP database systems were made available from the Utrecht region in the Netherlands. The total number of patients in the dataset amounted to 219.447. Data is available regarding a patient's age, gender, details of GP consults (> 5.5 million), drug prescriptions (> 6.6 million), specialist referrals (> 0.7 million), comorbidity (> 66.000), and lab test outcomes (> 7.6 million). Each consult is associated with an ICPC (International Classification of Primary Care) code, a standard describing symptoms and diseases in patients. Similarly, drug prescription records make use of the ATC (Anatomic Therapeutical Chemical) classification system. The comorbidity data is a list of chronic conditions a patient currently has, e.g. hypertension or even pregnancy. The period covered in the dataset lies between 01-07-2006 and 31-12-2011.

For conventional data mining algorithms, a single instance is typically represented as a one-dimensional fixed size input vector. In our case, an instance equals a single patient. It is not possible to represent the data described above as a fixed-size input vector 'as is'; number of prescriptions, consults, etc. differ too much for this among patients. In the paragraphs below, we describe the data preparation.

Obtaining the Target Value. The presence or absence of CRC in a patient is investigated using a patient's consulting history. The ICPC code for CRC is D75. The data is divided in two sets: the set of patients which have been diagnosed with CRC (i.e. their GP has classified a consult with a D75 ICPC code at least once), and the set of patients which have never been diagnosed with CRC. This makes for a highly imbalanced classification task, namely 808 CRC cases among 219.447 patients (0.37%). These numbers meet the expectation of specialists, and are consistent with Dutch national health studies (e.g. [14]).

Subsampling the Time Period. After consultation with specialists (Dutch GPs and gastro-enterologists), the choice was made to look at six-month periods per patient. For CRC cases, the period before the first recorded diagnosis of D75 was chosen. For non-CRC cases, a period was randomly chosen between 01-07-2006 and 31-12-2011. Any patient for which this was not possible, was purged. This occurs if a patient is registered with the GP shorter than six months, or when a CRC diagnosis occurred in the first six months of the 2006-2011 period. This resulted in 654 CRC cases among 202.126 patients (0.32%).

Selection by Age. The data is further subsampled by age (≥ 30 only). This split was chosen largely to be in line with related research [7,11]. After pruning patients with invalid time periods and ages, the dataset contained 651 CRC cases among 127.304 patients (0.51%).

Extracting Standard Attributes. Attributes are abstracted from the data by counting the occurrences of events. All rows but the last in Table 1 summarise this strategy. Note that this table partially overlaps with the table in [8] (indicated by *), of which the research presently described is a continuation.

HB, cell volume, and blood in the stool measurements are known CRC predictors [11]). These values stem from the lab result data. The reason for not currently utilising additional lab results is because of the sparseness of the lab result records; minimum and maximum threshold values are often not recorded, and the units of the values are ambiguously defined (e.g. mL, mmol, g, etc.).

Discovering Temporal Patterns. The final row of Table 1 requires some extra attention. The other attributes ignore a potentially important aspect of the data: its temporality. Thus, a temporal pattern mining approach based on is used Batal et al. [2]. The general idea of this approach is described below.

We can view each timestamped record in the dataset as an event occurring on a timeline. For example, if a patient consults the GP on 28-01-2009 with abdominal pain (ICPC D01), a 'consult event' will be generated stating that the patient exhibited ICPC D01 on 28-01-2009. An event sequence is the entire sequence of events for a specific patient.

A pattern is a set of events which may occur in patients. Pairs of events are mutually related to each other using the *(s)*uccession or *(c)*o-occuring relations. Consider a pattern with events ICPC D01, ICPC D12, and ATC A06, with relations ICPC D01 *(s)* ICPC D12; ICPC D01 *(s)* ATC A06; ICPC D12 *(c)* ATC 06. This pattern expresses a sequence in which a patient has abdominal

Table 1. List of attributes extracted. Overlap with [8] indicated by asterisks (*)

Attribute	Value	Description
*age	Integer	The age of a patient.
*gender	M/F	The gender of a patient.
*ICPC A01, ..., ICPC Z29	Integer	720 attributes, each representing the number of times a consult ended up in a classification of ICPC i for a patient.
ATC A01, ..., ATC V0	Integer	86 attributes, each representing the number of times medication with code ATC i was prescribed for a patient.
*ref kno, ..., ref wvk	Integer	94 attributes, each representing the number of times a patient was referred to a specialist of the category ref i.
comor angina pectoris, ..., comor pregnancy	Integer	33 attributes, each representing whether or not a patient is currently in a certain (medical) condition comor i.
HB inside thresh, HB outside thresh	Integer	Number of times a patient's haemoglobin value was inside/outside the desired range.
cell volume normal, cell volume abnormal	Integer	Number of times a patient's cell volume value was inside/outside the desired range.
blood in stool, no blood in stool	Integer	Number of times blood was found / was not found in a patient's stool.
temporal pattern P_1, ..., P_n	Binary	Indicates whether or not a patient's medical history contains a certain temporal pattern P_i.

pain (D01), succeeded by a co-occurrence of constipation (D12) and a laxative prescription (A06). If a patient history includes the pattern above (e.g. ICPC D01 on 28-01-2009, ICPC D12 on 30-01-2009, ATC A06 on 30-01-2009), the pattern is said to cover the patient.

The mining algorithm is based on the apriori algorithm [1]. As with standard apriori, the records are scanned first to create frequent patterns of size 1, *1-patterns*. These patterns are used to generate successively larger patterns, i.e. k-patterns are used to obtain frequent $k+1$-patterns. Generating a $k+1$-pattern is, however, more elaborate than for standard apriori, because the generated candidate patterns need to accommodate for multiple possible *(s)* and *(c)* relations. This results in more $k+1$-patterns being tested for frequency than with standard apriori, increasing the complexity. An entire explanation of the algorithm is beyond the scope of this paper. An in-depth description of the algorithm including many optimisations is available in [2]. To maximise the likelihood of finding predictive patterns, the algorithm is run on CRC and no CRC cases separately. The resulting patterns for both cases are then assembled into a single list. Each pattern discovered using the described method can now be used as an attribute. The attribute is binary, indicating the absence (0) or presence (1) of the pattern in the patient's medical history.

3 Methodology

Our experiments serve four main purposes, namely to investigate

1. whether or not the dataset is able to predict the occurrence of CRC at all;
2. the potential advantage of using advanced ML techniques;
3. the potential added value of including temporal information;
4. the predictors found by the algorithms in relationship to known predictors, in order to validate or disprove the generated models.

These four purposes are achieved by selecting five subsets, and applying four ML algorithms to them in a 5-fold cross validation fashion. The first three purposes are investigated quantitatively, latter purpose more qualitatively.

Creating Subsets. Subsets are made to investigate the dataset's predictive capability. First, as a benchmark, we investigate a gender/age-only subset. This is compared to non-temporal and temporal subsets, and a combination of both. Results of generating this temporal subset are presented in Section 4 prior to discussing the results of the model generation. Finally, we produce a knowledge-driven subset, consisting of the 31 known predictors as described in [11].[1] The resulting subsets are summarised in Table 2.

Table 2. The attributes contained within each subset

Subset	Description
non-temporal	941 non-temporal attributes + age/gender.
temporal	n temporal patterns + age/gender.
all	$941 + n$ + age/gender.
knowledge-driven	31 attributes as described in [11] + age/gender.
age/gender	Benchmark; age and gender only.

Learning Algorithms. Marshall et al. [11] obtain a high performance (area under ROC curve of 0.829) using the classification method logistic regression (LR) for predicting CRC. We compare this to the transparent CART decision tree algorithm, and two less transparent algorithms, namely RF and SVMs.

Existing implementations in the Python Scikit-Learn package were used for each of the algorithms. After extensive tuning, parameters were chosen as follows. For LR, the regularisation parameter L2 was chosen. For CART, we selected the Gini impurity measure as a splitting criterion, a maximum tree depth of 5, and the minimum number of samples at a leaf node equal to 50. Changing the splitting criterion did not alter results, whereas increasing the tree depth and reducing the minimum number of samples resulted in tremendous overfitting. For RF, identical settings as for CART were chosen for the same reasons, in conjunction with a forest size of 100. Further increasing the forest size did not alter the performance, whereas we did notice a decrease in performance upon reduction of the forest size. Finally, for SVM we set RBF as the kernel type. Attempts with a polynomial kernel type resulted in either worse results or unreasonable computation time, depending on the degree of the polynomial.

In an attempt to consolidate the quantitative results, we extract the predictors (averaged over all folds of the cross validation) from the LR and RF algorithms. Analysing these in a qualitative way may shed a different light on the quantitative results, or may provide additional insights. The same is done for the decision tree resulting from the CART algorithm.

---

[1] These consist of ICPC codes B80, 81, 82; D01, 02, 06, 08, 11, 12, 15, 16, 18, 24, 93; K93, 94; T07, 08, 82, 89, 90, 92; ATC codes G04; A06, 07; B03; and multiple variations of haemoglobin, cell volume, and blood in stool measurements.

4   Results

Temporal Data Mining. The temporal data mining algorithm was run with a minimum support of 0.1. This resulted in the discovery of 94 patterns: 29 *1*-patterns, 51 *2*-patterns, and 14 *3*-patterns. Three example patterns are presented in Table 3. These patterns are at this point only discovered - no conclusion is made regarding their predictive value for the occurrence of CRC. The reason for also including 1-patterns in our investigation is simple: single events may already be of great importance for GPs. It is unfair to give the temporal subset a disadvantage by ignoring potential predictors such as blood in the stool.

During experimentation, various support values were attempted, but only for an extremely low minimum support (< 0.025) did the algorithm find patterns for more than three states. However, such patterns would be very specific to the dataset, increasing the likelihood of overfitting were they to be used.

The 94 resulting temporal patterns are dominated by ATC (i.e. drug prescription) states. One cause may be that the prescriptions are well recorded in the dataset, a well known fact according to the specialists. In addition, recurring prescriptions for chronic diseases are relatively common, so it should be no surprise the algorithm finds such patterns.

Table 3. Three example temporal patterns of various sizes

Pattern	Meaning
ICPC D16	Presence of rectal bleeding (= ICPC D16).
ATC A06 *(c)* ICPC D12	Presence of a prescription of laxatives (= ATC A06) *co-occurring* with constipation (= ICPC D12).
ICPC T90 *(s)* ICPC T90 *(s)* ICPC T90	Presence of diabetes (= ICPC T90) occurring in *succession*.

Quantitative Analysis. For each algorithm applied to each of the five subsets, the AUC (area under the ROC curve) and 95% confidence interval (CI; as described in [6]) was recorded. The results of the runs are shown in Table 4.

We observe performances better than random for each subset-algorithm combination. This confirms the first purpose highlighted in Section 3. The benchmark performance is relatively high, a common occurrence for medical prediction tasks. Particularly the age attribute is known to be a good predictor for CRC. Additionally, the most complete part of the dataset is the age and gender of a patient. Other potential predictors (e.g. blood in the stool, or abdominal pain) may therefore be suppressed, since they occur less consistently in the data.

For the second purpose, we compared the various algorithms. The results show that RF performs significantly better than LR in the non-temporal, temporal, and knowledge-driven subsets (shown in **bold**). SVM and CART do not perform significantly better than LR. Thus, RF can be an improvement over LR for large (*non-temporal* and *all*) or knowledge-driven subsets.

For the third purpose, we compared the non-temporal and temporal subsets. The results improve using the temporal compared to the non-temporal subset. This is the case amongst all algorithms, except RF. Furthermore, the temporal subset provides us with the best overall performance (using LR, shown in *italics*), barring the biased knowledge-driven subset. The ROC curves resulting from applying CART to the temporal and non-temporal subsets are shown in Figure 1. This selection is made both to avoid clutter and to highlight the results of mining temporal data. It is evident that the temporal subset outperforms the non-temporal subset. Thus, the temporal information is of added value for prediction in this case. IF we view the temporal and knowledge-driven subsets as a kind of feature selection, their performances may lead us to believe that other feature selection methods are potentially helpful for the algorithms. However, performing such methods on the subsets did not alter their performances (results not shown).

Regarding computational efficiency, the temporal and non-temporal subset contain 94 and 941 attributes, respectively. This makes the learning process for the temporal subset much faster, while at the same time resulting in a better performance using all algorithms, with the exception of RF.

Table 4. AUCs and 95% CIs for all algorithm-subset combinations, established using 5-fold cross validation. The subsets are non-temporal *(NT)*, temporal *(T)*, all *(A)*, knowledge-driven *(KD)*, and the age/gender benchmark *(B)*.

Subset	LR	RF	SVM	CART
NT	0.792 (0.771 − 0.813)	**0.883** (0.866 − 0.900)	0.804 (0.784 − 0.824)	0.819 (0.799 − 0.839)
T	*0.893* (0.877 − 0.909)	0.882 (0.865 − 0.899)	0.861 (0.843 − 0.879)	0.863 (0.845 − 0.881)
A	0.796 (0.775 − 0.817)	**0.881** (0.864 − 0.898)	0.832 (0.813 − 0.851)	0.818 (0.798 − 0.838)
KD	0.854 (0.836 − 0.872)	**0.896** (0.880 − 0.912)	0.867 (0.849 − 0.885)	0.860 (0.842 − 0.878)
B	0.844 (0.825 − 0.863)	0.838 (0.819 − 0.857)	0.862 (0.844 − 0.880)	0.828 (0.808 − 0.848)

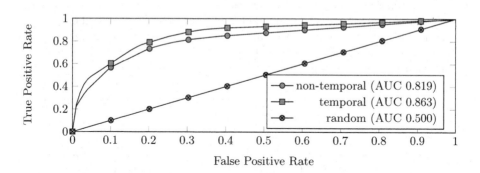

Fig. 1. ROC curves applied to several subsets of the data. To avoid clutter, only the curves for CART applied to the non-temporal and temporal subsets are shown.

Qualitative Analysis. We now investigate whether the resulting predictors for each algorithm are meaningful or likely incidental (the fourth purpose of the experiments). We highlight the *all* subset in this section since it is the only one which can show potentially *any* of the described attributes.

Linear Regression. The first column in Table 5 shows the top 5 predictors for the *all* subset using LR. The temporal patterns mostly indicate drugs for acid-related disorders (ATC A02), usually used for the treatment of abdominal complaints or pain together with non-steroidal anti-inflammatory drugs. Hypertension (second on list) occurs as a top 10 predictor resulting from applying LR and RF to the *non-temporal* and *all* subsets. Similar results were also observed in [9], in which it is noted this may be related to the metabolic syndrome. Rectal bleeding (third on list) is a predictor corresponding to Marshall et al.'s known predictors [11]. The orthopaedic referral is likely incidental.

Table 5. Predictors for the *all* subset for *LR* and *RF*. ATC codes are: A02 = drugs for acid-related disorders; B01 = antithrombotic agents; C10 = lipid modifying agents.

LR	RF
Pattern: ATC A02 *(s)* ATC C10	Psoriasis comorbidity
ICPC K86 (hypertension)	ATC J01 (antibacterials)
ICPC D16 (rectal bleeding)	Pattern: ATC A02 *(s)* ATC A02
Orthopaedic specialist referral	Pattern: ATC A02 *(s)* ATC C10
Pattern: ATC B01 *(s)* ATC A02	ICPC S29 (skin complaint)

Random Forest. The second column in Table 5 shows the best predictors for RF. The first and second (psoriasis, a skin disease; and ATC J01) are likely incidental. The relevance of the third and fourth is unclear, as in the previous paragraph. The final predictor, ICPC S29, may be related to psoriasis. The uncertainty in these predictors is likely due to the low number of CRC patients. This causes each tree in the forest to be specialized for a few dozen CRC patients only, whom are similar to each other with respect to disorders unrelated to CRC such as psoriasis.

Decision Tree. Figure 2 shows a partial decision tree generated with CART using the *all* subset. Each node occurs in the list of predictors by Marshall et al. [11]. Of particular interest is rectal bleeding, also occurring as an LR predictor.

In summary, the models generated by CART show predominantly known predictors, as opposed to the predictors found by LR and RF. This pattern holds for all subsets, with the obvious exception of the knowledge-driven subset and the benchmark. Furthermore, symptoms related to the metabolic syndrome were observed as CRC predictors, as in [9].

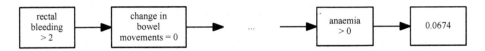

Fig. 2. A single traversable path of the decision tree generated by the CART algorithm using the *all* subset. The leaf node indicates the probability for a patient to have CRC.

5   Discussion

Current methods of detecting colorectal cancer in its early stages are sub-optimal. In an attempt to improve the detection rate, we generated risk models which

1. are able to accurately predict the occurrence of CRC in patients;
2. in doing so, can be (in the case of RF) more effective compared to traditional models in related research for larger amounts of data;
3. include temporal aspects of the data which improve performance (except in the case of RF);
4. are largely validated through the resulting predictors, particularly CART. This indicates that a transparent risk model is a competitive choice for incorporation in the current CRC diagnosis chain.

The present study may have resulted in the discovery of a new predictor, metabolic syndrome. This result needs to be validated in other datasets. Finding new predictors or correlations between events using data mining is not unheard of. For example, negative interaction among the drugs pravastatin and paroxetine was found in [13]. We attempted to analyse the data using temporal pattern mining based on Batal et al. [2]. Our results are consistent with that study and that of others (e.g. [12]), namely that temporal attributes can provide additional insights. However, the dataset used was different in that the data of Batal et al. was more tailored towards the target value to be predicted, and it was smaller in size. Thus, our study acts as a validation for the method, suggesting it is both robust and scalable. Finally, we move beyond the models proposed in [8] as we take temporal aspects into account and utilize more state-of-the-art algorithms.

For future work, we are working towards semantic integration of the dataset with medical ontologies (e.g. SNOMED) to improve the models while allowing for more insight. As an example how this could work, a collection of ICPC codes may all be classified as a new abstract attribute, 'infection'. In addition, we aim to include all lab results as opposed to the limited selection we presently used. Finally, we aim to enrich the current dataset with genetic and nutritional data. Ideally, the described work and the above future goals will accumulate into a predictive model implemented in the diagnosis cycle of actual GP practices.

Acknowledgements. This project has been partially funded by VGZ, a Dutch Health Care Insurer, under project number P6500/D3932. We thank the GPs from the Julius network who provided us with the datasets. Furthermore, we want to thank Scamander Solutions for providing the data management support.

References

1. Agrawal, R., Srikant, R. et al.: Fast algorithms for mining association rules. In: Proc. 20th Int. Conf. Very Large Data Bases, VLDB, vol. 1215, pp. 487–499 (1994)
2. Batal, I., Valizadegan, H., Cooper, G.F., Hauskrecht, M.: A temporal pattern mining approach for classifying electronic health record data. ACM Transactions on Intelligent Systems and Technology (TIST) 4(4), 63 (2013)
3. Breiman, L.: Random forests. Machine Learning 45(1), 5–32 (2001)
4. Breiman, L., Friedman, J., Olshen, R., Stone, C., Steinberg, D., Colla, P.: Cart: Classification and regression trees, Wadsworth, Belmont, CA, p. 156 (1983)
5. Ferlay, J., Parkin, D., Steliarova-Foucher, E.: Estimates of cancer incidence and mortality in europe in 2008. European Journal of Cancer 46(4), 765–781 (2010)

6. Hanley, J.A., McNeil, B.J.: The meaning and use of the area under a receiver operating characteristic (roc) curve. Radiology 143(1), 29–36 (1982)
7. Hippisley-Cox, J., Coupland, C.: Identifying patients with suspected colorectal cancer in primary care: derivation and validation of an algorithm. British Journal of General Practice 62(594), e29–e37 (2012)
8. Hoogendoorn, M., Moons, L.M.G., Numans, M.E., Sips, R.-J.: Utilizing data mining for predictive modeling of colorectal cancer using electronic medical records. In: Ślęzak, D., Tan, A.-H., Peters, J.F., Schwabe, L. (eds.) BIH 2014. LNCS, vol. 8609, pp. 132–141. Springer, Heidelberg (2014)
9. Koning, N., Moons, L., Buchner, F., ten Teije, A., Numans, M., Hesper, C.: Identification of patients at risk for colorectal cancer in primary care: An explorative study using routine health care data. In: NACPRG Annual Meeting. NACPRG (2014)
10. Lehman, L.-W., Saeed, M., Long, W., Lee, J., Mark, R.: Risk stratification of icu patients using topic models inferred from unstructured progress notes. In: AMIA Annual Symposium Proceedings, vol. 2012, p. 505. American Medical Informatics Association (2012)
11. Marshall, T., Lancashire, R., Sharp, D., Peters, T.J., Cheng, K.K., Hamilton, W.: The diagnostic performance of scoring systems to identify symptomatic colorectal cancer compared to current referral guidance. Gut 60(9), 1242–1248 (2011)
12. Patnaik, D., Butler, P., Ramakrishnan, N., Parida, L., Keller, B.J., Hanauer, D.A.: Experiences with mining temporal event sequences from electronic medical records: initial successes and some challenges. In: Proceedings of the 17th ACM SIGKDD International Conference on Knowledge Discovery and Data Mining, pp. 360–368. ACM (2011)
13. Tatonetti, N., Denny, J., Murphy, S., Fernald, G., Krishnan, G., Castro, V., Yue, P., Tsau, P., Kohane, I., Roden, D., et al.: Detecting drug interactions from adverse-event reports: Interaction between paroxetine and pravastatin increases blood glucose levels. Age (mean±SD) 63(10.1), 55–61
14. van der Linden, M., Wester, G., de Bakker, D., Schellevis, F.: (dutch) tweede nationale studie naar ziekten en verrichtingen in de huisartspraktijk: klachten en aandoeningen in de bevolking en in de huisartspraktijk. Huisarts en Wetenschap 46 (2004)
15. Vapnik, V., Kotz, S.: Estimation of dependences based on empirical data. Springer (2006)

Identifying Chemotherapy Regimens in Electronic Health Record Data Using Interval-Encoded Sequence Alignment

Haider Syed[1,2](✉) and Amar K. Das[1,3]

[1] Social Computing & Health Informatics Lab, Dartmouth College, Hanover, NH, 03755, USA
[2] Department of Computer Science, Dartmouth College, Hanover, NH, 03755, USA
[3] Department of Biomedical Data Science, Geisel School of Medicine at Dartmouth
Hanover, NH, 03755, USA
{haider.syed@cs.dartmouth.edu,amar.das@dartmouth.edu}

Abstract. Electronic health records (EHRs) play an essential role in patient management and guideline-based care. However, EHRs often do not encode therapy protocols directly, and instead only catalog the individual drug agents patients receive. In this paper, we present an automated approach for protocol identification using EHR data. We introduce a novel sequence alignment method based on the Needleman-Wunsch algorithm that models variation in treatment gaps. Using data on 178 breast cancer patients that included manually annotated chemotherapy protocols, our method successfully matched 93% of regimens based on the top score and had 98% accuracy using the top two scored regimens. These results indicate that our sequence alignment approach can accurately find chemotherapy plans in patient event logs while measuring temporal variation in treatment administration.

Keywords: Clinical guidelines · Plan recognition · Practice variation · Sequence alignment · Electronic health records · Cancer care

1 Introduction

The widespread adoption of electronic health records (EHRs) offers unprecedented opportunities to examine real-world treatment practices and outcomes. Many EHR systems, however, lack the internal ability to capture and monitor treatment plans, and may catalog the drug agents received by patients without encoding regimens directly. There is a need for robust computational methods to identify plan choice, adherence, and outcomes using EHR data, which can support research on quality of care, clinical practice variation and comparative effectiveness.

In this paper, we present a method for identifying cancer chemotherapy plans, which consist of patterns of single and multiple drug agents administered to patients in cyclical patterns known as treatment cycles. Physicians generally follow these chemotherapy protocols since they ensure standardized, evidence-based care with potentially toxic drugs. However, practice variations may result from delayed or dropped cycles.

© Springer International Publishing Switzerland 2015
J.H. Holmes et al. (Eds.): AIME 2015, LNAI 9105, pp. 143–147, 2015.
DOI: 10.1007/978-3-319-19551-3_17

A major open question in cancer care is determining which regimens are used in the current clinical practice and whether regimen variation affects efficacy. To address this challenge, we propose an autonomous treatment regimen identification method using known chemotherapy protocols. The approach models patient treatment histories and recommended treatment regimens as temporal sequences that encode the time interval of elapsed time between sequential events. Patient histories are compared to the treatment regimens using the proposed sequence alignment algorithm, which assigns a similarity score between the patient and protocol sequence. We present our method and evaluate it against a standard sequence alignment approach using institutional EHR data on chemotherapy administration.

2   Related Work

The use of sequence alignment methods to identify treatment regimens is a relatively new field of research. Lee et al. uses a local sequence alignment to detect HIV regimens of two sequential drug combinations [1], and a global alignment method without gaps to match patients to chemotherapy protocols with 68% accuracy [2]. Bourfa and Dankelman [3] use multi-sequence alignment to determine consensus procedural workflows in surgical activity logs, specifically for laparoscopy videos, and compare specific cases against the established consensus. Clinical workflow methods, such as [4, 5], have augmented classical edit distance to deal with temporal constraints.

3   Methods

Patient event logs were extracted, on November 1, 2014, from the EHR of Dartmouth-Hitchcock Medical Center, which was deployed on April 2, 2011. We selected all female patients who had invasive breast cancer diagnosed by the tumor registrar one year prior to November 1, 2014 and who had received NCCN (National Comprehensive Cancer Network, www.nccn.org) recommended chemotherapy agents for breast cancer based on medication administration records. We found 178 patients who met these criteria.

By reviewing the NCCN guidelines for breast cancer from 2011 through 2014, the author AD, who is a physician and has experience encoding protocols, identified 44 unique protocols. He manually matched the treatment sequences for the 178 patients to one of the 44 protocols. 115 patients received clearly identifiable NCCN recommended protocols while the rest received incomplete treatments or combinations of agents not recommended by NCCN guidelines. The patient and regimen data are encoded into event sequences, whereby chemotherapy agents are represented as single letter codes, with transition times between drug events appended to the letter codes as part of the proposed temporal extension for sequence alignment. Drugs given concurrently are cascaded sequentially, followed by the transition time.

Needleman-Wunsch Algorithm

The Needleman-Wunsch algorithm (NW) is a global sequence alignment algorithm (NW) [18]. The method guarantees the optimal alignment for a given scoring schema, which quantifies similarity for all possible event pairings. The alignment can include event gaps, which carry a scoring penalty; the alignment score is the sum of scores for aligned events between the sequences. We use a scoring scheme that assigns exact matching events a score of 1 and mismatching events a score of -1; gaps are penalized 0.5. More complex and continuous scoring schemes can also be used. Multiple drugs administered concomitantly, such as TC, are treated as single events; partial matches of the constituent agents are treated as mismatches; therefore, TC and T receive a score of - 1. This scoring choice signifies that missing agents in drug combinations indicate different treatment recommendations.

NW ignores timing between events and aligns sequences encoded without timing. For the NW method, we encoded treatment sequences that had the same series of treatment events but different intra-event distances as a single type of sequence since NW cannot distinguish between sequences with different intra-event interval lengths.

Interval-Encoded Needleman-Wunsch Algorithm

The Interval-encoded Needleman-Wunsch Algorithm   (IENW) algorithm uses temporally-ordered events and the interval time between events to incorporate timing information into NW without modifying the algorithm itself; instead, temporal information is handled using a novel scoring scheme. We introduce the idea of *temporal concepts* or *temporal events* whereby a drug or drug combination followed by its' associated transition time are defined to be a single temporal event. For example, we encode four bi-weekly cycles of concurrent Docetaxel (T) and Cyclophosphamide (C) as TC.14 TC.14 TC.14 TC.14, which contains a single temporal event, TC.14. Aligning the sequence to a hypothetical patient sequence of TC.21 TC.21 TC.21 TC.21, the algorithm scores TC.14 and TC.21. By contrast, the NW algorithm ignores the timing and scores TC and TC directly. Since all medication administration events in the data set are time stamped with dates, we have chosen to measure the time distance between events at the granularity of days.

The IENW uses the static NW scoring scheme and a user-defined temporal penalty that accounts for temporal variations. For events $A.t_A$ and $B.t_B$ where A and B are drug events and t_A and t_B are their respective transition times, we define the temporal scoring function, S_t:

$$S_t(A.t_A, B.t_B) = \begin{cases} S(A,B) - T_P \dfrac{|t_A - t_B|}{\max(t_A, t_B)} = 1 - T_P \dfrac{|t_A - t_B|}{\max(t_A, t_B)}, \forall A \equiv B \\ S(A,B) \qquad\qquad\qquad = -1.1 \qquad\qquad\quad, \forall A \neq B \end{cases}$$

where S(A, B) is the static similarity score between events A and B used in the traditional NW algorithm, TP is a heuristic representing the maximum temporal penalty that can be imposed on the score for temporal discrepancies, we set Tp to 0.3. In cases where drug events match, a temporal penalty dependent on the percentage difference between the timing of the events in question, is applied. IENW requires the scoring scheme to hold scores for every event-timing combination that can be encountered in sequences; for event X and transition times [0, N], the scoring scheme must hold scores for X.0, X.1

through X.N. For K events, the IENW holds scores for K(N + 1) events while the static-NW scoring scheme holds scores for K events.

4   Experiments and Results

For the 115 patients that were manually matched to recommended protocols, the NW and IENW were used to score the patients against protocols; the scores were normalized by dividing the raw score by the number of events in the protocol sequences. Results against the manual annotations show that the NW and IENW correctly identify a patient's protocol with 93% accuracy using the top-scoring protocol as the prediction, and 98% using the two matches as the prediction. Using Lee's [2] gapless global sequence alignment algorithm has a 54% accuracy.

5   Discussion

Our proposed IENW method identifies the treatments of breast cancer patients based on known protocols with high accuracy. Although the accuracies of the IENW and NW are the same, the standard NW algorithm does not compare sequences using inter-event timings, and thus could not distinguish the correct regimens in 24 cases, which we rated as a tie. By contrast, IENW treats such protocols as distinct regimens and can successfully match patients to the exact protocol. The patient histories misclassified by both NW and IENW did not complete the drug cycles at the end of the regimens, so they were matched to similar, shorter protocols. For patients that were correctly classified by the IENW, the range of scores was 5 to 100, the mean score was 77 and the median score was 89.

The IENW approach has several limitations. It cannot support continuous or an infinite number of transition times. As we derive timing between drugs using encounter dates, we only have discrete times available. Another shortcoming of the IENW is that it always uses the timing appended to an event to compute the temporal penalty; however, when gaps are introduced, the total timing across the gaps should also be used in computing the penalty. Future work will present an algorithm that overcomes this problem.

Identifying treatment plans based on medical events has been an active area of research in artificial intelligence in medicine for the past two decades. Tu et. al. [7] proposed generated therapy advice using a patient's treatment information. Probabilistic-topic modeling [8, 9, 10] and process mining approaches [9, 10] can abstract patterns from events logs and summarize clinical pathways but cannot match clinical pathways to recommended chemotherapy protocols. Bhatia and Levy [11] create a chemotherapy-plan detection method for EHR data that was found to perform poorly on complex patterns. Therapy-plan recognition for data containing intervals has also been studied extensively [12, 13]. Other work has also been done [14, 15]. Our approach is distinct from prior work in using a novel temporal sequence alignment method that measures variation from recommended treatment protocols based on timing and completeness of drug administration.

6   Conclusions

Automated chemotherapy-protocol identification is an important challenge as adherence to clinical guidelines ensures standardized and optimal-care for patients. In the clinical setting, the specific regimen patients receive is not always recorded in their medical record or may be mis-recorded. Abstracting the regimen from the patient's event log manually can be time-consuming and challenging. However, this information is pivotal when deciding what treatments patients actually receive in clinical practice. We have shown that using an interval-encoded sequence alignment as an approach for identifying chemotherapy regimens can provide high accuracy.

References

1. Lee, W.N., Das, A.K.: Local alignment tool for clinical history: temporal semantic search of clinical databases. In: AMIA Annu. Symp. Proc., pp. 437–441 (2010)
2. Lee, W.N.: Evaluating clinical practice variation using a knowledge-based temporal sequence alignment framework. Ph.D. Thesis. Stanford University: U.S.
3. Bouarfa, L., Dankelman, J.: Workflow mining and outlier detection from clinical activity logs. J. Biomed. Inform. 45(6), 1185–1190 (2012)
4. Combi, C., Gozzi, M., Oliboni, B., Juarez, J., Marin, R.: Temporal similarity measures for querying clinical workflows. Artificial Intelligence in Medicine 46, 37–54 (2009)
5. Montani, S., Leonardi, G.: Retrieval and clustering for supporting business process adjustment and analysis. Information Systems 40, 128–141 (2014)
6. Needleman, S.B., Wunsch, C.D.: A general method applicable to the search for similarities in the amino acid sequence of two proteins. Journal of Molecular Biology 48(3), 443–453 (1970)
7. Tu, S.W., Musen, M.A.: Episodic refinement of episodic skeletal-plan refinement. International Journal of Human–Computer Studies 48, 475–497 (1998)
8. Huang, Z., Dong, W., Ji, L., Gan, C., Lu, X., Duan, H.: Discovery of clinical pathway patterns from event logs using probabilistic topic models. J. Biomed. Inform. 47, 39–57 (2014)
9. Huang, Z., Lu, X., Duan, H.: On mining clinical pathway patterns from medical behaviors. Artif. Intell. Med. 56, 35–50 (2012)
10. Van der Aalst, W., Weijters, T., Maruster, L.: Workflow Mining Discovering Process Models from Event Logs. IEEE Trans. Knowl. Data Eng. 16(9), 1128–1142 (2004)
11. Hares, B., Levy, M.: Automated plan-recognition of chemotherapy protocols. In: AMIA Annu. Symp. Proc., pp. 108–114 (2011)
12. Batal, I., Fradkin, D., Harrison, J., Moerchen, F., Hauskrecht, M.: Mining Recent Temporal Patterns for Event Detection in Multivariate Time Series Data. In: Proceedings of Knowledge Discovery and Data Mining (KDD), Beijing, China (2012b)
13. Sacchi, L., Larizza, C., Combi, C., Bellazi, R.: Data mining with temporal abstractions: learning rules from time series. Data Mining and Knowledge Discovery (15) (2007)
14. Combi, C., Franceschet, M., Peron, A.: Representing and Reasoning about Temporal Granularities. Journal of Logic and Computation 14(1), 51–77 (2004)
15. Juárez, J.M., Guil, F., Palma, J.T., Marín, R.: Temporal similarity by measuring possibilistic uncertainty in CBR. Fuzzy Sets and Systems 160(2), 214–230 (2009)

An Evaluation Framework for the Comparison of Fine-Grained Predictive Models in Health Care

Ward R.J. van Breda[1]([✉]), Mark Hoogendoorn[1], A.E. Eiben[1],
and Matthias Berking[2]

[1] VU University Amsterdam, Department of Computer Science De Boelelaan 1081,
1081 HV Amsterdam, The Netherlands,
{w.r.j.van.breda,m.hoogendoorn,a.e.eiben}@vu.nl
[2] Friedrich-Alexander University Erlangen-Nuremberg, Germany
matthias.berking@fau.de

Abstract. Within the domain of health care, more and more fine-grained models are observed that predict the development of specific health (or disease-related) states over time. This is due to the increased use of sensors, allowing for continuous assessment, leading to a sharp increase of data. These specific models are often much more complex than high-level predictive models that e.g. give a general risk score for a disease, making the evaluation of these models far from trivial. In this paper, we present an evaluation framework which is able to score fine-grained temporal models that aim at predicting multiple health states, considering their capability to describe data, their capability to predict, the quality of the models parameters, and the model complexity.

1 Introduction

Predictive modeling is of utmost importance in health care and has potential to be the basis for prevention strategies, especially, early and highly personalized interventions. Predictive models can vary greatly in their level of granularity, ranging from relatively coarse-grained models, that e.g. provide a general risk disease score, to highly fine-grained ones that predict detailed developments of disease and/or disease-relevant states over time. The latter is received more and more attention due to the improvements in measurement capabilities.

The evaluation of fine-grained models is unfortunately far from trivial as they often are of a temporal nature, predict multiple states, have parameters with which the model can be personalized, et cetera. In order to make informed decisions during model development, or when comparing models, there is a need to understand how model quality can be evaluated in a rigorous way.

In this paper, we present an evaluation framework for fine-grained predictive models. The framework considers the following aspects: (1) the descriptive capability; (2) predictive capability; (3) parameter sensitivity, and (4) model complexity. The weight of each of these criteria can be set according to the characteristics of the specific disease or health aspects under consideration.

J.H. Holmes et al. (Eds.): AIME 2015, LNAI 9105, pp. 148–152, 2015.
DOI: 10.1007/978-3-319-19551-3_18

2   Evaluation Framework

Scope of Framework. The framework we describe is meant for domains with temporal data over a number of attributes $a_1, \ldots, a_m$ for a number of patients $b_1, \ldots, b_n$. Attributes represent an aspect of the health state of a patient, and we denote the domain of a_i by A_i. At any give time t, the state of a patient b is a vector $s(b, t) \in A_1 \times \ldots \times A_m$. To designate the specific value of an attribute we use the notation $s(b, t, i) \in A_i$.

We assume a dataset that contains a state for each patient for a number of time instances $t_1, \ldots, t_{end}$. These measured data are contained in the matrix Z, where at any give time t_j ($j = 1, \ldots, end$) the observed state of patient b is a vector $z(b, t_j) \in A_1 \times \ldots \times A_m$.

Furthermore, we consider models composed from rules for state transition and assume one rule for each of the given attributes that describes the value of $a_i(t + 1)$ based on $a_i(t)$ and possibly some other attributes. Formally, we have $r_i : A_1 \times \ldots \times A_m \to A_i$. Obviously, a transition rule for attribute i may not need all other attributes, only a few of them; in the extreme case only a_i itself.

A model M is then a composed entity that can predict the consecutive states of any give patient. Thus, $M : A_1 \times \ldots \times A_m \to A_1 \times \ldots \times A_m$ and given a state $s(b, t)$ of patient b at time t we can denote the predicted state at time $t + 1$ by $M(s(b, t))$. Each model is equipped with parameters, a model instance is a model for which a value has been assigned to each parameter denoted as M_p where $p \in P$ and P is the set of possible parameter value vectors. To employ a model M for predicting a full sequence of states for a patient b it needs to be applied to the first observed state $z(b, t_1)$ and then iteratively to the outcomes. To avoid an unnecessarily heavy notation, we define these predicted states interactively as follows. Given a patient b and a model instance M_p, the predicted state at the start is the observed state

$$s_{M_p}(b, 1) = z(b, 1)$$

and for all $t = 1, \ldots, \ end - 1$

$$s_{M_p}(b, t + 1) = M_p(s_{M_p}(b, t))$$

The goal of the model instance is to minimize the difference between the predicted and observed states. The error of a model M for a patient b over the full observation period is then

$$e(b, M_p) = \sum_{t=t_1}^{t_{end}} (D(z(b, t), s_{M_p}(b, t))$$

where D is some application specific measure of difference between two states.

Furthermore, we define $e(b, M_p, i)$ defines the error the model makes on an attribute i. Throughout this paper, the Mean Squared Error (MSE) is assumed to be the error measure.

Descriptive Capability. To express the quality of a model M for a given patient b we consider the error $e(b, M, a_i)$ on each attribute a_i. This implies a multi-objective optimization (MOO) problem, where each objective corresponds to one attribute. In the sequel we assume that we have and use a multi-objective optimization algorithm that searches in the space of model instances M_p based on a training set. For examples of MOO algorithms, see [2], [3]. Given a patient b, the output of one run of the algorithm is a set of non dominated model instances, where dominance is defined in the usual manner: M_p dominates $M_{p'}$, if for each attribute a_i the error $e(b, M_p, i)$ is lower or equal than $e(b, M_{p'}, i)$ and there is at least one attribute a_j where the error $e(b, M_p, j)$ is lower than $e(b, M_{p'}, j)$. Because each model instance corresponds to one point in the space of model parameter vectors, the set non-dominated model instances forms a Pareto front in this vector space.[1]

Due to the typical stochastic nature of the algorithms to find such assignments it is assumed that multiple runs of the algorithm are performed per patient. Each run r delivers a Pareto front of q non-dominated model instances $\{M_{p_{1,r}}, ..., M_{p_{q,r}}\}$ and each model instance $M_{p_{i,r}}$ has a corresponding m-dimensional error vector $\langle e(b, M_{p_{i,r}}, 1), ..., e(b, M_{p_{i,r}}, m)\rangle$, where m is the number of attributes. Each of these q vectors can be plotted using an attainment surface [1]. Given such an attainment surface its dominated hypervolume can be calculated, which is the volume above each attainment surface, related to an error reference point, set to 1 for each objective, based on the assumption that all error values are scaled to an interval of [0,1]. For more details, see [1].

We use the notation $nh_M(b, r)$ to denote the dominated hypervolume for run r of the MOO algorithm to optimize model M for patient b. Executing r_{max} runs of the MOO algorithm, we obtain r_{max} attainment surfaces and r_{max} values of $nh_M(b, r)$. Taken all runs into account we now can define model quality by averaging the values of the non-dominated hypervolumes:

$$nh_M(b) = \sum_{r=1}^{r_{max}} \frac{nh_M(b,r)}{r_{max}}$$

Each patient has its own unique value, and we therefore end up with a vector of n values: $\langle nh_M(b_1), ..., nh_M(b_n)\rangle$. The final score of the criterion is then defined as multiplication of the mean μ_{nh_M} with 1 minus the standard deviation σ_{nh_M} of the values in this vector since a high mean is good in combination with a small standard deviation:

$$descriptive\_score_M = \mu_{nh_M}(1 - \sigma_{nh_M})$$

Predictive Capability. Next to a good descriptive capability, we also want the model to perform well on the test set, i.e. have a good predictive capability. Hereto, we define two measurements: (1) we define the absolute predictive performance on the test set, and (2) we quantify the relationship between how well the model performs on the training and test set, we would prefer these to go hand-in-hand and call this the relative predictive performance. Concerning absolute predictive performance, for a model M we calculate the mean $\mu_{e_M(j)}$ and the standard deviation $\sigma_{e_M(j)}$ over the set of errors belonging to attribute j for the q model instances per run and r_{max} runs, for all patients (i.e. 1 to n), resulting in a set size of $q \cdot r_{max} \cdot n$ errors. We then take the average of the mean

---

[1] The dimensionality of this vector space depends on the number of model parameters.

and standard deviation over all m attributes: μ_{e_M} and σ_{e_M}. Then, the absolute predictive performance score becomes:

$$absolute\_pred\_score_M = (1 - \mu_{e_M})(1 - \sigma_{e_M})$$

To measure the relation between the errors on training and test set, for the q model instances per run and r_{max} runs we end up with a total of $q \cdot r_{max}$ model instances with specific parameter vectors per patient b. For each attribute j we determine the correlation between the error of each of the $q \cdot r_{max}$ model instances on the training and the test set for each individual patient (whereby the training set is the first period of data and the test set the second, later, period): $e_{train}(b, M_{p_{i,r}}, j)$ and $e_{test}(b, M_{p_{1,r}}, j)$. Hereto, we use the correlation (note $training$ and $test$ to tr and te respectively) for a specific model M:

$$cor_M(b,j) = \frac{\sum\limits_{i=1}^{q}\sum\limits_{r=1}^{r_{max}}\left(e_{tr}(b,M_{p_{i,r}},j) - \overline{e_{tr}(b,M_{p_i},j)}\right)\left(e_{te}(b,M_{p_{i,r}},j) - \overline{e_{te}(b,M_{p_i},j)}\right)}{\sqrt{\sum\limits_{i=1}^{q}\sum\limits_{r=1}^{r_{max}}\left(e_{tr}(b,M_{p_{i,r}},j) - \overline{e_{tr}(b,M_{p_i},j)}\right)^2}\sqrt{\sum\limits_{i=1}^{q}\sum\limits_{r=1}^{r_{max}}\left(e_{te}(b,M_{p_{i,r}},j) - \overline{e_{te}(b,M_{p_i},j)}\right)^2}}$$

Then, we calculate the average μ_{cor_M} across the set of all correlations of all patients (i.e. 1 to n) and criteria (i.e. 1 to m): $\langle cor_M(b_1, a_1), ..., cor_M(b_n, a_1), ..., cor_M(b_n, a_m)\rangle$ as well as the standard deviation $(\sigma_{cor_M})^2$:

$$relative\_pred\_score_M = max(\mu_{cor_M}, 0)(1 - \sigma_{cor_M})$$

Given weights w_1 and w_2 a final evaluation score for model M is calculated:

$$predictive\_score_M = w_1 \cdot absolute\_pred\_score_M + w_2 \cdot relative\_pred\_score_M$$

Parameter Sensitivity. The parameter sensitivity is the most complex metric. In the current version we keep it as simple as possible. We want to avoid meaningless parameters, that do not have any influence on the performance of the model. Therefore we look at the relationship between parameters and the various evaluation objectives. Assuming we define $p_{i,r,b}(u)$ as the value for parameter u for model instance i from during run r of patient b, we define correlation between a parameter and the resulting error on an attribute j for model M as follows:

$$cor_M(b,j,k) = \frac{\sum\limits_{i=1}^{q}\sum\limits_{r=1}^{r_{max}}\left(e_{tr}(b,M_{p_{i,r,b}},j) - \overline{e_{tr}(b,M_p,j)}\right)\left(p_{i,r,b}(k)) - \overline{p_b(k)}\right)}{\sqrt{\sum\limits_{i=1}^{q}\sum\limits_{r=1}^{r_{max}}\left(e_{tr}(b,M_{p_{i,r,b}},j) - \overline{e_{tr}(b,M_p,j)}\right)^2}\sqrt{\sum\limits_{i=1}^{q}\sum\limits_{r=1}^{r_{max}}\left(p_{i,r,b}(k)) - \overline{p_b(k)}\right)^2}}$$

If a parameter always has a correlation close to zero (for different evaluation criteria and patients) this is considered bad. Thus, we look for the maximum of the absolute value of the correlation found in the set of all patients and criteria, which gives an indication whether a parameter has a use (i.e correlation) in at least one patient/model instance combination. We define a correlation as useless (or weak) if it falls under a boundary of 0.35 [4].

$$useful_{M,p(k)} = \begin{cases} 1 & max_{b\in[1,n], j\in[1,m]}(|cor_M(b,j,k)|) \geq 0.35 \\ 0 & otherwise \end{cases}$$

---

[2] Note that with respect to the mean a cutoff point of 0 is used (via the max operator) as we consider all correlations below 0 equally bad.

Finally, we calculate the fraction of useless parameters in a model as its score for the parameter sensitivity (where $|P|$ is the number of elements in the parameter vector and is the highest parameter number of the model):

$$sensitivity\_score_M = \frac{\sum_{k=1}^{|P|} \left(useful_{M,p(k)}\right)}{|P|}$$

Model Complexity. The model complexity counts the number of states and parameters:

$$complexity\_score_M = 1 - \frac{(|A_M|+|P_M|)}{max_{mo \in Models}(|A_{mo}|+|P_{mo}|)}$$

The score is scaled according to the maximum complexity of the models that are subject to evaluation.

3   Discussion

This paper has introduced a framework which is able to evaluate fine-grained temporal predictive models for health care. Hereto, several criteria have been introduced which can be combined by taking a weighted sum of the different scores, thereby selecting weights depending on the importance of the criterion for the case at hand. Initial experiments suggest that the framework is able to generate important insights in the properties of the models.

For future work we want to test and refine the framework by further investigating the usefulness and performance of the different criteria and related metrics. Furthermore, we want to use the framework as a fitness function for automatically generating predictive dynamic models using genetic programming techniques.

Acknowledgements. This research has been performed in the context of the EU FP7 project E-COMPARED (project number 603098).

References

1. Deb, K.: Multi-objective optimization using evolutionary algorithms, vol. 16. John Wiley & Sons (2001)
2. Deb, K., Pratap, A., Agarwal, S., Meyarivan, T.: A fast and elitist multiobjective genetic algorithm: Nsga-ii. IEEE Transactions on Evolutionary Computation 6(2), 182–197 (2002)
3. Mlakar, M., Petelin, D., Tušar, T., Filipič, B.: Gp-demo: Differential evolution for multiobjective optimization based on gaussian process models. European Journal of Operational Research (2014)
4. Taylor, R.: Interpretation of the correlation coefficient: a basic review. Journal of Diagnostic Medical Sonography 6(1), 35–39 (1990)

A Model for Cross-Platform Searches in Temporal Microarray Data

Guenter Tusch$^{(\boxtimes)}$, Olvi Tole , and Mary Ellen Hoinski

Grand Valley State University, Allendale, MI, USA
tuschg@gvsu.edu,{toleo,hoinskim}@mail.gvsu.edu

Abstract. Even with the advance of next-generation sequencing, microarray technology still has its place in molecular biology. There is a large body of information available through a growing number of studies in public repositories like NCBI GEO and ArrayExpress. Software is now developed to allow for cross-platform comparison. An important part of temporal translational research is based on stimulus response studies and includes searching for particular time pattern like peaks in a set of given genes across studies and platforms. This study explores the feasibility based on a statistical model and temporal abstraction using our SPOT software.

Keywords: Temporal and spatial representation and reasoning · Translational research · Statistical · Logic-based · Decision support · Microarrays

1   Introduction

Today RNA-seq technology is readily available, but DNA microarrays still have its importance in assessing gene expression in molecular biology, esp. for diagnostic and prognostic purposes (genotyping). In many aspects microarray analysis can compete in terms of result with RNA-seq at a significantly lower cost. Researchers studying different model-systems or organisms have compared the two technologies (microarrays and RNA-Seq) and reached the conclusion that when the objective is to evaluate the differential expression the results offered by both types of methods are comparable (see, e.g., [1]). Currently, microarray studies are still by far the majority of data accessible online, for instance, the US National Center for Biotechnology Information Gene Expression Omnibus (NCBI GEO) has data of more than 1.2 Mio samples, ArrayExpress from the European Molecular Biology Laboratory has more than 1.5 Mio assays. Therefore, we will focus on that technology. A growing number of those are stimulus response studies based on time series data. Peaks in gene profiles (identified, e.g., by a significant change from one time point to the next) in temporal microarray studies can represent a biological effect that is reversed over time. In temporal translational research a researcher typically obtains a fold change profile and tries to retrieve similar profiles in a set of genes or gene products in microarray databases or clinical databases (that more frequently include microarray data, whole-genome sequencing, or other next-generation sequencing data).

© Springer International Publishing Switzerland 2015
J.H. Holmes et al. (Eds.): AIME 2015, LNAI 9105, pp. 153–158, 2015.
DOI: 10.1007/978-3-319-19551-3_19

Standard query languages like SQL are not well suited for this kind of queries because they do not support a sufficient time model. A very flexible approach is Knowledge-based Temporal Abstraction, which has been implemented in a number of proprietary systems [2]. We use for temporal modeling knowledge-based temporal abstraction that allows for the conversion of quantitative data to an interval-based qualitative representation that can utilize Allen's approach of temporal relationships [3]. We developed SPOT [4] to make KBTA more readily available for translational research.

2   Challenges Comparing Temporal Microarray Studies

Assume a researcher conducted a temporal study where she discovered peaks in a set of genes might be found in the same pathway. She now wants to see if finding the same effect in related studies can extend her hypothesis. Although different studies address similar questions a comparative search through the database is impeded by the use of heterogeneous microarray platforms and analysis methods. Researchers who perform high throughput gene expression assays often deposit their data in public databases, although the heterogeneity of platforms leads to challenges for the combination and search of these data sets. However, the quality and comparability of data from different studies has improved over time and will continue to improve. Older publications have suggested that some of the variability in cross-platform studies was due to annotation problems that made it difficult to reconcile which genes were measured by specific probes (see, e.g., [5]).

These issues have been resolved recently (e.g., [6]), but only for future applications. Some issues can be overcome by carefully selecting high quality datasets, as has been done for select problems on the INMEX website (http://www.inmex.ca). A challenge here is cross platform normalization where nine different methods are currently available, and no rigorous comparison exists. Furthermore, software for the selected method must be obtained and incorporated into each data analysis workflow. Several packages and tools are currently available, for instance the virtualArray software package in Bioconductor (http://www.bioconductor.org/) can combine raw data sets using almost any chip types based on current annotations from NCBI GEO. No such tool is currently available for temporal studies. We chose a different approach based on the inherent information of time oriented data sets.

3   Methodology

An overview over the current SPOT architecture is depicted in figure **Error! Reference source not found.**. The researcher (user) can define biological patterns, e.g., peaks, and then search for studies or experiments with that concept in the microarray research subset database.

To represent those patterns, we use knowledge-based temporal abstraction, i.e. transforming the time-stamped data points into an interval-based representation. Each interval represents a specific trend (gradient abstraction), e.g., "increasing", "decreasing", or "stable", defined by statistical significance. A "peak" can be defined as an increasing interval immediately followed by a decreasing one. Thus peaks can be found even if not all experiments use the same time points. If as in our example a researcher tries to extend the finding in a local dataset by searching for similar public datasets "similarity" would mean that a peak could be found in a specified time interval, i.e., first 24 hours. The entire interval data file can be loaded into Protégé, and in the SWRL Tab more complex temporal patterns can be created using Allen's time logic and executed.

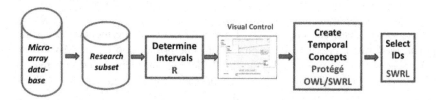

Fig. 1. The SPOT design

Here are the steps to determine a trend for an interval:
1. We select the normalized dataset according to the normalization chosen by the experimenter.
2. All gene expression data are averaged for each time point and gene.
3. Each time point average is standardized by dividing by the baseline mean (average at time point 0) – only for experiments with baseline. This is for graphical representation purposes.
4. As a first approach, we assume that biological significance is measured by statistical significance. This is typically not always the case and poses a problem, but most researchers take the same approach. In particular, if the expression values for one gene at two consecutive time points show a significant difference then the interval is considered "increasing" or "decreasing" depending on the difference of means, otherwise constant.

The significance does not change if the expression values are not divided by the baseline mean, but if so, the starting value is always 1, which aligns and adjusts the curves for easy graphical comparison and assessment by the researcher.

One key advantage of using temporal abstractions is that the transformation from the expression values at the time points of the experiment into the interval space makes it independent of the particular time points that the experimenter chose for his/her study. For example, if one experiment has time points at 2, 4, 6, and 12 hours with a peak at time 4 and another at 3, 6, 9, and 24 hours with peak at 6, a peak in between time 4 or 6 still will be found in both experiments because the categorization into a limited number of trends makes the data independent of a particular set of time points. This becomes more apparent if more complex time patterns are used. Based on our above stated assumptions the levels "increasing" or "decreasing" immediately translate into the presence of a biological signal is present. We now can compare across different microarray platforms, i.e., chips from the same or different manufacturer using the same or different technology, if they have the same genes assuming that the same biological signal is expressed on each microarray independent of the used technology. This should be the case because it only depends on statistical significance not actual values. The here-described approach should not be confused by meta-analysis of non-temporal data (see for instance [6]).

A major challenge in this model is that the p-value depends on the actual sample size of the study. For instance, if there are more samples (chips) in study A than in study B and both studies have the same expression patterns, then you'll find more likely significant p-values in study A than in B simply because of the sample size. A standard way to deal with challenges of this kind is to use the moderated t-statistics [7]. The moderated t-statistic for a particular gene is the ratio of the M-value to its standard error. (The M-value is the log2-fold change, or sometimes the log2-expression level for that gene.) This has the same interpretation as an ordinary t-statistic only standard errors being moderated across genes, borrowing information from the ensemble of genes to aiding with inference about each individual gene.

Another major challenge for similar time course gene expression studies across different platforms is probe mapping. Here the MicroArray Quality Consortium (FDA supported) evaluated the concordance of measurements across seven platforms [8]. The dataset collected has been validated by alternative quantitative gene expression platforms for humans. One finding is that data from different platforms can be compared under certain precautions by mapping probes to the RefSeq or AceView databases. The third phase of the MAQC project (MAQC-III), also called Sequencing Quality Control (SEQC), aims at assessing the technical performance of next-generation sequencing platforms.

4   Implementation and Application to Microarray Data

SPOT supports statistical packages (R/S-Plus®) and knowledge representation standards using the open source Semantic Web tool Protégé-OWL [9]. The implementation uses open source and standardized tools: the Web Ontology Language (OWL; http://www.w3.org/TR/owl-features), the Semantic Web Rule Language (SWRL; http://www.daml.org/2003/11/swrl), Protégé plug-ins; http://protege.stanford.edu/, and open source statistical software (R; http://www.r-project.org/). Ontologies are used in OWL to formally specify meaning of annotations by providing a vocabulary of patterns. Combining existing ones the researcher can form new patterns. SWRL allows users to write rules that can be expressed in terms of OWL concepts and that can reason about OWL individuals. In the microarray application, we use a temporal ontology implementing the valid time model.

R is an interactive environment for data analysis. The Protégé OWL plug-in allows to easily building ontologies that are backed by OWL code. A Java program interfaces R and Protégé. All statistical and GEO access functionality is implemented in R and Bioconductor using the Bioconductor package GEOmetadb to access GEO.

The platform SPOT connects the user through a web interface hosted on a Fedora Linux account and utilizing R and a MySQL database. The web application supports multiple user accounts using PHP, database technology and JavaScript. The user can interrupt the search process any time, to later return to the position where she left off. We evaluated our approach on a set of 644 temporal GDS with 171 different platforms from NCBI GEO. Preliminary results indicate that if you choose gene ensembles large enough the approach has significant potential.

5   Discussion and Future Aspects

The reported research shows that SPOT is a feasible approach to use open source and standards based software. Currently, concept intervals are passed from OWL/SWRL through a Java interface. The next step is of connection using the Protégé APIs for easy access to an online rule editor (see e.g. [10]).

The here-described methodology can directly be applied to temporal RNA-seq data as well because it uses only the statistical features of the biological signal. RNA-seq data can be found recently and more and more extensively in public repositories, e.g., NCBI GEO. It is exploratory in nature and not intended for modelling (see e.g. [11]).

Acknowledgments. We would like to thank the following individuals without whose support this study would not have been possible:
Dr. Amar Das (Dartmouth), Martin O'Connor, Tania Tudorache,
Dr. Mark Musen (Stanford U),
Dr. Mary Winn (VAI), Vincent K. Sam, Lakshmi Mammidi, Yuka Kutsumi (GVSU)

References

1. Rudy, J., Valafar, F.: Empirical comparison of cross-platform normalization methods for gene expression data. Bmc Bioinformatics 12(1), 467 (2011)
2. Shahar, Y., Musen, M.A.: Knowledge-based temporal abstraction in clinical domains. Artif. Intell. Med. 8(3), 267–298 (1996)
3. Allen, J.F.: Towards a general theory of action and time. Artif. Intell. 23(2), 123–154 (1984)
4. Tusch, G., Bretl, C., O'Connor, M., Das, A.: SPOT – towards temporal data mining in medicine and bioinformatics. In: AMIA Annu. Symp. Proc., p. 1157 (2008)
5. Morris, J.S., Wu, C., Coombes, K.R., Baggerly, K.A., Wang, J., Zhang, L.: Alternative probeset definitions for combining microarray data across studies using different versions of affymetrix oligonucleotide arrays. In: Meta-Analysis in Genetics, pp. 1–214. Chapman-Hall, New York (2006)
6. Ramasamy, A., Mondry, A., Holmes, C.C., Altman, D.G.: Key Issues in Conducting a Meta-Analysis of Gene Expression Microarray Datasets. PLoS Med. 5(9), e184 (2008)
7. Smyth, G.: Linear models and empirical Bayes methods for assessing differential expression in microarray experiments. Statistical Applications in Genetics and Molecular Biology 3, Article 3 (2004)

8. MAQC Consortium: The MicroArray Quality Control (MAQC) project shows inter- and intraplatform reproducibility of gene expression measurements Nat. Biotechnol. 24(9), 1151–1161 (2006)
9. O'Connor, M.J., Shankar, R.D., Parrish, D.B., Das, A.K.: Knowledge-Data Integration for Temporal Reasoning in a Clinical Trial System. Int. J. Med. Inform. 78(1), S77-S85 (2009)
10. Orlando, J.P., Rivolli, A., Hassanpour, S., O'Connor, M.J., Das, A.K., Moreira, D.A.: SWRL Rule Editor - A Web Application as Rich as Desktop Business Rule Editors. In: ICEIS (2) pp. 258–263 (2012)
11. Sacchi, L., Larizza, C., Magni, P., Bellazzi, R.: Precedence Temporal Networks to represent temporal relationships in gene expression data. Journal of Biomedical Informatics 40(6), 761–774 (2007)

Uncertainty and Bayesian Networks

Risk Assessment for Primary Coronary Heart Disease Event Using Dynamic Bayesian Networks

Kalia Orphanou[1(✉)], Athena Stassopoulou[2], and Elpida Keravnou[3]

[1] Department of Computer Science, University of Cyprus, Nicosia, Cyprus
korfan01@cs.ucy.ac.cy
[2] Department of Computer Science, University of Nicosia, Nicosia, Cyprus
stassopoulou.a@unic.ac.cy
[3] Department of Electrical and Computer Engineering and Computer Science, Cyprus University of Technology, Limassol, Cyprus
Rector@cut.ac.cy

Abstract. Coronary heart disease (CHD) is the leading cause of mortality worldwide. Primary prevention of CHD denotes limiting a first CHD event in individuals who have not been formally diagnosed with the disease. This paper demonstrates how the integration of a Dynamic Bayesian network (DBN) and temporal abstractions (TAs) can be used for assessing the risk of a primary CHD event. More specifically, we introduce basic TAs into the DBN nodes and apply the extended model to a longitudinal CHD dataset for risk assesment. The obtained results demonstrate the effectiveness of our proposed approach.

Keywords: Temporal abstraction · Temporal reasoning · Dynamic bayesian networks · Risk assessment · Primary coronary heart disease

1 Introduction

Coronary heart disease (CHD) is the most common cause of death in many countries. CHD is generally caused by atherosclerosis and often develops over years. The principle goal of this paper is to estimate the risk of CHD in middle-aged men, without an established CHD.

A number of models have been introduced in the literature for CHD risk assessment [8, 4]. However, the novelty of our proposed approach is the usage of patients' medical history in order to assess the risk of a potential CHD event. Our methodology employs the development of an extended Dynamic Bayesian network which is the integration of a regular DBN with basic temporal abstractions. Temporal abstraction (TA) is a heuristic process which interprets time point data into interval-based concepts based on background knowledge. The derived high-level abstract concepts have been shown to be helpful in various clinical tasks and domains such as summarizing and managing patient data. Dynamic Bayesian networks (DBNs) [6] are temporal extensions of Bayesian networks, which are graphical models representing explicitly probabilistic relationships among variables. DBNs have been applied in many clinical domains for various tasks such as prognosis and diagnosis. A detailed survey on TA and DBN applied to medicine and the benefits of their potential integration can be found in our recent work in [7].

© Springer International Publishing Switzerland 2015
J.H. Holmes et al. (Eds.): AIME 2015, LNAI 9105, pp. 161–165, 2015.
DOI: 10.1007/978-3-319-19551-3_20

The paper is organized as follows: In Sect. 2, we describe the methods used for the development and deployment of an extension of a DBN model and our evaluation dataset. In Sect. 3, we give an extensive discussion of the undertaken experiments and their results. Finally, conclusions and future work are presented in Sect. 4.

2 DBN Model Overview

The benchmark dataset used for this study is the longitudinal STULONG dataset [1] which includes middle-age men who were monitored for about 24 years. By selecting a temporal range of 21 years, patients whose total observation period is less than 21 years are neglected from this study. The target group is further reduced by removing records of patients who had a history of CHD event, since in this study we are going to focus on the primary prevention of coronary heart disease. The key features which are the risk factors of CHD are selected based on expert domain knowledge. The incorporation of the key features in the network are described in the next two subsections.

2.1 Basic Temporal Abstractions

Temporal abstraction (TA) techniques are divided into two categories: basic and complex TAs. In this study we are concerned with basic TA techniques such as: state, trend and persistene. The chosen time interval period for the derived abstractions is three years. This period is selected since at least two examinations are needed in order to have any abstractions. It is noted that the finer granularity of the dataset is one year, however, most cases do not have examinations on an annual basis.

The state abstractions determine the state (value) of a parameter over a time period based on categories predefined by clinical experts. All state TAs are displayed in Table 1. Trend abstractions of a feature are generated by observing the changes between their

Table 1. State TAs variables and their values. Variable code is the variable name in the DBN model

Variable	Variable Code	Value = 1	Value = 2	Value = 3
Smoking	Smoking	Non Smoker	Current Smoker	
Hypertension Medicines	medBP	Taken	Not taken	
Dyslipidemia Medicines	medCH	Taken	Not taken	
Hypertension	HT	No Hypertension	Well Controlled	Poorly Controlled
Dyslipidemia	Dyslipidemia	Absent	Present	
Obesity	Obesity	Absent	Present	
Age	AGE	Normal	High	Very High
Diet	DIET	Following a Diet	Not Following a Diet	
Exercise	Exercise	Exercising	Not Exercising	

values during an interval period. In our approach, we used a combination of trends

---

[1] The data resource is on: http://euromise.vse.cz/challenge2004/ [Date accessed: 26 March 2015]

and state abstractions such as: i) 'Abnormal' (A) when the variable state is abnormal and increasing over time or remaining steady, ii) 'AbnormalDecreasing' (AD) when the variable state is abnormal and decreasing, iii) 'NormalIncreasing' (NI) when the variable state is normal and increasing and iv) 'Normal' (N) when the variable state is normal and decreasing or remaining steady. It should be noted that, contrary to the rest of the variables, HDL is considered as a CHD risk factor when its levels are low, thus its trend values are: 'Abnormal' (A), 'AbnormalIncreasing' (AI), 'NormalDecreasing' (ND) and 'Normal' (N). The resulting trend abstractions are displayed in Table 2.

Table 2. Trend TAs variables and their values. Variable code is the variable name in the DBN model

Variable Name	Variable Code	Value = 1	Value = 2	Value = 3	Value =4
Low-density lipoprotein cholesterol	LDL	A	AD	NI	N
Triglycerides	TRIG	A	AD	NI	N
High-density lipoprotein cholesterol	HDL	A	AI	ND	N
Total Cholesterol	TCH	A	AD	NI	N

Persistence TA techniques derive maximal intervals showing the temporal persistence of the state of a parameter. The resulting persistence TAs are displayed in Table 3.

Table 3. Persistence TAs variables and their values. Variable code is the variable name in the DBN model

Variable Name	Variable Code	Value = 1	Value = 2
Diabetes	Diabetes	Present	Absent
Family History	FH	Present	Absent
History of Hypertension	HHT	Present	Absent

2.2 Constructing the Dynamic Bayesian Network

The most popular temporal extension of a Bayesian network is the Dynamic Bayesian network (DBN) which represents the change of variable states at different time points. A node in a DBN represents a temporal process and its possible states. Arcs represent the local or transitional dependencies among variables. The construction of the extended DBN consists of building the network structure and learning the parameters of the network.

The network structure, as displayed in Fig. 1, is designed by incorporating prior information elicited from medical experts. The derived basic temporal abstractions described in Sect. 2.1 form the nodes of our DBN. The model consists of 17 variables, out of which 15 are observed and two are hidden.[2] Hidden variables are: the class attribute Pred_Event, representing the risk of a primary CHD at $t = 6$, and the Dyslipidemia

---

[2] The model presented in this paper was created and tested using the SMILE inference engine and GeNIe available at: https://dslpitt.org/genie/ [Date accessed: 26 March 2015]

node. The Pred_Event variable is represented outside of the temporal network and it is only connected to its parents in the last time-slice of the unrolled network [2].

The first time slice ($t = 0$) in the network represents the time period starting from the patients' entry examination and ending three years after the entry examination. All of the network parameters are learned from data using the expectation-maximization (EM) algorithm [5]. For performing risk assessment, the DBN is unrolled for seven time slices $t = [0, ..., 6]$ in order to represent the observation period of 21 years. It then derives the belief in the class variable Pred_Event given the evidence at the last time slice ($t = 5$).

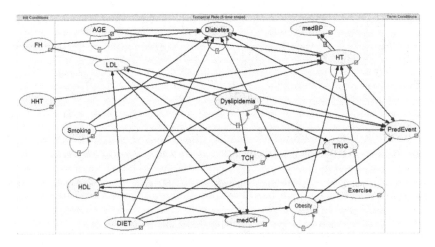

Fig. 1. The structure of the extended DBN model representing the basic temporal abstractions. An arc labeled as 1 between the variables denotes an influence that takes one time step.

3   Experimental Results and Analysis

In this section, we present the experiments performed in order to apply our methodology and evaluate the performance of our extended DBN model for predicting the risk of a primary event. For the evaluation of the performance of our model, we split the dataset into two-third training (70%) and one-third testing (30%) datasets.

One important problem in the data mining field is how to deal with imbalanced datasets [1]. The imbalance problem is usually addressed using resampling methods such as random oversampling and undersampling. In the current dataset, individuals who did not suffer a primary CHD event during the last three years of their monitoring period are many more than those who suffered with a CHD event. In our training dataset, we apply the clustering oversampling technique [1] to overcome the imbalanced probem.

We have used various metrics commonly applied to imbalanced datasets to evaluate the performance of our model, namely: Specificity, Sensitivity (Recall), Precision and

F_1 score. Table 4 shows the obtained results after applying clustering oversampling and normalizing [3]. Results prove the good prognostic performance of our model.

Table 4. The evaluation results for our model

Evaluation Metrics	Clustering Oversampling Dataset
Specificity	0.73
Sensitivity (Recall)	0.75
Precision	0.74
F_1 score	0.74

4   Conclusions and Future Work

In this paper, we applied our proposed integration of temporal abstractions with Dynamic Bayesian networks for primary CHD risk assessment using a longitudinal dataset. Our system has successfully handled class imbalance in the training and evaluation stages. The high performance accuracy of our model proves the effectiveness of our proposed methodology in estimating the risk of primary CHD. Our results provide a promising direction for future work. We are currently investigating the introduction of complex temporal abstractions to the extended DBN model in order to achieve greater functionality.

References

[1] He, H., Garcia, E.A.: Learning from imbalanced data. IEEE Transactions on Knowledge and Data Engineering 21(9), 1263–1284 (2009)

[2] Hulst, J.: Modeling physiological processes with Dynamic Bayesian networks. Master's thesis, Man-machine interaction group Delft University of Technology, Delft, Netherlands (2006)

[3] Jeni, L.A., Cohn, J.F., De La Torre, F.: Facing imbalanced data–recommendations for the use of performance metrics. In: Humaine Association Conference on Affective Computing and Intelligent Interaction (ACII). pp. 245–251. IEEE Computer Society (2013)

[4] Kurt, I., Ture, M., Kurum, A.T.: Comparing performances of logistic regression, classification and regression tree, and neural networks for predicting coronary artery disease. Expert Systems with Applications 34(1), 366–3744 (2008)

[5] Moon, T.K.: The Expectation-Maximization algorithm. IEEE Signal Processing Magazine 13(6), 47–60 (1996)

[6] Murphy, K.P.: Dynamic Bayesian Networks: Representation, Inference and Learning. Ph.D. thesis, Department of Computer Science, UC Berkeley (2002)

[7] Orphanou, K., Stassopoulou, A., Keravnou, E.: Temporal abstraction and temporal Bayesian networks in clinical domains: A survey. Artificial Intelligence in Medicine 60(3), 133–149 (2014)

[8] Rao, V.S.H., Kumar, M.N.: Novel approaches for predicting risk factors of atherosclerosis. IEEE Journal of Biomedical and Health Informatics 17(1), 183–189 (2013)

Uncertainty Propagation in Biomedical Models

Andrea Franco, Marco Correia, and Jorge Cruz[(⊠)]

NOVA Laboratory for Computer Science and Informatics, DI/FCT/UNL, Lisboa, Portugal
{andreafrfranco,marco.v.correia}@gmail.com jcrc@fct.unl.pt

Abstract. Mathematical models are prevalent in modern medicine. However, reasoning with realistic biomedical models is computationally demanding as parameters are typically subject to nonlinear relations, dynamic behavior, and uncertainty. This paper addresses this problem by proposing a new framework based on constraint programming for a sound propagation of uncertainty from model parameters to results. We apply our approach to an important problem in the obesity research field, the estimation of free-living energy intake in humans. Complementary to alternative solutions, our approach is able to correctly characterize the provided estimates given the uncertainty inherent to the model parameters.

1 Introduction

Uncertainty and nonlinearity play a major role in modeling most real-world continuous systems. In this work we use a probabilistic constraint approach that combines a stochastic representation of uncertainty on the parameter values with a reliable constraint framework robust to nonlinearity. The approach computes conditional probability distributions of the model parameters, given the uncertainty and the constraints.

The potential of our approach to support clinical practice is illustrated in a real world problem from the obesity research field. The impact of obesity on health is widely documented and the main cause for the "obesity pandemics" is the energy unbalance caused by an increased calorie intake associated to a lower energy expenditure.

Many biomedical models use the energy balance approach to simulate individual body weight dynamics. Change of body weight over time is modeled as the rate of energy stored (or lost), which is a function of the energy intake (from food) and the energy expended. The inability to rigorously assess the energy intake hinders the success and adherence to individual weight control interventions. The correct evaluation of such interventions will be highly dependent on the precision of energy intake estimates and the assessment of the uncertainty inherent to those estimates. We show how the probabilistic constraint framework can be used in clinical practice to characterize such uncertainty given the uncertainty of the underlying biomedical model.

2 Energy Intake Problem

The mathematical models that predict weight change in humans are usually based on the energy balance equation, $R = I - E$, where R is the energy stored or lost (kcal/d), I is the energy intake (kcal/d) and E is the energy expended (kcal/d). Several models have

© Springer International Publishing Switzerland 2015
J.H. Holmes et al. (Eds.): AIME 2015, LNAI 9105, pp. 166–171, 2015.
DOI: 10.1007/978-3-319-19551-3_21

been applied to provide estimates of individual energy intake [10]. Our paper focus on the EI model [6] that computes the energy intake based on the differential equation:

$$cf\frac{dF}{dt} + cl\frac{dFF}{dt} = I - (DIT + PA + R\dot{M}R + SPA) \tag{1}$$

The left hand side of eq. (1) represents the change in body's energy stores (R) and is modeled through the weighted sum of the changes in Fat mass (F) and Fat Free mass (FF). Differently from other models, that express the relationship between F and FF using a logarithmic model $FF^{log}(F)$ [9], or linear model [16], the EI model uses a 4th-order polynomial $FF^{poly}(F, a, h)$ to estimate FF as a function of F, the age of the subject a, and its height h. The rate of energy expended (E) is the total energy spent in several physiological processes: Diet Induced Thermogenesis (DIT); Physical Activity (PA); Resting Metabolic Rate (RMR); Spontaneous Physical Activity (SPA).

3   Constraint Programming

Continuous constraint programming [13,7] has been widely used to model safe reasoning in applications where uncertainty on parameter values is modeled by intervals including all their possibilities. A Continuous Constraint Satisfaction Problem (CCSP) is a triple $\langle X, D, C \rangle$ where X is a tuple of n real variables $\langle x_1, \cdots, x_n \rangle$, D is a Cartesian product of intervals $D(x_1) \times \cdots \times D(x_n)$ (a box), where each $D(x_i)$ is the domain of x_i and C is a set of numerical constraints (equations or inequalities) on subsets of the variables in X. A solution of the CCSP is a value assignment to all variables satisfying all the constraints in C. The feasible space F is the set of all CCSP solutions within D.

Continuous constraint reasoning relies on branch-and-prune algorithms [12] to obtain sets of boxes that cover the feasible space F. These algorithms begin with an initial crude cover of the feasible space (D) which is recursively refined by interleaving pruning and branching steps until a stopping criterion is satisfied. The branching step splits a box from the covering into sub-boxes (usually two). The pruning step either eliminates a box from the covering or reduces it into a smaller (or equal) box maintaining all the exact solutions. Pruning is achieved through an algorithm that combines constraint propagation and consistency techniques based on interval analysis methods [14].

The direct application of classical constraint programming to biomedical models suffers from two major pitfalls: system dynamics modeled through differential equations cannot be represented and integrated within the constraint model; the interval representation of uncertainty is inadequate to distinguish between consistent scenarios.

Differential Equations. The behavior of many systems is naturally modeled by a system of Ordinary Differential Equations (ODEs). A parametric ODE system, with parameters p, represented as $y' = f(p, y, t)$, is a restriction on the sequence of values that y can take over t. A solution within interval T, is any function that satisfies the equation for all values of $t \in T$. An Initial Value Problem (IVP) is characterized by an ODE system together with the initial condition $y(t_0) = y_0$ and its solution is the unique function that is a solution of the ODE system and satisfies the initial condition.

Several extensions to constraint programming [5,3,4] were proposed for handling differential equations based on interval methods for solving IVPs [14] which verify the existence of unique solutions and produce guaranteed error bounds for the solution trajectory along an interval T. They use interval arithmetic to compute safe enclosures for the trajectory, explicitly keeping the error term within safe bounds.

In this paper we use an approach similar to [5]. The idea is to consider an IVP as a function Φ where the first argument are the parameters p, the second argument is the initial condition to be verified at time point t_0 (third argument) and the last argument is a time point $t \in T$. A relation between the values at two time points t_0 and t_1 along the trajectory is represented by the equation $y(t_1) = \Phi(p, y(t_0), t_0, t_1)$. Using variables x_0 and x_1 to represent respectively $y(t_0)$ and $y(t_1)$, the equation is integrated into the CCSP as a constraint $x_1 = \Phi(p, x_0, t_0, t_1)$ with specialized constraint propagators to safely prune both variable domains based on a validated solver for IVPs [15].

Probabilistic Constraint Programming. An extension of the classical constraint programming paradigm is used to support probabilistic reasoning. Probabilistic constraint programming [2] associates a probabilistic space to the classical CCSP by defining an appropriate density function. A probabilistic constraint space is a pair $\langle \langle X, D, C \rangle, f \rangle$, where $\langle X, D, C \rangle$ is a CCSP and f a p.d.f. defined in $\Omega \supseteq D$ such that: $\int_\Omega f(\mathbf{x})d\mathbf{x} = 1$. The constraints C can be viewed as an event $\mathcal{H}$ whose probability can be computed by integrating f over its feasible space. The probabilistic constraint framework relies on continuous constraint reasoning to get a box cover of the region of integration $\mathcal{H}$ and compute the overall integral by summing up the contributions of each box in the cover.

Monte Carlo methods [11] are used to estimate the integrals at each box. The success of this technique relies on the reduction of the sampling space where a pure Monte Carlo method is not only hard to tune but also impractical in small error settings.

4   Probabilistic Constraints for Solving the EI Problem

Let t be the number of days since the beginning of treatment of a given subject, $F(t)$ the fat mass at time t, $w(t)$ the weight observed at time t, and I the subject's energy intake, which is assumed to be a constant parameter between consecutive observations [6]. The energy balance equation and total body mass are related through the model:

$$F'(t) = g(I, F(t), t) \qquad w(t) = FF(a, h, F(t)) + F(t) \qquad (2)$$

where g is obtained by solving equation (1) with respect to $F'(t)$.

Let $i \in \{0, \dots, n\}$ denote the i'th observation since beginning of treatment, occurred at time t_i, and let F_i and w_i be respectively the fat mass and the weight of the patient at time t_i (with $t_0 = 0$). The EI model may be formalized as a CCSP $\langle X, \mathbb{R}^{2n+1}, C \rangle$ with a set of variables $X = \{F_0\} \bigcup_{i=1}^{n} \{F_i, I_i\}$ representing the fat mass F_i at each observation and the energy intake I_i between consecutive observations (at t_{i-1} and t_i), and a set of constraints $C = \{b_0\} \bigcup_{i=1}^{n} \{a_i, b_i\}$ enforcing eqs. (2):

$$a_i \equiv [F_i = \Phi(I_i, F_{i-1}, t_{i-1}, t_i)] \qquad b_i \equiv [w_i = FF^M(a, h, F_i) + \epsilon_i + F_i]$$

where uncertainty inherent to FF estimation is integrated by considering that the true value of FF is the model given FF^M plus an error term $\epsilon_i \sim \mathcal{N}(\mu = 0, \sigma_\epsilon)$. Additionally, bounding constraints are considered for each observation: $3\sigma_\epsilon \leq \epsilon_i \leq 3\sigma_\epsilon$.

If we assume that the FF model errors over the $n + 1$ distinct observations are independent, then each solution has an associated probability density value given by the joint p.d.f. $\prod_{i=0}^{n} f_i (\epsilon_i)$ where f_i is the normal distribution associated with the error ϵ_i. A more realistic alternative to errors independence, explicitly represents the deviation between error ϵ_i and the previous error ϵ_{i-1} as a normally distributed random variable $\delta_i \sim \mathcal{N} (\mu = 0, \sigma_\delta)$, resulting in the joint p.d.f. $\prod_{i=0}^{n} f_i (\epsilon_i) \prod_{i=1}^{n} h_i (\epsilon_i - \epsilon_{i-1})$ where f_i and h_i are the normal distributions associated with the errors ϵ_i and δ_i respectively.

Method. We developed an incremental method to efficiently solve the problem. It starts by computing the probability distribution of F_0 given the initial weight w_0 subject to the constraint b_0 and the bounding constraints for ϵ_0. This distribution, $P^{\boxplus} (F_0)$, is discretized on a grid over $D (F_0)$ computed through probabilistic constraint programming. Given a sampled point $\dot{F}_0$, value $\dot{\epsilon}_0$ is determined by the constraint b_0, and its p.d.f. value is $f(\dot{F}_0) = f_0 (\dot{\epsilon}_0)$. Similarly, the joint probability $P^{\boxplus} (F_1, I_1)$, is computed through probabilistic constraint programming by considering the constraints associated with observation 1, the observed weight w_1, and $P^{\boxplus} (F_0)$. Given a sampled point $(\dot{F}_1, \dot{I}_1)$, the values $\dot{F}_0$ and $\dot{\epsilon}_1$ are determined by constraints a_1 and b_1, and assuming errors independence, its p.d.f. is $f_0 (\dot{\epsilon}_0) f_1 (\dot{\epsilon}_1)$. However, we replace the computation of $f_0 (\dot{\epsilon}_0)$ with the value of the probability $P^{\boxplus}(\dot{F}_0)$ computed in the previous step providing an approximation that converges to the correct value when the number of grid subdivisions goes to infinity: $f(\dot{F}_1, \dot{I}_1) \approx P^{\boxplus}(\dot{F}_0) f_1 (\dot{\epsilon}_1)$. If the alternative p.d.f. is used, the approximation is: $f(\dot{F}_1, \dot{I}_1) \approx P^{\boxplus}(\dot{F}_0) f_1(\dot{\epsilon}_1) h_1(\epsilon_i - \epsilon_{i-1})$. Finally, the $P^{\boxplus} (F_1, I_1)$ is marginalized to obtain $P^{\boxplus} (F_1)$, and the process is iterated for the remaining observations.

5   Experimental Results

This section demonstrates how the approach may be applied to complement EI model predictions with measures of confidence. The algorithm was implemented in C++ and used for obtaining the probability distribution approximations $P^{\boxplus} (F_i, I_i)$ of a 45 years old woman over the course of the 24-week trial (CALERIE Study phase I [8]). The runtime was about 2 minutes per observation on an Intel Core i7 @ 2.4 GHz.

Fat Free mass is estimated using two distinct models: FF^{poly}[6], and FF^{log}[9]. Both models were initially fit to a set of 7278 North American women resulting in the standard deviation of the error, $\sigma_\epsilon^{poly} = 3.35$ and $\sigma_\epsilon^{log} = 5.04$. This data set was collected during NHANES surveys (1994 to 2004) and is available online [1]. We considered both assumptions regarding independence of the error. Due to space reasons we only show the results of the FF^{poly} model assuming a correlated error with $\sigma_\delta = 0.5$.

Joint Probability Distributions. Figure 1(left) plots the results regarding the first observation showing the correlation between the uncertainty on F and I. Experiments with the error independence assumption clarify its negative repercussion on the predicted distribution of I. Experiments with the FF^{log} model revealed that the improved accuracy of FF^{poly} model ($\sigma_\epsilon^{poly} < \sigma_\epsilon^{log}$) does not seem to impact the estimation of I.

Marginal Probability Distributions with Confidence Intervals. Figure 1(right) shows the estimated I_i over time. Each box depicts the most probable value (marked in the center

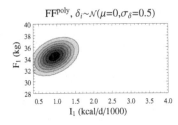
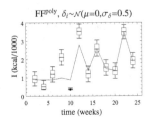

Fig. 1. Joint probabilities on the 1st observation (left). Confidence intervals for I over time (right)

of the box), the union hull of the 50% most probable values (rectangle), and the union hull of the 82% most probable values (whiskers). Additionally, the plot overlays the estimates obtained from the algorithm published by the author of the EI model.

6 Conclusions

The standard practice for characterizing confidence on the predictions resulting from a complex model is to perform controlled experiments to assess its fitness statistically. However, controlled experiments are not always practical or have associated high costs. Contrary to the empirical, black-box approach, this paper proposes to characterize the uncertainty on the model estimates by propagating the errors stemming from each of its parts. The approach extends constraint programming to integrate probabilistic reasoning and dynamic behavior, offering a mathematically sound and efficient alternative.

The application field of the presented approach is quite broad: it targets models which are themselves composed of other (sub)models, for which there is a known characterization of the error. The selected EI model is a fairly complex model including dynamic behavior and nonlinear relations, and integrates various (sub)models with associated uncertainty. The experimental section illustrated how different choices for one of these (sub)models, the FF model, impacts the error of the complete EI model, providing valuable information that can be integrated in a decision making support tool.

References

1. National health and nutrition examination survey, http://www.cdc.gov/nchs/nhanes.htm
2. Carvalho, E.: Probabilistic Constraint Reasoning. PhD thesis, FCT/UNL (2012)
3. Cruz, J.: Constraint Reasoning for Differential Models. IOS Press (2005)
4. Cruz, J., Barahona, P.: Constraint reasoning in deep biomedical models. Artificial Intelligence in Medicine 34(1), 77–88 (2005)
5. Goldsztejn, A., Mullier, O., Eveillard, D., Hosobe, H.: Including ordinary differential equations based constraints in the standard CP framework. In: Cohen, D. (ed.) CP 2010. LNCS, vol. 6308, pp. 221–235. Springer, Heidelberg (2010)
6. Thomas, D., et al.: A computational model to determine energy intake during weight loss. Am. J. Clin. Nutr. 92(6), 1326–1331 (2010)
7. Benhamou, F., et al.: CLP(intervals) revisited. In: ISLP, pp. 124–138. MIT Press (1994)
8. Redman, L., et al.: Effect of calorie restriction with or without exercise on body composition and fat distribution. J. Clin. Endocrinol. Metab. 92(3), 865–872 (2007)

9. Forbes, G.: Lean body mass-body fat interrelationships in humans. Nut. R. 45, 225–231 (1987)
10. Hall, K.D., Chow, C.C.: Estimating changes in free–living energy intake and its confidence interval. Am. J. Clin. Nutr. 94, 66–74 (2011)
11. Hammersley, J., Handscomb, D.: Monte Carlo Methods. Methuen London (1964)
12. Van Hentenryck, P., Mcallester, D., Kapur, D.: Solving polynomial systems using a branch and prune approach. SIAM J. Num. Analysis 34, 797–827 (1997)
13. Lhomme, O.: Consistency techniques for numeric CSPs. In: IJCAI, pp. 232–238 (1993)
14. Moore, R.: Interval Analysis. Prentice-Hall, Englewood Cliffs (1966)
15. Nedialkov, N.: Vnode-lp a validated solver for initial value problems in ordinary differential equations. Technical report, McMaster Univ., Hamilton, Canada (2006)
16. Thomas, D., Ciesla, A., Levine, J., Stevens, J., Martin, C.: A mathematical model of weight change with adaptation. Math. Biosci. Eng. 6(4), 873–887 (2009)

A Bayesian Network for Probabilistic Reasoning and Imputation of Missing Risk Factors in Type 2 Diabetes

Francesco Sambo[1]([✉]), Andrea Facchinetti[1], Liisa Hakaste[2], Jasmina Kravic[3], Barbara Di Camillo[1], Giuseppe Fico[4], Jaakko Tuomilehto[5], Leif Groop[3], Rafael Gabriel[6], Tuomi Tiinamaija[2], and Claudio Cobelli[1]

[1] University of Padova, Padua, Italy
sambofra@dei.unipd.it
[2] FolkhälsanResearch Centre, Helsinki, Finland
[3] Lund University Diabetes Centre, Malmö, Sweden
[4] Life Supporting Technologies, Technical University of Madrid, Madrid, Spain
[5] National Institute for Health and Welfare, Helsinki, Finland
[6] Instituto IdiPAZ, Hospital Universitario La Paz,
University of Madrid, Madrid, Spain

Abstract. We propose a novel Bayesian network tool to model the probabilistic relations between a set of type 2 diabetes risk factors. The tool can be used for probabilistic reasoning and for imputation of missing values among risk factors.

The Bayesian network is learnt from a joint training set of three European population studies. Tested on an independent patient set, the network is shown to be competitive with both a standard imputation tool and a widely used risk score for type 2 diabetes, providing in addition a richer description of the interdependencies between diabetes risk factors.

Keywords: Bayesian networks · Type 2 diabetes · Probabilistic reasoning · Missing values imputation

1 Introduction

Complex diseases, such as type 2 diabetes (T2D), arise from the interaction of several physiological, lifestyle and environmental risk factors. Complete information on all risk factors, however, is often not available or expensive to acquire. Bayesian networks can be used for reasoning even in the presence of missing information and for providing probabilistic estimates of missing values.

A Bayesian network (BN [7]) is a probabilistic graphical model which represents the joint probability distribution of a set of random variables with two components: a direct acyclic graph (DAG), where each node corresponds to a variable and each edge to a conditional dependence between variables, and a probability distribution of each node given its parents in the DAG.

© Springer International Publishing Switzerland 2015
J.H. Holmes et al. (Eds.): AIME 2015, LNAI 9105, pp. 172–176, 2015.
DOI: 10.1007/978-3-319-19551-3_22

In this paper, we propose a Bayesian network tool for reasoning and inference in type 2 diabetes in the presence of missing risk factors. The network structure and distributions parameters are learned from a joint dataset of three population studies. On an independent test set, the Bayesian network is shown to be effective in estimating the probability distribution of missing values and competitive with a state-of-the-art risk score in detecting the T2D condition.

2   Datasets

The datasets exploited in this paper come from the Botnia Prospective Study (BPS [5]), the Prevalence, Prediction and Prevention of Diabetes Botnia study (PPP [3]) and the Variability of Insulin with Visceral Adiposity study (VIVA [8]). All three studies comprise a screen visit for a population of non-diabetic subjects and a second, follow-up visit 5 to 15 years later. The number of subjects involved in each study is 3331 for BPS, 2000 for PPP and 2476 for VIVA.

All studies include anthropometric data, information on co-morbidities, lifestyle habits, fasting blood test measures and an Oral Glucose Tolerance Test (OGTT). The latter is required for a complete diagnosis of Type 2 Diabetes, defined as fasting plasma glucose $\geq$ 6.9 mmol/l or glucose at 120 minutes of the OGTT $\geq$ 11.1 mmol/l.

3   Data Pre-Processing

The three datasets are initially processed by identifying all common T2D risk factors with overall missingness below 30% and by aligning their definitions and unit of measures. The risk factors we select as variables are gender (SEX), education (EDU), current profession (PROF), ethnicity (ETHN), current smoker (C_SMK), history of habitudinal smoke (H_SMK), physical demanding work (PHY_W), physical activity in leisure time (PHY_F), history of cardio-vascular event (H_CVD), stroke (H_STR) or high blood glucose (H_HBG), body mass index (BMI), waist circumference (WAIST), systolic (SBP) and diastolic blood pressure (DBP), use of anti-hypertensive (AHT_M) and lipid-lowering medication (LLO_M), cholesterol (CHOL), triglycerides (TRIG), high-density lipoprotein (HDL), fasting insulin (INS0), fasting glucose (GL0), metabolic syndrome (MS) and 120-min OGTT glucose (GL120).

A test set is then obtained by sampling 10% of the patients at random from each of the three datasets, stratifying for gender, age, BMI and incident T2D at the follow-up visit. Defining a *record* the observation of all variables for a patient in one of the two visits, we obtain a training set by merging all the 13237 records for the patients not in the test set. Missing values in the training set are then imputed with the k-Nearest Neighbour (kNN) algorithm, with $k = 10$ and using the Heterogeneous Euclidean Overlap Metric as a measure of distance between records [1]. After imputation, continuous variables are quantized according to meaningful clinical thresholds, when available in the literature, or according to tertiles across all records in the follow-up visit otherwise.

4   Bayesian Network Learning

The most probable Bayesian network structure given a dataset without missing values can be obtained by searching the space of all possible DAGs for the one with the maximum likelihood, computed as the Bayesian Dirichlet equivalent score with uniform priors (BDeu, [2]). To search for the best BN structure given the training data we exploit the Max-Min Hill-Climbing algorithm (MMHC [9]). We further limit the search space by dividing the set of variables in *layers* and by allowing each node to only have children in the same or subsequent layers.

The probability distribution of each node given its parents is then estimated based just on data from the follow-up visit: the rationale of this choice is to learn the probabilities from a medical visit investigating the presence of T2D, for a patient with a former non-diabetic profile.

5   Network Performance

We assessed the reasoning and inference accuracy of the Bayesian network in the hypothetical scenario of a citizen using a questionnaire-based self screening tool at home: in this case, the *unobserved* variables are SBP, DBP, TRIG, CHOL, HDL, GL0, INS0, MS and GL120. For one patient at a time from the test set, we exploit the Junction Tree [7] inference algorithm to query the network for the *marginal* probability distribution of the unobserved variables, both providing some evidence on the values of the observed variables (*posterior distribution*) and without any evidence (*prior distribution*).

We first assess the ability of the network in providing correct probability estimates for unobserved variables. Given the actual value of each unobserved variable in each test subject, we measure the error as one minus the probability assigned to that value by the network. For a variable of cardinality c, we further normalize the error dividing it by $(1 - 1/c)$: this is meant to make it equal to 1 in case the estimate is a uniform probability distribution, which corresponds to a completely random assignment of values to the variable.

Figure 1 reports the median, first and third quartile of the normalized error measure across all test subjects, for all unobserved variables and for both the prior (squares) and posterior (dots) probability estimates. The dotted line indicates the uniform random estimate, identically equal to 1 thanks to the normalization of the error measure. From the figure one can observe that the estimated posterior probabilities across the test set are always significantly better than both the random estimates (Wilcoxon sign-rank test, all p-values $< 10^{-17}$) and the prior probabilities (all p-values $< 10^{-9}$).

We then assess the ability of the Bayesian network in imputing missing values in the test set, comparing the imputation obtained by both the prior and posterior probability estimates with the one obtained by the k-Nearest Neighbour algorithm, with $k = 10$. Table 1 reports the imputation accuracy, as fraction of correctly imputed missing values, for all unobserved variables and all subjects in the test set. In all but one case, the best accuracy is obtained by the posterior probability estimate (bold values).

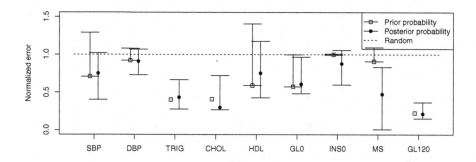

Fig. 1. Median (dot/square), first and third quartile (whiskers) of the normalized error for prior (squares) and posterior (dots) probabilities estimated by the Bayesian network. The dashed line indicates the error of the uniform random estimate.

Table 1. Imputation accuracy obtained by the Bayesian network using prior and posterior probabilities and by the k-Nearest Neighbour algorithm

	SBP	DBP	TRIG	CHOL	HDL	GL0	INS0	MS	GL120
prior probabilities	0.630	0.551	**0.813**	0.803	**0.701**	0.640	0.278	0.559	**0.839**
kNN	0.704	0.629	0.785	**0.806**	0.685	0.643	0.360	0.794	0.837
posterior probabilities	**0.735**	**0.632**	**0.813**	0.803	**0.701**	**0.655**	**0.571**	**0.817**	**0.839**

Finally, we assess the performance of the Bayesian network in detecting T2D, defined as in Section 2, in the aforementioned scenario. This allows us to fairly compare our tool with one of the most widely used questionnaire-based T2D risk score, the FINDRISC score [4]. Given the observed variables, by the rules of probability calculus the posterior probability of a patient being type 2 diabetic is: $p_{T2D} = p_{(GL0=high)} + p_{(GL120=high)} - p_{(GL0=high \wedge GL120=high)}$.

We compare our probability estimates with a variant of the FINDRISC score computed from the quantized variables measured in our datasets. The area under the the ROC curve obtained from the probability estimates results 0.79, slightly higher than the one of the FINDRISC score, 0.77, but not significantly different (DeLong's test p-value 0.26).

6 Conclusions and Future Directions

In this paper, we presented a Bayesian network tool for reasoning and imputation in type 2 diabetes in the presence of missing values. The network structure and probability distributions are learnt from a training set, obtained by merging three European population studies, and the network performance is assessed on an independent test set, sampled from the original joint set.

We introduced the scenario of a citizen querying the network with a questionnaire-based self screening tool and showed that, in such a scenario, our

BN outperforms the k-Nearest Neighbour algorithm in imputing missing values in almost all cases. The network was also shown to be competitive with the widely adopted FINDRISC risk score in detecting the T2D condition. In addition, the Bayesian network provides a rich description of each unobserved variable, in terms of a probability distribution across all its possible values, and an accessible representation of the interdependencies between risk factors. Compared to other Bayesian tools for reasoning in type 2 diabetes ([6,10]), our model includes a wider set of risk factors, providing a richer description of the patients and possibly leading to the definition of more personalized interventions.

All computations have been carried out with the R package bnstruct[1] and the analysis pipeline is sufficiently general to be easily applied to other complex diseases. The tool has been developed as part of the activities of the European FP7 project MOSAIC (MOdels and Simulation techniques for discovering dIAbetes influence faCtors, Grant N. 600914). The tool will be further validated on several external datasets, in order to assess its generalization ability on different populations.

References

1. García-Laencina, P.J., Sancho-Gómez, J., Figueiras-Vidal, A.R.: Pattern classification with missing data: A review. Neural Comput. Appl. 19(2), 263–282 (2010)
2. Heckerman, D., Geiger, D., Chickering, D.: Learning Bayesian networks: The combination of knowledge and statistical data. Machine Learning 20, 197–243 (1995)
3. Isomaa, B., et al.: A family history of diabetes is associated with reduced physical fitness in the Prevalence, Prediction and Prevention of Diabetes (PPP)-Botnia study. Diabetologia 53(8), 1709–1713 (2010)
4. Lindström, J., Tuomilehto, J.: The diabetes risk score: A practical tool to predict type 2 diabetes risk. Diabetes Care 26(3), 725–731 (2003)
5. Lyssenko, V., et al.: Predictors of and longitudinal changes in insulin sensitivity and secretion preceding onset of type 2 diabetes. Diabetes 54(1), 166–174 (2005)
6. Park, H.S., Cho, S.B.: Evolutionary attribute ordering in bayesian networks for predicting the metabolic syndrome. Expert Systems with Applications 39(4), 4240–4249 (2012)
7. Sambo, F., Ferrazzi, F., Bellazzi, R.: 12 - Probabilistic Modelling with Bayesian Networks. In: Carson, E., Cobelli, C. (eds.) Modelling Methodology for Physiology and Medicine, 2nd edn., pp. 257–280. Elsevier, Oxford (2014)
8. The DECODE study group: Comparison of three different definitions for the metabolic syndrome in non-diabetic europeans. The British Journal of Diabetes and Vascular Disease 5(3), 161–168 (2005)
9. Tsamardinos, I., Brown, L.E., Aliferis, C.F.: The Max Min Hill Climbing Bayesian Network Structure Learning Algorithm. Machine Learning (65), 31–78 (2006)
10. Watabe, T., Okuhara, Y., Sagara, Y.: A hierarchical bayesian framework to infer the progression level to diabetes based on deficient clinical data. Computers in Biology and Medicine 50, 107–115 (2014)

---

[1] https://github.com/sambofra/bnstruct

Causal Discovery from Medical Data: Dealing with Missing Values and a Mixture of Discrete and Continuous Data

Elena Sokolova[1(✉)], Perry Groot[1], Tom Claassen[1], Daniel von Rhein[2], Jan Buitelaar[2], and Tom Heskes[1]

[1] Faculty of Science, Radboud University, Nijmegen, The Netherlands
`e.sokolova@cs.ru.nl`
[2] Donders Institute for Brain, Cognition and Behaviour, Radboud University Medical Center, Nijmegen, The Netherlands

Abstract. Causal discovery is an increasingly popular method for data analysis in the field of medical research. In this paper we consider two challenges in causal discovery that occur very often when working with medical data: a mixture of discrete and continuous variables and a substantial amount of missing values. To the best of our knowledge there are no methods that can handle both challenges at the same time. In this paper we develop a new method that can handle these challenges based on the assumption that data is missing completely at random and that variables obey a non-paranormal distribution. We demonstrate the validity of our approach for causal discovery for empiric data from a monetary incentive delay task. Our results may help to better understand the etiology of attention deficit-hyperactivity disorder (ADHD).

Keywords: Causal discovery · Missing data · Mixture of discrete and continuous data · ADHD

1 Introduction

In recent years, the use of causal discovery in the field of medical research has become increasingly popular. Existing algorithms deal reasonably well with models that contain only discrete variables or only Gaussian variables, while real-world data often contains mixture variables, where continuous variables are not Gaussian. To tackle the problem of mixture variables, several approaches have been developed, including partial correlation tests [7], Mercer kernels [2], and neural networks [8]. Existing algorithms for causal discovery mainly start from the assumption that the data is complete, whereas in practice, medical data sets often have missing values. For example, some tests are often performed only for part of the patients, the quality of some data is poor, participants drop out etc. Several methods have been proposed to deal with missing values for causal discovery, including imputation methods, expectation maximization algorithms, and importance sampling [6,9]. However, these methods usually rely on the assumption that data is either discrete or continuous Gaussian. To the best of our

© Springer International Publishing Switzerland 2015
J.H. Holmes et al. (Eds.): AIME 2015, LNAI 9105, pp. 177–181, 2015.
DOI: 10.1007/978-3-319-19551-3_23

knowledge there are no methods that can handle both a mixture of discrete and continuous variables as well as missing values for directed graphical models. An ad hoc solution would be to apply standard methods and ignore all missing values. However, when the percentage of missing values is significant one can end up with the insufficient data to learn a causal structure.

We propose a method that can handle missing values and mixture variables based on the ideas for undirected graphical models presented in [12,1]. As a prototypical example we apply our algorithm to a data set of patients with Attention-deficit/hyperactivity disorder (ADHD). The data set is ideal for our purposes because it provides all characteristics of a typical medical data set: it describes relationships between various possible factors of the disease such as genes, age, gender, and different types of symptoms and behavioral characteristics. Moreover, it has a mixture of discrete and continuous variables and approximately 10% of missing data.

The rest of the paper is organized as follows. Section 2 explains the proposed method. Section 3 presents the results for ADHD data. Section 4 provides our conclusion and future work.

2   Proposed Method

In this section we propose a causal discovery algorithm that can deal with both a mixture of discrete and continuous variables and missing data. In the first two steps of this algorithm we estimate the correlation matrix for mixed data with missing values, based on the ideas proposed in [12,1]. In the third step, we use this correlation matrix as an input into a causal discovery algorithm to infer the causal structure. We use the BCCD algorithm for this purpose, one of the state-of-the-art algorithms in causal discovery. Claassen and Heskes [3] showed that BCCD outperforms reference algorithms in the field, such as FCI and Conservative PC. Moreover, BCCD provides an indication of the reliability of the causal links that makes it easier to interpret the results and compare alternative models. We rely on the assumption that data is missing completely at random and that variables obey a non-paranormal distribution.

Step 1 Mixture of discrete and continuous variables
   To deal with mixed data we propose to use a Gaussian copula. For each variable X_i we estimate the rescaled empirical distribution

$$\hat{F}_i(x) = \frac{1}{n+1} \sum_{i=1}^{n} \mathcal{I}\{X_i < x\}, \tag{1}$$

and then transform the data into Gaussian normal scores $\hat{X}_i = \hat{\Phi}_i^{-1}(\hat{F}(X_i))$. In this step missing values are ignored.

Step 2 Correlation matrix with missing data
   New variables now have a Gaussian distribution, so we can use Pearson correlation to estimate dependencies between variables. Since our data has

missing values, we propose to first use the expectation maximization algorithm to estimate the correlation matrix, since this algorithm provides an unbiased estimate of parameters and their standard error [4].

Step 3 Apply BCCD

Having the correlation matrix we can use it in the BCCD algorithm to estimate the causal structure of the graph. A more detailed description can be found in [3,10]. The core part of the algorithm BCCD is the estimation of the reliability of the causal relations, based on the marginal likelihood of data given graphical structure $p(\mathbf{D}|\mathcal{G})$. We approximate the logarithm of the marginal likelihood $\log(p(\mathbf{D}|\mathcal{G}))$ using the Bayesian Information Criterion (BIC), which depends on the correlation matrix computed in Step 2:

$$BICscore(\mathbf{D}|\mathcal{G}) = M \sum_{i=1}^{n} -\frac{1}{2} \log \frac{|\Sigma|}{|\Sigma_{Pa_i}|} - \frac{\log M}{2} \mathrm{Dim}[\mathcal{G}] \ , \qquad (2)$$

where n is the number of variables, M is the sample size, $\mathrm{Dim}[\mathcal{G}]$ is the number of parameters in the model corresponding to graph $\mathcal{G}$, Pa_i are the parents of node X_i, and Σ_{Pa_i} is a correlation matrix between the parents of variable X_i. Having all the causal relations, BCCD ranks them in decreasing order of reliability and uses logical deduction with transitivity and acyclicity to derive additional causal statements. If there is a conflict, it picks the causal statement that has a higher reliability.

3   ADHD Data

In a future paper we will analyze the performance of our method on simulated data, where we know the ground truth. Here we describe an application of our algorithm to the ADHD data set that was collected as a part of the NeuroIMAGE study [11]. This study investigated the brain response during reward anticipation and receipt with a monetary incentive delay (MID) task in a large sample of adolescents and young adults with ADHD, their unaffected siblings and healthy controls. The brain activation was measured in ventral striatum (VS) and orbitalfrontal cortex (OFC) brain areas during the anticipation of the reward cue and feedback after reward cue. During the experiments the difference in reaction time was measured when there was and there was no reward cue (Reaction time difference). The data set contained 189 probands with ADHD, 104 unaffected siblings, and 116 age-matched controls. Since the presence of the unaffected siblings can blur the effect of the genes, we did not include them in our study and consider only ADHD patients and healthy controls.

The goal of our study is to identify the endophenotypic model [5] that explains the relationships between genes, brain functioning, behaviors, and disease symptoms. To apply causal discovery to this data set, we selected 12 variables that represent genes, brain functioning in different regions of the brain, symptoms, and general factors. We included the prior knowledge that no variable in the network can cause gender, and the endophenotypic assumption from [5] that symptoms are the consequence of the brain functioning problems.

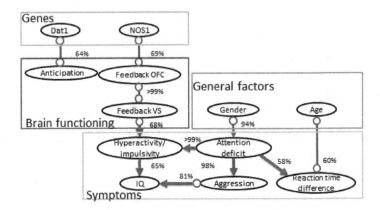

Fig. 1. The causal graph representing causal relationships between variables for the ADHD data set. The graph represents a PAG, where edge directions are marked with " − " and " >" for invariant edge directions and with "o" for non-invariant edge directions. The reliability of an edge between two variables is depicted with a percentage value near each edge.

A causal network learned from the data is presented in Figure 1. This figure includes only edges with a reliability of a direct causal link higher than 50%. The graph built by BCCD shows an effect of genes on brain functioning, the effect of brain functioning and general factors on disease symptoms, and an interaction between these symptoms. The relationships between variables found by BCCD are in line with several other studies in ADHD that considered mainly pairs of variables [13]. An additional advantage of this study is that interactions are visualized in a single graph that makes it easy to interpret the results.

4   Conclusions and Discussion

The contribution of this paper is the presentation of an algorithm for causal discovery and application of it to real-world data describing ADHD. The results of the algorithm were corroborated by medical experts and literature. As any statistical approach, methods for causal discovery have to rely on assumptions. In this paper we relaxed standard assumptions on, for example, Gaussianity and the absence of missing values. By doing this we open up the application of causal discovery to a much wider class of data sets. However, we obviously rely on some other assumptions such as data being missing completely at random, monotonic interactions between variables, and absence no cycles. As future work we would like to consider data sets with more complex interactions between variables and relax in particular the assumption that data is missing completely at random.

Acknowledgments. This work was supported by NIH Grant R01MH62873 (to Stephen V. Faraone), NWO Large Investment Grant (1750102007010 to Jan Buitelaar), NWO Brain & Cognition grants (056-13-015 and 433-09-242 to Jan Buitelaar), and grants from

Radboud University Nijmegen Medical Center, University Medical Center Groningen and Accare and VU University Amsterdam. The research leading to these results also received support from the EU FP7 project TACTICS under grant agreement n°278948, the NWO grants MoCoCaDi (612.001.202) and CHILL (617.001.451).

References

1. Abegaz, F., Wit, E.: Penalized EM algorithm and copula skeptic graphical models for inferring networks for mixed variables. Statistics in Medicine (2014)
2. Bach, F.R., Jordan, M.I.: Learning graphical models with Mercer kernels. In: Proceedings of the NIPS Conference, pp. 1009–1016 (2002)
3. Claassen, T., Heskes, T.: A Bayesian approach to constraint based causal inference. In: Proceedings of the UAI Conference, pp. 207–216 (2012)
4. Dempster, A.P., Laird, N.M., Rubin, D.B.: Maximum likelihood from incomplete data via the EM algorithm. Journal of the Royal Statistical Society. Series B (Methodological), pp. 1–38 (1977)
5. Franke, B., Neale, B.M., Faraone, S.V.: Genome-wide association studies in ADHD. Human Genetics 126(1), 13–50 (2009)
6. Friedman, N.: The bayesian structural EM algorithm. In: Proceedings of the Fourteenth
   Conference on Uncertainty in Artificial Intelligence, pp. 129–138. Morgan Kaufmann Publishers Inc. (1998)
7. Harris, N., Drton, M.: PC algorithm for nonparanormal graphical models. Journal of Machine Learning Research 14, 3365–3383 (2013)
8. Monti, S., Cooper, G.F.: Learning hybrid Bayesian networks from data. Technical Report ISSP-97-01, Intelligent Systems Program, University of Pittsburgh (1997)
9. Riggelsen, C., Feelders, A.: Learning bayesian network models from incomplete data using importance sampling. In: Proc. of Artificial Intelligence and Statistics, pp. 301–308 (2005)
10. Sokolova, E., Groot, P., Claassen, T., Heskes, T.: Causal discovery from databases with discrete and continuous variables. In: van der Gaag, L.C., Feelders, A.J. (eds.) PGM 2014. LNCS, vol. 8754, pp. 442–457. Springer, Heidelberg (2014)
11. von Rhein, D., Mennes, M., van Ewijk, H., Groenman, A.P., Zwiers, M.P., Oosterlaan, J., Heslenfeld, D., Franke, B., Hoekstra, P.J., Faraone, S.V.: et al. The NeuroIMAGE study: a prospective phenotypic, cognitive, genetic and MRI study in children with attention-deficit/hyperactivity disorder. Design and descriptives. European Child & Adolescent Psychiatry, 1–17 (2014)
12. Wang, H., Fazayeli, F., Chatterjee, S., Banerjee, A., Steinhauser, K., Ganguly, A., Bhattacharjee, K., Konar, A., Nagar, A.: Gaussian copula precision estimation with missing values. Biotechnology Journal 4(9) (2009)
13. Willcutt, E.G., Pennington, B.F., DeFries, J.C.: Etiology of inattention and hyperactivity/impulsivity in a community sample of twins with learning difficulties. J. Abnorm. Child Psychol. 28(2), 149–159 (2000)

Modeling Coronary Artery Calcification Levels from Behavioral Data in a Clinical Study

Shuo Yang[1(✉)], Kristian Kersting[2], Greg Terry[3], Jefferey Carr[3],
and Sriraam Natarajan[1]

[1] Indiana University, Bloomington, USA
{shuoyang,natarasr}@indiana.edu
[2] TU Dortmund, Dortmund, Germany
[3] Vanderbilt University, Nashville, USA

Abstract. Cardiovascular disease (CVD) is one of the key causes for death worldwide. We consider the problem of modeling an imaging biomarker, Coronary Artery Calcification (CAC) measured by computed tomography, based on behavioral data. We employ the formalism of Dynamic Bayesian Network (DBN) and learn a DBN from these data. Our learned DBN provides insights about the associations of specific risk factors with CAC levels. Exhaustive empirical results demonstrate that the proposed learning method yields reasonable performance during cross-validation.

1 Introduction

Cardiovascular disease (CVD) is one of the key causes of death worldwide. It is well known that successful and established lifestyle intervention and modification can result in prevention of the development of cardiovascular risk factors. In this work-in-progress, we consider a clinical study, Coronary Artery Risk Development in Young Adults (CARDIA), to model the development of Coronary Artery Calcification (CAC) amounts, a measure of subclinical Coronary Artery Disease [1]. For modeling this risk factor development in adults, we employ the use of temporal-probabilistic models called Dynamic Bayesian Networks (DBNs) [3]. We employ standard optimization scoring metrics [3] – Bayesian Information Criterion (BIC), Bayesian Dirichlet metric (BDe) and mutual information (MI) – for learning these temporal models. We combine the different probabilistic networks resulting from different metrics and evaluate their predictive ability through cross-validation.

One aspect of our work is that in order to learn these DBNs, we consider non-clinical data. We use only basic socio-demographic information and health behaviour information for predicting the incidence of CAC-levels as the individual ages from early to middle adult life. Our results indicate that these behavioral features are reasonably predictive of the occurrence of increased CAC-levels. They allow us to potentially identify potential life-style and behavioral changes that can minimize cardiovascular risks. In addition, the interpretative nature of the learned probabilistic model allows us to easily present the learned models to domain experts (physicians) who could potentially interact with the model and modify/refine the learned model based on their experience/expertise.

J.H. Holmes et al. (Eds.): AIME 2015, LNAI 9105, pp. 182–187, 2015.
DOI: 10.1007/978-3-319-19551-3_24

2   Background

One of the questions that the CARDIA study tries to address is to identify the risk factors in early life that have influence on the development of clinical CVD in later life. It is a longitudinal population study started in 1985-86 and performed in 4 study centers in the US and includes 7 subsequent evaluations (years 2, 5, 7, 10, 15, 20, 25). It includes various clinical and physical measurements and in-depth questionnaires about sociodemographic background, behavior, psychosocial issues, medical and family history, smoking, diet, exercise and drinking habits. We consider the demographic and socio-economic features to predict the CAC-level as a binary prediction task. Specifically, we consider these features (with their number of categories in the following parentheses) – participant's education level(9), full time(3)/part time(3) work, occupation(8), income(6), marriage status(8), number of children(3), alcohol usage(3), tobacco usage(3) and physical activities(6) during the last year – to model the development of CAC level (High($CAC > 0$)/Low($CAC = 0$)) in each year of study.[1]

3   Proposed Approach

The first issue with this study is that there are several missing values. Preprocessing is required for matching the solutions for missing values across study centers. While the participant retention rate is relatively high (91%, 86%, 81%, 79%, 74%, 72%, and 72%, respectively for each evaluation), there are still at least 10 percent of the data are missing from the records. When a subject is absent from a certain subsequent test, we fill in the missing values using the values from his/her previous measurement. For the missing entries due to other unknown reasons, we treat them as a special class.

Another issue is the evolution of the evaluation measurements and the survey design. Some of the questions related to a certain aspect of the sociodemographic background may be divided into multiple questions or combined into one question in the follow up evaluations. For example, since year 15, the question related to the participant's marriage status has an option as "living with someone in a marriage-like relationship" which is a separate question from year 0 to year 10.

Given these challenges, we employed a purely probabilistic formalism of dynamic Bayesian networks (DBNs) that extend Bayesian networks (BNs) to temporal setting. They employ a factorized representation that decreases the dimension from exponential in the total number of features to exponential in the sizes of parent sets. They also handle the longitudinal data by using a BN fragment to represent the probabilistic transition between adjacent time slots which allows both intra-time-slice and inter-time-slice arcs. Finally, cyclic dependencies in time are allowed. For instance, treatment of a disease in the current time can influence the incidence of the disease in the next time which in turn can influence the treatment in the next time step.

---

[1] For detailed information about the features, please refer to CARDIA online resource at http://www.cardia.dopm.uab.edu/exam-materials2/data-collection-forms.

In most literature, the probabilistic influence relationships of the DBN (particularly the temporal influences) are pre-specified and only the parameters are learned. However, since we are interested in determining how the CAC-levels evolve as a function of 10 other risk factors, we instead learn the influences by adapting standard BN structure learning algorithms. The most popular approaches for learning BNs are to employ a greedy local search such as hill climbing based on certain decomposable local score functions. We consider three different scoring functions – Bayesian Dirichlet (BDe) scores, Bayesian information criterion (BIC) and Mutual Information Test (MIT).Before discussing the scoring functions, we present the high-level overview of our framework in Figure.1.

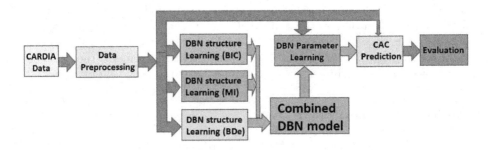

Fig. 1. Flow Chart of the Proposed Model. The blue arrows denote the flow of data and the grey arrows denote the flow of the model.

After preprocessing, we run three hill-climbing algorithms using the three different scoring metrics. First, we transfer the multi-series dynamic data into a training set by extracting every pair of sequential study measurements of every patient as a training instance. After this step, we got 5114 ($|subjects|$) $*5$ ($|paired\ time\ slices|$) instances in total. Using these training instances, we learn three models using the three metrics. We also combine these models by using the union of all the edges to construct a new unified model[2]. The goal is to introduce more dependencies and evaluate if a more complex model is indeed more accurate. For this new unified model, we learn the parameters and perform 5-fold cross-validation for evaluation.

Returning to the scoring function, the first row of Table.1 presents the general form of the decomposable penalized log-likelihood (DPLL) [4] for a BN $\mathcal{B}$ given the data $\mathcal{D}$. $\mathcal{D}_{il}$ is the instantiation of X_i in data point D_l , and PA_{il} is the instantiation of X_i's parent nodes in D_l. So the general form of DPLL is the sum of individual variable scores which equal to the loglikelihood of the data given the local structure minus a penalty term for the local structure. Note that BIC and BDe mainly differ in the penalty term. The penalty term for BIC is presented in the second row where q_i is the number of possible values of PA_i, r_i is the number of possible values for X_i and N is number of examples (5114×5). Hence the BIC penalty is linear in the number of independent parameters and logarithmic in the

---

[2] When the combination induces intra-slice cycles, we randomly remove one edge.

number of instances. BDe penalty is presented in third row where $\mathcal{D}_{ijk}$ is the number of times $X_i = k$ and $PA_i = j$ in $\mathcal{D}$, and $\alpha_{ij} = \sum_k \alpha_{ijk}$ with $\alpha_{ijk} = \frac{\alpha}{q_i r_i}$ in order to assign equal scores to different Bayesian network structures that encode the same independence assumptions. Ignoring the details, the key is that the complexity of BIC score is independent of the data distribution, and only depend on the arity of random variables and the arcs among them while the BDe score is dependent on the data and controlled by the hyperparameters α_{ijk}. For more details, we refer to [3]. Instead of calculating the log-likelihood, MIT score (Table.1 last row) uses mutual information to evaluate the goodness-of-fit [5]. $I(X_i, PA_i)$ is the mutual information between X_i and its parents. $\chi_{\alpha, l_{i\sigma_i(j)}}$ is chi-square distribution at significance level $1 - \alpha$. We refer to [5] for more details.

Table 1. The different scoring functions

$DPLL(\mathcal{B}, \mathcal{D})$	$DPLL(\mathcal{B}, \mathcal{D}) = \sum_i^n [\sum_l^N \log P(\mathcal{D}_{il}\|PA_{il}) - Penalty(X_i, \mathcal{B}, \mathcal{D})]$
	$Penalty_{BIC}(X_i, \mathcal{B}, \mathcal{D}) = \frac{q_i(r_i - 1)}{2} \log N$
	$Penalty_{BDe}(X_i, \mathcal{B}, \mathcal{D}) = \sum_j^{q_i} \sum_k^{r_i} \log \frac{P(\mathcal{D}_{ijk}\|\mathcal{D}_{ij})}{P(\mathcal{D}_{ijk}\|\mathcal{D}_{ij}, \alpha_{ij})}$
$DPMI(\mathcal{B}, \mathcal{D})$	$S_{MIT}(\mathcal{B}, \mathcal{D}) = \sum_{i, PA_i \neq \emptyset} 2N * I(X_i, PA_i) - \sum_{i, PA_i \neq \emptyset} \sum_j^{q_i} \chi_{\alpha, l_{i\sigma_i(j)}}$

4 Experiments

For the DBN DPLL-structure learning, we extended the BDAGL package of Murphy et al. [2] to allow learning from multi-series dynamic data and to support learning with BIC score function. We also adapted DPMI-structure learning by exploiting the GlobalMIT package which was used to model multi-series data from gene expression [5]. The learned DBN structure is shown in Figure.2. Note that all three score metrics learned the self-link for every variable. This shows that many socio-demographic factors are influenced by previous behavior(5 years backward). Observe that both BIC and BDe learned the inter-slice dependency between "Smoke" and "CAC" level. Both BIC and MI returned a temporal correlation between "Exercise" and "CAC", which indicates that previous health behaviors have strong influence on the risk of CAC in current time.

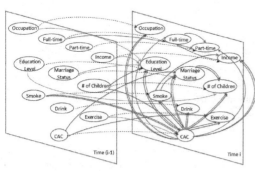

Fig. 2. Combined DBN model. The blue arcs are learned by DPLL-BDe; reds by DPLL-BIC; greens by DPMI; black dash lines are self-links are learned by all three.

Then we combined the structure from the different learning approaches into a comprehensive model for learning parameters. We applied this DBN to test data and predict the CAC score based on the variables in the current and previous time steps. As CAC score from previous time-steps is highly predictive of future values, we hid the CAC-scores in the test set for fair evaluation.

We calculated the accuracy, AUC-ROC as well as F measure[3] to evaluate the independent and mixed models learned by different score functions. The results are shown in Table.2. As the table shows, the model learned by BDe score has the best performance while the MI the worst. We also performed t-test on the five folds results, which shows the BDe is significantly better than MI with P-values at $0.0014(AUC)$, $0.0247(Accuracy)$ and $5.7784 \times 10^{-6}(F)$. In order to rule out the possibility that the better performance of BDe is resulted from the non-temporal information which MI does not have, we also experimented on BNs with intra-slice arcs only as well as DBNs with inter-slice arcs only. And the results showed that the difference between them is not statistically significant at 5% significance level, in other word, the temporal information is as important as the non-temporal information in predicting the CAC level. Compared to BDe alone, the combined model has deteriorated performance. This is probably because the combined model has more arcs which exponentially increases the parameter space and the limited amount of training data cannot guarantee the accurate training for such high dimension model (possibly overfitting).

Table 2. Model Evaluation Results

	MI	BIC	BDe	MI+BIC	MI+BDe	BIC+BDe	MI+BIC+BDe	Inter-s	Intra-s
Accuracy	0.5774	0.6558	**0.6805**	0.6482	0.6715	0.6701	0.6600	0.5774	0.5853
AUC-ROC	0.4870	0.6979	**0.7139**	0.6473	0.6809	0.7092	0.6581	0.6013	0.6489
F measure	0	0.5417	**0.6144**	0.4640	0.5632	0.5880	0.5244	0.0005	0.0501

Future Work: While our work generatively models all the variables across the different years, extending this work to predict CAC-levels discriminatively remains an interesting direction. Considering more risk factors and more sophisticated algorithms which allows learning temporal influence jumping through multiple time slices is another direction. The end goal is the development of interventions that can reduce the risk of CVDs in young adults.

Acknowledgments:. The Coronary Artery Risk Development in Young Adults Study (CARDIA) is supported by contracts HHSN268201300025C, HHSN268201300026C, HHSN268201300027C, HHSN268201300028C, HHSN268201300029C, and HHSN268200900041C from the National Heart, Lung, and Blood Institute (NHLBI), the Intramural Research Program of the National Institute on Aging (NIA), and an intra-agency agreement between NIA and NHLBI (AG0005). SY and SN gratefully acknowledge National Science Foundation grant no. IIS-1343940.

---

[3] Accuracy $= (TP+TN)/(P+N)$; $F = 2TP/(2TP+FP+FN)$

References

1. Detrano, R., Guerci, A.D., Carr, J.J., et al.: Coronary calcium as a predictor of coronary events in four racial or ethnic groups. New England Journal of Medicine 358(13), 1336–1345 (2008)
2. Eaton, D., Murphy, K.: Bayesian structure learning using dynamic programming and MCMC. In: UAI (2007)
3. Koller, D., Friedman, N.: Probabilistic Graphical Models: Principles and Techniques. MIT Press (2009)
4. Liu, Z., Malone, B.M., Yuan, C.: Empirical evaluation of scoring functions for bayesian network model selection. BMC Bioinformatics 13(S-15), S14 (2012)
5. Vinh, N.X., Chetty, M., Coppel, R.L., et al.: Globalmit: learning globally optimal dynamic bayesian network with the mutual information test criterion. Bioinformatics 27(19), 2765–2766 (2011)

Running Genome Wide Data Analysis Using a Parallel Approach on a Cloud Platform

Andrea Demartini[1](✉), Davide Capozzi[2,4], Alberto Malovini[1,2,3]
and Riccardo Bellazzi[1,2,3]

[1] University of Pavia, Pavia, Italy
andrea.demartini01@universitadipavia.it
[2] Biomeris s.r.l., Pavia, Italy
[3] IRCCS Fondazione Salvatore Maugeri, Pavia, Italy
[4] Spindox s.p.a., Milano, Italy

Abstract. Hierarchical Naïve Bayes (HNB) is a multivariate classification algorithm that can be used to forecast the probability of a specific disease by analysing a set of Single Nucleotide Polymorphisms (SNPs). In this paper we present the implementation of HNB using a parallel approach based on the Map-Reduce paradigm built natively on the Hadoop framework, relying on the Amazon Cloud Infrastructure. We tested our approach on two GWAS datasets aimed at identifying the genetic bases of Type 1 (T1D) and Type 2 Diabetes (T2D). Both datasets include individual level data of 1,900 cases and 1,500 controls with ~ 420,000 SNPs. For T2D the best results were obtained using the complete set of SNPs, whereas for T1D the best performances were reached using few SNPs selected through standard univariate association tests. Our cloud-based implementation allows running genome wide simulations cutting down computational time and overall infrastructure costs.

Keywords: Map reduce · Cloud computing · Data mining algorithm · Genome-wide association studies

1 Introduction

In the last few years, the term "Big Data" has been extensively used in the field of genomics; as a matter of fact, thanks to the novel high throughput sequencing techniques, huge amounts of data can be quickly generated from a single individual. However, due to the high computational capacity required to process this type of data, the majority of the analytical approaches are still based on the use of feature selection techniques aimed at reducing the problem dimensionality allowing to perform data mining analyses on a much smaller set of attributes. This approach is often not appropriate, in particular when studying complex traits diseases, since their clinical expression can be considered as the consequence of multiple causes, meaning that every measured variable may give an even small contribution to the overall impact on the phenotype. Recently, we proposed a multivariate classification algorithm to deal with

© Springer International Publishing Switzerland 2015
J.H. Holmes et al. (Eds.): AIME 2015, LNAI 9105, pp. 188–192, 2015.
DOI: 10.1007/978-3-319-19551-3_25

complex–trait diseases, called Hierarchical Naïve Bayes (HNB) [1]. The HNB is able to forecast the individual-level probability of a specific disease, based on the analysis of a set of Single Nucleotide Polymorphisms (SNPs). To test the usefulness of exploiting genetic information collected from the whole genome, we decided to apply the HNB to the analysis of two Genome Wide Association Studies (GWAS) datasets, each characterized by more than 400K SNPs.

In this paper we describe the parallel approach we developed for HBN implementation. With this approach it has been possible to distribute the computational load among a cluster of machines, greatly reducing the overall time needed for the analysis. Since the IT infrastructures needed to run parallel computation are very expensive, we exploited the services offered by a cloud computing platform.

2   Methods

2.1   Classification Algorithm

The Hierarchical Naïve Bayes (HNB) is an extension of the traditional Naïve Bayes classifier. HNB uses a multivariate approach thanks to its hierarchical structure that introduces a further abstraction level. The individual SNPs are not used as independent predictors, but they are grouped into blocks according to their structural correlation. To this end, SNPs with strong structural correlation ($r2>0.8$) and localized at a maximum pairwise distance of 500kb are grouped into blocks. The idea behind this approach is that variables belonging to the same block can be considered as replicates generated by the same information source. The SNPs are thus modeled as random variables having the same probability distribution, whose parameters are sample-related and thus called individual parameters. Individual parameters related to subjects belonging to the same class (e.g. cases or controls) are seen, in turn, as random variables having the same distribution, whose parameters (hyperparameters) are population-related. Therefore, the algorithm is made up of a training phase and a test phase. The estimation of the hyperparameters corresponding to each class and block is performed during the training phase, while during the test phase each block provides a contribution to the marginal likelihood (and thus to the posterior probability) of the subjects under analysis.

2.2   Parallel Algorithm Implementation

Our implementation of HNB algorithm is based on the Map-Reduce paradigm [2], a well-known programming model that allows distributing the computation on different cores of a network of machines. According to this approach, the data have to be split into fragments of more or less equivalent size, each passed as an input to a software object named Mapper. Many Mappers can run simultaneously on different machines since there are no dependencies among them. Input files are seen as key-value pairs and, for each of them, the Mappers can generate one or more key-value pairs as output. After an aggregation phase, each of the newly generated keys, with all its associated values, is passed as input to other software objects, named Reducers, which operate the final processing.

The distribution of the tasks among the cluster is operated by a special and unique node named master, instead all the other cores, the ones who actually make the computation, are called slaves.

The parallel implementation of HNB is a sequence of three steps, each one carried out through a sequence of Map-Reduce tasks (Figure 1). Since the 10-fold cross-validation was adopted as the model validation strategy, the program is designed to first partition the input data into 10 parts of approximately equivalent size. This operation has been implemented through 2 Map-Reduce tasks.

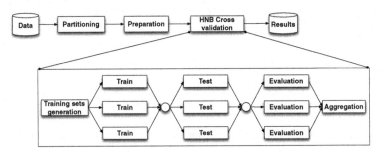

Fig. 1. Flowchart showing the main steps of the program, with focus on the parallelization of the cross validation step

Since both training and testing steps need variables aggregated on the basis of a block definition, a preparation step was introduced, composed of a single Map Reduce task. The newly generated dataset was then used as input of the HNB algorithm. In order to maximize parallelism the program has been designed to perform simultaneous calculations for all the folds. To parallelize the training steps, the first task executed during this phase is the generation of the training sets, obtained by merging all the possible combination of nine out of ten folds. All the parameters are then estimated in parallel through a Map-Reduce task that properly exploits the key-value mechanism to also keep track of the folds association. The following steps are the test task, focused on the computation of the posterior probabilities for each example, and the evaluation task, during which the classification performances of the model are assessed for each fold. Finally, an aggregation step is performed to compute the averages and the confidence intervals of all the statistics previously calculated on the single folds.

For the implementation of the program described above, we used the Hadoop framework [3], one of the most common implementations of the Map-Reduce paradigm. It consists of a set of Java libraries, produced by the Apache Software Foundation, that deal with the distribution and management of the individual map and reduce tasks, providing mechanisms for balancing the workload among all the cluster nodes. Therefore, our work was focused on the definition of the single Map-Reduce steps and on the implementation of the single map and reduce functions in Java.

2.3   Program Deploying

As regards the computational resources, we exploited the Amazon Web Services (AWS), a cloud computing platform that allows the user to get computation resources on demand with high performance and high IT security standards. Both input data and source code were uploaded on a bucket of the Amazon Simple Storage Service (S3). Exploiting the Amazon Elastic Map-Reduce service (EMR), it has been possible to build on demand a custom Hadoop cluster in few minutes. In this way, it has been possible to deploy the algorithm on an un-expensive parallel computational infrastructure without the need of owning a physical cluster of machines.

3   Results

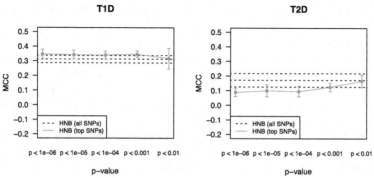

Fig. 2. Results for T1D and T2D in terms of MCC, filtering the datasets with different p-values

We tested our approach on two real GWAS datasets generated by the Wellcome Trust Case Control Consortium (WTCCC) and aimed at identifying the genetic bases of Type 1 Diabetes (T1D) and Type 2 Diabetes (T2D) respectively. Both datasets were represented by individual level data regarding approximately 1,900 cases and 1,500 controls, characterized by 420,000 SNPs (for details about data quality control the reader is referred to [1]). The mean Matthews correlation coefficient (MCC) estimated over the 10 test sets was 0.312 (95% CI = 0.286, 0.338) for the T1D and 0.171 (95% CI = 0.125, 0.217) for the T2D dataset. These results were compared to the ones obtained by running the same analyses after filtering the whole genome set of SNPs according to different significance thresholds, from $p < 10\text{-}6$ to $p < 0.01$, based on standard univariate association tests performed on each training set (Figure 2). Results from the analysis of T1D data show that the best classification performances are reached using few SNPs passing $p < 10\text{-}6$ (MCC = 0.347, 95% CI = 0.315 - 0.379). On the opposite, results from T2D data show that the highest MCC is obtained by considering the complete set of SNPs, even if very close performances can be reached by considering the SNPs passing $p < 0.01$ (MCC = 0.166, 95% CI = 0.124-0.208). The program was tested both on a local computer and on the AWS cloud platform.

As regards the first solution, a laptop with a 2.2 GHz Intel Core i7 processor and 8 GB of RAM was used, which took nearly 13 hours to complete a single simulation. On the AWS platform, 2 instance types were used. In particular, for the master we chose the m1.small instance (1 virtual CPU and 1.7 GB of RAM) and for the slave we chose the m3.xlarge instance (4 virtual CPU and 15 GB of RAM). Two different simulations were evaluated, using a different number of slave cores: 2 and 5. With 2 slaves, the cluster took 5.5 hours, for a total cost of 4.53$, while with 5 slaves it took 2.5 hours, for an overall cost of 5.42$.

4   Discussion

In this work we have shown the possibility of running analysis on complete SNP set coming from whole genome studies using a parallel implementation of the HNB classification algorithm. From the biological point of view, results highlighted a different behavior in the two analyzed datasets. In the case of the T1D dataset the results seem to worsen by adding variables showing weak univariate statistical association, whereas for T2D the overall classification performance improve if all the variables are included in the model. These results suggest that adding more variables may increase the discriminative power of classification models for complex-trait diseases but it can also add more noise, especially when the majority of the information is contained in few variables, as in the case of T1D.

From a technological perspective, our implementation based on a distributed approach shows the feasibility of analyzing this type of data using all the information available and thus without the necessity of a pre-processing step for feature selection. Moreover we showed how the need for computational resources can be easily fulfilled by a cloud computing platform. Relying on a cloud solution allows users to run complete analysis in a short time, on a secure and not expensive infrastructure and without the need of buying a physical cluster of machines.

Acknowledgements. This study makes use of data generated by the WTCCC. A full list of the investigators who contributed to the generation of the data is available from http://www.wtccc.uk. Funding for the project was provided by the Wellcome Trust under award 076113. Cloud resources have been supported by Amazon Web Services in Education Research Grant award.

References

1. Malovini, A., et al.: BMC Bioinformatics (13 suppl.14), S6 (2012)
2. Dean, J., Ghemawat, S.: MapReduce: simplified data processing on large clusters. Communications of the ACM 51(1), 107–113 (2008)
3. Shvachko, K., et al.: The hadoop distributed file system. In: 2010 IEEE 26th Symposium on Mass Storage Systems and Technologies (MSST). IEEE (2010)

Text Mining

Extracting Adverse Drug Events from Text Using Human Advice

Phillip Odom[1(✉)], Vishal Bangera[1], Tushar Khot[2], David Page[3],
and Sriraam Natarajan[1]

[1] Indiana University Bloomington, Bloomington, USA
phodom@indiana.edu
[2] Allen Institute of AI, Seattle, USA
[3] University of Madison-Wisconsin, Madison, USA

Abstract. Adverse drug events (ADEs) are a major concern and point of emphasis for the medical profession, government, and society in general. When methods extract ADEs from observational data, there is a necessity to evaluate these methods. More precisely, it is important to know what is already known in the literature. Consequently, we employ a novel relation extraction technique based on a recently developed probabilistic logic learning algorithm that exploits human advice. We demonstrate on a standard adverse drug events data base that the proposed approach can successfully extract existing adverse drug events from limited amount of training data and compares favorably with state-of-the-art probabilistic logic learning methods.

1 Introduction

Adverse drug events (ADE) are one of the major causes of death in the world. For instance, nearly 11% of hospital admissions of older adults in US are attributed to ADEs [5]. Consequently there has been an increase in focus and application of statistical learning algorithms for detecting ADEs from data such as Electronic Health Records (EHRs) and clinical studies [16]. While there is a plethora of research on detecting them from clinical data, there are not many methods that can validate the output of these algorithms except for manually scanning through the ADEs. In this case, the burden is on the expert to evaluate these extracted ADEs by knowing all the ones published in the literature.

We explore the use of published medical abstracts to serve as ground truth for evaluation and present a method for effectively extracting the ADEs from published abstracts. To this effect, we adapt and apply a recently successful machine learning algorithm [15] that uses a human expert (say a physician) as more than a "mere labeler", i.e., the human expert in our system is not restricted to merely specify which of the drug event pairs are true ADEs. Instead, the human expert would "teach" the system much like a human student by specifying patterns that he/she would look for in the papers. These patterns are employed as advice by the learning system that seamlessly integrates this advice with training examples to learn a robust classifier.

© Springer International Publishing Switzerland 2015
J.H. Holmes et al. (Eds.): AIME 2015, LNAI 9105, pp. 195–204, 2015.
DOI: 10.1007/978-3-319-19551-3_26

More precisely, given a set of ADE pairs (drug-event pairs), we build upon an NLP pipeline [12] to rank the ADE pairs based on the proof found in the literature. Our system first searches for PubMed abstracts that are relevant to the current set of ADE pairs. For each ADE pair, these abstracts are then parsed through a standard NLP parser (we use Stanford NLP parser [3], [10]) and the linguistic features such as parse trees, dependency graphs, word lemmas and n-grams etc. are generated. These features are then used as input to a relational classifier for learning to detect ADEs from text. The specific relational classifier that we use for this purpose is called Relational Functional Gradient-Boosting (RFGB) classifier [14]. The advantage of employing this classifier over standard machine learning classifiers such as decision-trees [11], SVMs [2] and boosting [17] is that RFGB does not assume a flat-feature vector representation for learning. This is important in our current setting as it is unreasonable to expect the same number of abstracts for each ADE pair. More importantly, it is not correct to expect the same type of parse trees and dependency graphs for each article (as each set of authors can have a different style). The presence of this diverse set (and number) of features necessitates the use of a classifier that can leverage a richer representation that is more natural to model the underlying data. Needless to say, relational representations have been successful in modeling the true nature of the data and we adapt the state-of-the-art relational learning algorithm.

While powerful, standard learning will not suffice for the challenging task of extracting ADEs as we will show empirically. The key reason is that we do not have sufficient number of training examples to learn a robust classifier. Also, the number of linguistic features can be exponential in the number of examples and hence learning a classifier in this hugely imbalanced space can possibly yield sub-optimal results. To alleviate this imbalance and guide the learner to a robust prediction model, we explore the use of human guidance as advice to the algorithm. This advice could be in terms of specific patterns in text. For instance it is natural to say something like, "if the phrase *no evidence* is present between the drug and event in the sentence then it is more likely that the given ADE is not a true ADE". The learning algorithm can then identify the appropriate set of features (from the dependency graph) and make the ADE pair more likely to be a negative example. As we have shown in non-textual domains [15], this type of advice is robust both to noisy training examples as well as for a small number of training examples. We adapt and extend the previous work for textual data.

To summarize, we make several key contributions: first is that we develop a robust method that can automatically learn a classifier for detecting ADEs from text. This goes beyond current state-of-the-art methods that employ a hand-crafted classifier such as conditional random fields (CRF) [6]. Second, we lessen the burden on human experts by allowing them to provide some generalized advice instead of the mundane task of manually labeling a huge number of learning examples. Also, it removes the burden of designing a specific classifier such as CRF or a SVM for the task. Effectively, our expert is required to be a domain expert (who understands medical texts) instead of machine learning expert who needs to carefully design the underlying model and set the parameters. Finally, we evaluate the learning method on a corpus of available ADEs and empirically demonstrate the superiority of the proposed approach over the alternatives.

The rest of the paper is organized as follows: we present the background on the learning algorithms (with advice) next. We follow this with a discussion on how these algorithms are adapted to our specific task. We then present the empirical evaluations before concluding by outlining areas for future research.

2 Prior Work on Learning Relational Models

We now present our prior work on relational classifiers that we build upon in this work. We first present Relational Functional Gradient Boosting (RFGB) [14] and its extension to handle expert knowledge [15].

2.1 RFGB

Before outlining the algorithms that we employ, we will present them in the standard machine learning setting. Gradient ascent is the standard technique for learning the parameters of a model and typically starts with initial parameters θ_0 and computes the gradient (Δ_1) of an objective function w.r.t. θ_0. The gradient term is then added to the parameters θ_0 and the gradient ascent is performed for the new parameter value $\theta_1 = \theta_0 + \Delta_1$ and repeated till convergence. Friedman [4] proposed an alternate approach where the objective function is represented using a regression function ψ over the examples $\mathbf{x}$ and the gradients are performed with respect to $\psi(x)$. Similar to parametric gradient descent, the final function after n iterations of functional gradient-descent is the sum of the gradients, i.e., $\psi_n(x) = \psi_0(x) + \Delta_1(x) + \cdots + \Delta_n(x)$. Each gradient term (Δ_m) is a regression function over the training examples (E) and the gradients at the mth iteration can be represented as $\langle x_i, \Delta_m(x_i) \rangle$ where $x_i \in E$.

Rather than directly using $\langle x_i, \Delta_m(x_i) \rangle$ as the gradient function (memorization), functional gradient descent *generalizes* by fitting a regression function $\hat{\psi}_m$ (generally regression trees) to the gradients Δ_m. The $\hat{\psi}_m$ function uses the features of the example x to fit a regression function to $\Delta_m(x)$. For example, to predict the relationship between an example drug-effect pair in a sentence, the dependency paths and the words connecting the drug-effect pair would be the features used to learn the regression function. The final model $\psi_m = \psi_0 + \hat{\psi}_1 + \cdots + \hat{\psi}_m$ is a sum over these regression trees. Functional-gradient ascent is also known as functional-gradient boosting (FGB) due to this sequential nature of learning models based on the previous iteration.

But standard FGB assumes the examples have a flat feature representation. However, as mentioned earlier, each sentence can have structured features such as dependency path structure and parse trees leading to different number of features for every example in a flat representation. Relational models can handle data by using first-order logic representation. E.g., "prep_of" dependency between words "cause" and "MI" can be represented as prep_of(cause, MI).

FGB has been extended to relational models [14], [8], [9], [13] to simultaneously learn the structure and parameters of these models. Relational examples are groundings/instantiations (e.g. drug-event(aspirin, headache)) of the predicates/relations (e.g. drug-event) to be learned. The ψ function is represented by relational regression trees (RRT)[1] which uses the structured data as input in the trees. A standard objective function used in RFGB is the log-likelihood and the probability of an example is represented as a sigmoid over the ψ function [14]. They showed that the functional gradient of likelihood w.r.t. ψ is

$$\frac{\partial log P(\mathbf{X} = \mathbf{x})}{\partial \psi(x_i)} = I(y_i = 1) - P(y_i = 1; x_i, Pa(x_i)) \tag{1}$$

which is the difference between the true distribution (I is the indicator function) and the current predicted distribution. A sample relational regression tree for $target(X)$ is shown in Figure 1.

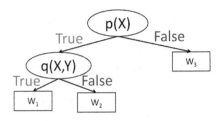

Fig. 1. Relational regression tree for a target predicate of interest, such as target(X) where p(X) and q(X, Y) are the features used. w_1 is the weight returned for target(x), if p(x) is true and q(x, Y) is true for some value of Y. X and Y are variables and can be instantiated with values such as "aspirin","headache" etc.

2.2   Relational Advice

While effective, the above method requires a large number of manually annotated examples. This translates to requiring a human to manually annotate every mention of a positive ADE pair and possibly several negatives. This is unreasonable and limits the human expert to be a *mere labeler*. It would be more practical for the human to provide some sort of advice. An example could be to "extract all positive ADEs even at the cost of some false positives". This is a cost-sensitive advice and we have explored this in the context of RFGB [18]. While effective, this advice is restricted to a trade-off between false positives and false negatives.

Human experts are capable of specifying richer advice. For instance, it is more reasonable to specify that *if the same sentence has an event word and a drug with a word cause somewhere in their path, then it is more likely that it is an adverse event*. We have recently developed a formulation based on RFGB that can handle such advice [15].

Our gradients contain an extra term compared to RFGB.

$$\Delta(x_i) = \alpha \cdot (I(y_i = 1) - P(y_i = 1; \psi)) + (1 - \alpha) \cdot [n_t(x_i) - n_f(x_i)]$$

where n_t is number of advice rules that prefer the example x_i to be true and n_f that prefer it to be false. Hence, the gradient consists of two parts: $(I - P)$ which is the gradient from the data and $(n_t - n_f)$ which is the gradient with respect to the advice.

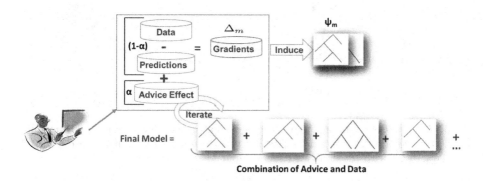

Fig. 2. Advice-based RFGB

Figure 2 presents the advice-based RFGB approach. Intuitively when the example label is preferred in more advice models than the avoided target, $n_t(x_i) - n_f(x_i)$ is set to be positive. This will result in pushing the gradient of these examples in the positive direction (towards $+\infty$). Conversely when the example label should be avoided in more advice models, $n_t(x_i) - n_f(x_i)$ is set to be negative which will result in pushing the gradient of this example in the negative direction (towards $-\infty$). Examples where the advice does not apply or has equally contradictory advice, $n_t(x_i) - n_f(x_i)$ is 0. Hence, this approach can also handle *conflicting advice for the same example*.

Consider the adverse drug event prediction task using the dependency paths from sentences. A sample advice in our formalism is:

$$object("cause", event) \land agent("cause", drug) \rightarrow adverse(drug, event)$$

where *adverse* is the preferred label for this advice[1].

3   Proposed Approach

Our approach aims to predict whether there is evidence in the medical literature that a drug is known to cause a particular event. As there are very few examples that we are provided with compared to the number of features, our system incorporates domain knowledge that could be employed to identify text patterns in sentences that suggest an event is caused by a given drug. As mentioned previously, such a system can be used by other ADE predictors to evaluate whether they have identified a previously known drug and event. This would

---

[1] $\land$ is used to represent AND in logic.

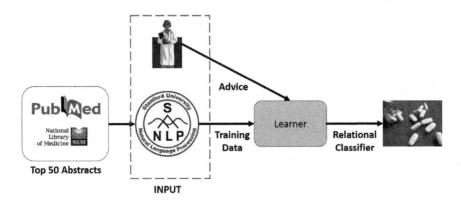

Fig. 3. Our proposed approach first finds medical abstracts that contain the drug and effect. Features are constructed by running them through the Stanford NLP parser. This data, along with the expert advice, is input to the learning algorithm.

allow a knowledge-base of known ADEs that is constantly updated with the latest medical knowledge.

Figure 3 shows the process of training a model to predict ADEs. The first step of this process starts with searching PubMed, the standard database of medical publications, for abstracts that contain names for both the drug as well as the event. A sample query that we use is "Angioedema Renal Failure". We collect the first 50 abstracts for our deeper analysis. Previous empirical analysis [12] showed that 50 publications were sufficient and going beyond 50 to 75 or 100 did not statistically improve the results. While PubMed contains many articles of varying degrees of quality, we restrict the search to only articles that have been verified by PubMed (MEDLINE). If a drug and event have more than 50 results, then only the top 50 are extracted.

The abstracts for these drug and events are then passed to the Stanford NLP parser that generates facts (relational features) that represent the known medical knowledge for these drug and events. The specific features that we extract are parse trees, dependency paths, word lemmas and bag-of-word features. These are the standard features used in NLP literature and hence we employ them as well. The key reason for considering a relational representation is that the chances of two parse trees and/or dependency paths to look similar is minimal. Instead of carefully standardizing the features, relational models allow for learning using their natural representations. To summarize, for every ADE pair, the top 50 abstracts are parsed through the NLP parser and the corresponding features are then given as training data to the next step – the relational learning algorithm.

The learning algorithm has two sources of input: the training data and the expert domain knowledge. The training data is generated from a database (described in Section 4) of drug and event pairs that are either known to or known not to be ADEs. The second source of input is the expert domain knowledge. This knowledge should capture the terminology by which medical experts express whether or not a drug and effect are related. For instance, "drug A causes event B" or "drug A is caused by event B" are two sample sentences that could have been used in abstracts. These are then used as advice to express that a drug causes a particular event. This knowledge is key to overcome the few training examples from which to learn. Note that soliciting advice is less costly than labeling more examples. We use 10 similar statements. For the purposes of this work, we as English speakers, served as the domain expert and wrote these rules. These rules were then used as advice by the learning algorithm for learning a set of relational regression trees that will serve as the model.

Once the learning phase is complete, the model can then be queried for inferring unseen ADEs from published, medical literature. This will become the test phase of our approach. Given, a new set of ADEs, the method automatically searches PubMed, constructs the NLP features and queries the model. The model in turn returns $P(ade(drug, event)|evidence)$ i.e., it returns the posterior probability of the drug-event pair being an ADE given the scientific evidence. Since all the evidence is observed, performing inference requires simply querying all the relational regression trees, summing up their regression values and returning the posterior estimates.

We must mention a few salient features of the proposed system (1) As more medical papers are published, the evidence of a drug causing an event can change and the system can automatically update its prediction resulting in an efficient refinement of medically known ADEs. (2) The nature of the formulation allows for contradicting and imprecise advice from domain experts. This allows for multiple experts to provide their inputs and our algorithm can automatically learn which of these are valid and which are not. (3) The use of richer advice enables for potentially weighing the different medical literature as well. For instance, it is possible to specify that "Journal X is more prestigious than Journal Y and hence trust it more than Y". This type of advice can also allow for specifying that more recent findings can potentially be more correct than older ones.

In summary, we have outlined a powerful system that allows for seamless human advice taking learning system that can automatically infer if a given drug-event pair has evidence in the literature to be an ADE.

4   Experiments

Our experimental results focus on three key questions:

Q1: How effective is the ADE extraction from text?

Q2: Can domain experts provide useful knowledge to extract evidence about ADEs from medical abstracts?

Q3: How effective is our method in incorporating advice into learned model?

Methods Considered: We compare our method (called *Adv-RFGB* in the results) to three different baseline approaches. Both approaches, *MLN-Boost* and *RDN-Boost*, learn only from the data without considering the expert knowledge. The third baseline that we considered is Alchemy[2], the state-of-the-art structure

---

[2] alchemy.cs.washington.edu

learning package for learning relational probabilistic models. The goal of this comparison is to establish the value of the expert knowledge (i.e., answer **Q2**).

Experimental Setup: The drug and event pairs come from Observational Medical Outcomes Partnership [3] 2010 ground truth, a manually curated database. To facilitate evaluation and comparison of methods and databases, OMOP established a common data model so that disparate databases could be represented uniformly. This included definitions for ten ADE-associated health outcomes of interest (HOIs) and drug exposure eras for ten widely-used classes of drugs.

Since this OMOP data includes very few positive examples (10 to be precise), we investigated other positive examples found in the literature to increase the training set. Our final dataset that we built contains 39 positive and 1482 negative examples (i.e.,39×38, the cross-product of all drug-effect pairs and obtained the ones that are not true ADE). The abstracts that we collected for the drug and event pairs contained 5198 sentences. Note that some drug and event pairs were not mentioned in any abstracts. In all experiments, we performed 4-fold cross validation. We compare both area under the curve for ROC and PR curves.

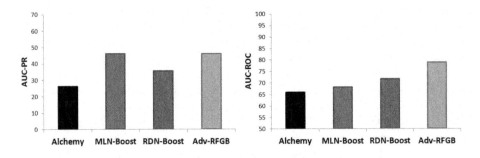

Fig. 4. Experimental results for predicting ADEs

Results: The results are presented in figure 4. The first three graphs present the results of using only data and employing standard relational learning methods. As can be seen, our proposed method that also employs "human advice" outperforms the three baselines that do not incorporate advice - (*RDN-Boost*, *MLN-Boost*, and *Alchemy*). This highlights the high value that the expert knowledge can have when learning with few training examples and thus answers **Q2**. **Q1** and **Q3** can also be answered affirmatively in that our proposed method is effectively learning with a high degree of accuracy to predict from the text abstracts. It is also clear that the advice is effectively incorporated when compared to merely using the data for learning and inference.

We investigated the differences between our predictions and the OMOP ground truth to understand whether our method was truly effective. One key example where our method predicted an ADE pair to be positive, but OMOP labeled it as a negative ADE pair was: **Bisphosphonate** causes **Acute Renal Failure**. Our

---

[3] http://omop.org/

method predicted it as an ADE with a high (98.5%) probability. We attempted to validate our prediction and were able to find evidence in the literature to support our prediction. As an example, PubMed article (PMID 11887832) contains the sentence:

Bisphosphonates have several important toxicities: **acute renal failure**, worsening renal function, reduced bone mineralization, and osteomalacia.

This suggests that our method (1) is able to find some evidence to support its prediction and (2) is capable of incorporating novel medical findings.

5   Discussion

Extracting ADEs from medical text has been an active area for recent research [7], [12]. Kang et al.'s method relied on a dictionary system to identify the drugs and effects in the sentence and a knowledge graph to semantically identify if any relationship was present between drug and effect. We allow human advice to guide our learning algorithm as opposed to using previously defined knowledge-bases. Natarajan et al. first use a human expert to define a full model that can just be queried and not learned. They use the expert advice as a prior and then refine that model according to the data. In comparison, we learn from human advice and training data jointly to learn a more robust model in the presence of noisy evidence. Our proposed approach builds upon a recently successful probabilistic learning algorithm that exploits domain knowledge. We adapted an NLP pipeline that allows for this learning method to search for PubMed abstracts, construct appropriate NLP features and learn a model by seamlessly taking human advice. Our experimental evaluation on the standard OMOP data set showed that this approach effectively and efficiently exploits human advice.

There are several possible directions for future work. In this work, we assume ADE pairs but extending this to multiple drugs and multiple events is not difficult and we plan to pursue this next. Also, we only consider abstracts but considering the full text of articles remains an interesting direction. As we have shown even with only abstracts, there is an imbalance in the number of examples vs the number of features. This dimensional disparity can potentially grow exponentially with full text. Extending our learning algorithms to handle this huge dimension is another direction. Finally, understanding if it is possible to unearth novel ADEs by "reading between lines" of text articles remains an exciting and potentially game-changing future direction of research.

Acknowledgements. SN and PO thank Army Research Office (ARO) grant number W911NF-13-1-0432 under the Young Investigator Program. SN gratefully acknowledges the support of the DARPA DEFT Program under the Air Force Research Laboratory (AFRL) prime contract no. FA8750-13-2-0039. Any opinions, findings, and conclusion or recommendations expressed in this material are those of the authors and do not necessarily reflect the view of the DARPA, ARO, AFRL, or the US government.

References

1. Blockeel, H.: Top-down induction of first order logical decision trees. AI Communications 12(1-2) (1999)
2. Cristianini, N.: Shawe-Taylor: An Introduction to Support Vector Machines and Other Kernel-based Learning Methods. Cambridge University Press (2000)
3. Finkel, J., Grenager, T., Manning, C.: Incorporating non-local information into information extraction systems by gibbs sampling. In: Proceedings of the 43rd Annual Meeting on Association for Computational Linguistics, ACL 2005, pp. 363–370. Association for Computational Linguistics (2005)
4. Friedman, J.: Greedy function approximation: A gradient boosting machine. In: Annals of Statistics (2001)
5. Gurwitz, J., Field, T., L, Harrold, R.J., Kebellis, K., Seger, A.: Incidence and preventability of adverse drug events among older persons in the ambulatory setting. JAMA 289 (2003)
6. Gutmann, B., Kersting, K.: TildeCRF: Conditional random fields for logical sequences. In: Fürnkranz, J., Scheffer, T., Spiliopoulou, M. (eds.) ECML 2006. LNCS (LNAI), vol. 4212, pp. 174–185. Springer, Heidelberg (2006)
7. Kang, N., Singh, B., Bui, C., Afzal, Z., van Mulligen, E.M., Kors, J.: Knowledge-based extraction of adverse drug events from biomedical text. BMC Bioinformatics 15 (2014)
8. Karwath, A., Kersting, K., Landwehr, N.: Boosting relational sequence alignments. In: ICDM (2008)
9. Kersting, K., Driessens, K.: Non-parametric policy gradients: A unified treatment of propositional and relational domains. In: ICML (2008)
10. Klein, D., Manning, C.: Accurate unlexicalized parsing. In: Proceedings of the 41st Annual Meeting on Association for Computational Linguistics, vol. 1, pp. 423–430. Association for Computational Linguistics (2003)
11. Mitchell, T.: Machine Learning. McGraw-Hill (1997)
12. Natarajan, S., Bangera, V., Khot, T., Picado, J.: et al.: A novel text-based method for evaluation of adverse drug event discovery. Journal of Biomedical Informatics (2015) (under review)
13. Natarajan, S., Joshi, S., Tadepalli, P., Kersting, K., Shavlik, J.: Imitation learning in relational domains: A functional-gradient boosting approach. In: IJCAI (2011)
14. Natarajan, S., Khot, T., Kersting, K., Gutmann, B., Shavlik, J.: Gradient-based boosting for statistical relational learning: The relational dependency network case. Machine Learning 86(1) (2012)
15. Odom, P., Khot, T., Porter, R., Natarajan, S.: Knowledge-based probabilistic logic learning. In: AAAI (2015)
16. Ryan, P., Welebob, E., Hartzema, A.G., Stang, P., Overhage, J.M.: Surveying us observational data sources and characteristics for drug safety needs. Pharmaceutical Medicine, 231–238 (2010)
17. Schapire, R., Freund, Y.: Boosting: Foundations and Algorithms. MIT Press (2012)
18. Yang, S., Khot, T., Kersting, K., Kunapuli, G., Hauser, K., Natarajan, S.: Learning from imbalanced data in relational domains: A soft margin approach. In: ICDM (2014)

An Analysis of Twitter Data on E-cigarette Sentiments and Promotion

Andreea Kamiana Godea[1](✉), Cornelia Caragea[1], Florin Adrian Bulgarov[1], and Suhasini Ramisetty-Mikler[2]

[1] Computer Science and Engineering, University of North Texas, Denton, TX, USA
{andreeagodea,florinbulgarov}@my.unt.edu, ccaragea@unt.edu
[2] Biostatistics and Epidemiology, University of North Texas Health Science Center, Fort Worth, TX, USA
Suhasini.Ramisetty-Mikler@Unthsc.edu

Abstract. We investigate general sentiments and information dissemination concerning *electronic cigarettes* or *e-cigs* using Twitter. E-cigs are relatively new products, and hence, not much research has been conducted in this area using large-scale social media data. However, the fact that e-cigs contain potentially dangerous substances makes them an interesting subject to study. In this paper, we propose novel features for e-cigs sentiment classification and create sentiment dictionaries relevant to e-cigs. We combine the proposed features with traditional features (i.e., bag-of-words and SentiStrength features) and use them in conjunction with supervised machine learning classifiers. The feature combination proves to be more effective than the traditional features for e-cigs sentiment classification. We also found that Twitter users are mainly concerned with sharing information (33%) and promoting e-cigs (22%). Although a low percentage of users share opinions, the majority of these users have positive opinions about e-cigs (11% positive, 3% negative).

Keywords: E-cigs · Sentiment analysis · Social networking sites · Twitter

1 Introduction

Much has been written concerning the effects of tobacco smoking on people's health. Research has shown that smoking is harmful to almost every organ in the human body and can cause people's deaths [1,2]. In particular, tobacco smoking results in more than 480,000 deaths every year in the United States [1,2,3]. Smoking is associated with many diseases such as cardiovascular and respiratory diseases, and cancer. Quitting smoking can help reduce the risk of such diseases and could boost people's lifespan. Electronic nicotine delivery systems (ENDS) such as *electronic cigarettes* or *e-cigs* have been recently introduced as an alternative way to using tobacco products. E-cigs provide a nicotine-containing aerosol to users by heating glycerol, nicotine, and flavoring agents [4].

It is not fully known yet if e-cigs are safer than tobacco cigarettes or if they are simply a way to develop addiction to nicotine, and hence, a gateway leading

© Springer International Publishing Switzerland 2015
J.H. Holmes et al. (Eds.): AIME 2015, LNAI 9105, pp. 205–215, 2015.
DOI: 10.1007/978-3-319-19551-3_27

non-smokers into smoking tobacco habits. However, recent progress has been made to reveal the negative effects of e-cigs on human health. For example, it has been shown that glycerol can produce mouth and throat irritation and dry cough [5]. Furthermore, despite that nicotine can help people feel calmer and more relaxed by reducing stress and anxiety, it has paradoxical effects, acting as a depressant [6]. Nicotine also has a negative impact on insulin resistance, which raises the risk of developing diabetes and heart diseases [7]. Despite these potentially negative effects of *e-cigs* on health, e-cigs have become a popular product in recent years. Their increasing popularity is in part due to the social context in which they occur (e.g., among friends), their availability in attractive flavors, and the perception of youth that e-cigs are safer than other nicotine products. The Centers for Disease Control and Prevention perform surveillance to monitor trends in the health of populations. National surveys such as National Youth Tobacco Survey and Youth Risk Behavior Surveys have recently begun to assess new and evolving health risk behaviors. However, trending behaviors are not comprised in such surveys, consequently resulting in the delay in recognizing the problem and its impact on the population health. Social networking sites appear to have embraced the attention in a unique way, being used as a tool for personal expression and freedom. Technological advancements allow online users to instantaneously share their experiences, sentiments and beliefs via blogs, micro-blogs (e.g., Twitter), discussion boards, etc., with peers and the public. Such social networking sites provide researchers a great opportunity to utilize alternate ways to analyze trending behaviors and sentiments shared by users.

In this study, we employ natural language processing and text-mining techniques to analyze the sentiment polarities expressed by Twitter users towards e-cigs and investigate how information is disseminated about these relatively new products. Twitter is now in the top 10 most visited Internet sites, which makes it an attractive platform to analyze sentiments and information spread.

2   Related Work

Sentiment analysis has been an actively researched area due to its importance in mining, analyzing and summarizing user opinions from online sites such as product review sites, forums, Facebook, and Twitter [8,9]. Sentiment analysis focuses on identifying the polarity (positive/negative) of a piece of text (often tied to a particular target). Here, we survey several sentiment analysis works.

Pang et al. [10] used supervised learning techniques on lexical features (e.g., unigrams, bigrams, part-of-speech tags) for sentiment analysis of movie reviews. Previous approaches based on lexicon rules exist that aim at aggregating sentiments for an entity [9,11]. Sentiment analysis has also been recently used in online health communities (OHCs). For example, Biyani et al. [12] performed sentiment classification of posts in a Cancer Survivors' Network to discover sentiment change patterns in its members and to detect factors affecting the change.

E-cigs have recently become the subject of several studies. For example, Bullen et al. [13] explored the effectiveness of e-cigs compared to nicotine patches in helping smokers to quit. The authors found no significant difference between e-cigs over nicotine patches. Popova and Ling [14] analyzed the correlation between e-cig usages among tobacco smokers and quit attempts. They found no substantiated evidence that e-cigs lead to smoking cessation. Myslín et al. [15] analyzed sentiments towards tobacco products from Twitter. They found that they are generally positive and are correlated with social image, personal experience, and recently popular products like hookah and e-cigs.

In contrast, our work is significantly different from the previous works. In this paper, we aim to study *"the voice of population"* concerning e-cigs by using Twitter data. Specifically, we seek to identify the general sentiments and information dissemination related to e-cigs, by implementing a supervised approach. For our task, we created domain-dependent sentiment dictionaries and designed new features based on polarity measures, user information and tweet structure.

3   Materials and Methods

Data Source and Analysis. For our study, we used Twitter data. We collected 105,605 tweets between March and April 2014 (using Twitter API), based on the following words: *e-cigs, electronic cigarette, vapor, vaping, e-juice, e-liquid and personal vaporizer*. We refer to these words as keywords throughout the paper. From the dataset, we manually annotated 1200 random tweets with the categories: *advertising, informational, opinion (positive and negative)* and *other*. The *advertising* category contains tweets shared with a commercial purpose, whereas the *informational* type refers to the ones providing general information. The *opinion* class was subdivided into *positive* and *negative* based on the overall sentiment about e-cigs. The *other* category consists of neutral or irrelevant tweets that could not be associated with any category above. Table 1 shows categories' names, the number of tweets in each category, the username and examples of tweets from each class. The keywords are encoded with bold.

Table 1. Examples of tweets from each category and categories distribution

Category	#Tweets	Username	Tweet content
Advertising	356	*TheVapeBook*	Great deals on Starter Kits. Save 10% - **Clearomizers** on Sale too! http://t.co/AMANIrXzte #ecig
Informational	339	*Forest_Smoking*	**E-cigs** now banned on all Dublin buses: "The news will come as a breath of fresh air for commuters"
Positive opinion	81	*SonnHardesty*	Oh how I enjoy the pleasure of **vaping**.
Negative opinion	54	*ksquarl*	**E-CIGS** ARE THE STUPIDEST THING I HAVE EXPERIENCED IN MY 15 YEARS OF EXISTENCE
Other	370	*Ernesto_Calva*	**Vaping** at the movies with the crew #BTC #betyoucandoitlikeme

Domain-Dependent Sentiment Dictionaries. Many previously proposed sentiment analysis approaches made use of dictionaries that contain words considered positive or negative in a general context (i.e. domain-independent dictionaries). However, our analysis indicated that many words that express a sentiment in a general context become neutral when used in the e-cigs context. Hence, using domain-independent dictionaries in our experiments may introduce noise. For example, the word *victory* is generally considered positive, but used in the e-cigs context, it does not express any sentiment. Considering this word to be positive will bring the tweet "Victory has the best flavors." closer to the positive class, although *victory* has no sentiment attached to it.

We built e-cigs dictionaries based on the tweets' contexts and the syntactical relationships obtained using Stanford Lexicalized Parser (SLP) [16]. We considered two steps: 1) extract opinion words associated with keywords by leveraging direct and indirect dependencies; 2) extract opinion words from hashtags (i.e., words/phrases prefixed with the character "#").

For the first step, we started with an empty set D. Words that are linked to keywords in a tweet via direct dependencies are added to D. Each tweet is represented as a dependency tree using SLP, based on the grammatical relationships between the words. From the resulting tree, we used the following direct relations: *nsubj (nominal subject), acomp (adjectival complement), dobj (direct object), xcomp (open causal complement), ccomp (clausal complement), prep_about (words linked through the preposition about), prep_in (preposition in), prep_of (preposition of)*. For example, the tweet "I enjoy the pleasure of vaping." contains two direct dependencies: [enjoy - pleasure]^{dobj} and [pleasure - vaping]$^{prep\text{-}of}$. We add "pleasure" to D due to its linkage with the keyword "vaping." Next, we used direct dependencies to find indirect dependencies between keywords and other words. Specifically, for each tweet, we identified two or (possibly) more direct dependencies that are linked by a word, such that at least one dependency contains a keyword. From these direct dependencies, we extracted all words that were not already in D. For the above example, from the direct dependencies [enjoy - pleasure]^{dobj} and [pleasure - vaping]$^{prep\text{-}of}$, linked by "pleasure," we inferred the indirect dependency [enjoy - vaping] and added "enjoy" to D. After extracting all the words using the above procedure (i.e., the compilation of D), we determined the polarity of each word in D using SentiStrength [17]. For each word, SentiStrength returns two scores: positive and negative. A word was added to a dictionary (positive or negative) based on the maximum absolute value between the scores; in case of equality, the word was considered neutral and was not added to the dictionaries. For example, "victory" has the SentiStrength scores 1 and -1 and is considered neutral, although it appears in domain-independent dictionaries. We ended this first step by using a domain-independent dictionary, developed by Hu and Liu [8]. Specifically, we added all word forms. For example, for the word *love*, different forms were added from the domain-independent dictionaries: *loved, loveliness, lovely, lover, loves*.

For the second step, we collected all the hashtags from the dataset and employed SentiStrength and the domain-independent dictionary to create positive and negative dictionaries. Finally, we concatenated the sentiment dictionaries obtained from both steps and acquired a positive dictionary of 260 words and a negative dictionary with 353 words. The dictionaries are available upon request.

Feature Engineering. We designed novel features and used them in conjunction with traditional sentiment features to improve the performance of sentiment classifiers targeted to e-cigarettes. These features, described in Table 2, are compiled based on polarity measures, user information and tweet structure.

Next, we provide some intuition that led to the design of several features as well as some implementation details. The features *noOfPositiveWords* and *noOfNegativeWords* were designed considering the negations, i.e., negations preceding the sentiment in a window of 2 words reverse the sentiment's polarity. For the feature *checkIfHasECigSenti*, we checked if there was a grammatical dependency between a keyword and sentiment words in a tweet. The intuition behind this feature is to identify if the sentiment is related to e-cigs.

Further, to identify user's opinions towards e-cigarettes, we created *personalECigSenti* feature. Specifically, we used dependency trees and checked if the subject of a sentence with a sentiment inside is a keyword or a first-person singular/plural pronoun; e.g., "I love vaping" and "E-cigs smell good." The sentiments shared in these tweets are those of the writer, and can express a personal opinion, based on his/her experience. On the contrary, a tweet such as "You love vaping" does not show the writer's opinion i.e., no personal sentiment is attached, but it reflects his/her opinion that someone else could possibly love e-cigs.

Features based on user information proved to be effective for our task. According to

Table 2. Features' description

FEATURES	DESCRIPTION
SENTIMENT FEATURES	
TRADITIONAL FEATURES	
noOfPositiveWords	Number of positive words.
noOfNegativeWords	Number of negative words.
noOfPositiveEmoticons	Number of positive emoticons.
noOfNegativeEmoticons	Number of negative emoticons.
SentiStrength − positive	Positive SentiStrength score.
SentiStrength − negative	Negative SentiStrength score.
+NEWLY DESIGNED	
checkIfHasECigSenti	Checks for opinions about e-cigs.
personalECigSenti	Checks if the opinion is personal.
+USER INFORMATION	
userHasKeyword	Checks if the username contains e-cigs' specific words.
noOfRetweetsOverAVG	Checks if the user has more retweets than the average.
+TWEET STRUCTURE	
hasQuestion	Checks the presence of questions.
noOfWords	Number of words in a tweet.
noOfKeywords	Number of e-cigs' related words.
hasLink	Checks if a tweet has a link.
hasHashtag	Checks if a tweet has hashtags.
hasNumbersAndQuantities	Checks the presence of product details (e.g., price, discounts).
hasRepeatingCharacters	Checks for repeating characters.
hasSlangWords	Checks slang words' presence.
oneSentenceAndLink	Checks if a tweet contains a sentence and link.

statistics from the labeled data, 85 out of 356 advertising tweets were posted by a user whose username contains a keyword. Therefore, the username can be a good indicator of advertising tweets and we seize this aspect through the *userHasKeyword* feature. Also, the statistics based on all 105,605 tweets show that many tweets represent retweets. Hence, we extracted information about highly re-tweeted users, encoded in the feature *noOfRetweetsOverAVG*.

Intuitively, the features based on the tweet structure can also be effective, because each category of tweets can have a specific structure. The *informational* tweets usually contain general-interest information and hyperlinks to further information; *advertising* tweets usually contain products' details and, often, external links. The *opinion* tweets are generally more informal than informational or advertising tweets, e.g., they contain slang words or repeating characters.

4   Experimental Setting

Our experiments are designed around the following questions:

1. *How do models trained only on the proposed features perform compared with other models for sentiment analysis such as those trained on bag-of-words and SentiStrength? Does the combination of bag-of-words, SentiStrength features and our features result in better performance compared with that obtained using each feature type individually?*
2. *What are the most informative categories of features for our task?*
3. *How can we characterize the entire dataset of 105,605 tweets in terms of informational, advertising, and opinion tweets, when automatically labeling them using our best classifiers?*

To answer the first question, we compared the performance of classifiers trained using our features with that of classifiers trained using bag-of-words (in a 10-fold cross-validation setting) and with SentiStrength [17] and report Precision, Recall and F1-score. SentiStrength [17] is an algorithm specifically designed to calculate sentiment strength of short informal texts in online social media. We experimented with four classifiers: Support Vector Machine (SVM), Naïve Bayes (NB), Random Forest (RF) and Decision Trees (DT). Although we show results only for SVM, NB and RF due to space constraints, DT followed the same trends in performance as the other studied classifiers. For bag-of-words, we removed stopwords, except pronouns, which were useful for our task. We used binary features, i.e., the presence/absence of a word from the vocabulary. Using SentiStrength, we identify tweet's polarity using positive and negative scores. We tested two multiplier values: 1.5 (SentiStrength's default) and 1 (equally weighting positive and negative scores) and obtained higher performance using the latter value. Therefore, a tweet was assigned to the class with the maximum absolute score and in case of equality, the tweet was neutral. Last, we combined all features and compared their performance with that of individual features, specifically, the proposed features, SentiStrength features and bag-of-words features.

To answer the second question, we incrementally added feature categories, starting with the traditional sentiment features. From the spectrum of these experiments, we show the classifiers' performance after the addition of a feature category, that yields an improvement in performance (from the smallest to the largest increase over the preceding setting).

To answer the third question, we employed our best performing classifiers trained on the combination of features to label the entire dataset and computed statistics with respect to each class.

5   Results

Classifiers' performance using various types of features. Table 3 shows the results obtained using our features in comparison with those obtained by bag-of-words and with their combination.

Table 3. Results obtained with our approach, bag-of-words and the combined method

Categories	Metrics	SVM			Naïve Bayes			Random Forest		
		Our approach	Bow	Bow+our approach	Our approach	Bow	Bow+our approach	Our approach	Bow	Bow+our approach
Informational	Precision	0.627	0.671	0.778	0.628	0.644	0.700	0.612	0.654	0.715
	Recall	0.587	0.723	0.809	0.606	0.682	0.761	0.652	0.717	0.817
	F1-score	0.603	0.693	**0.792**	0.614	0.660	**0.728**	0.628	0.680	**0.760**
Advertising	Precision	0.606	0.840	0.845	0.663	0.883	0.898	0.687	0.841	0.833
	Recall	0.691	0.772	0.822	0.659	0.661	0.715	0.703	0.717	0.749
	F1-score	0.642	0.803	**0.832**	0.659	0.753	**0.795**	0.692	0.772	**0.787**
Positive opinion	Precision	0.663	0.371	0.634	0.460	0.340	0.473	0.501	0.383	0.578
	Recall	0.315	0.267	0.545	0.551	0.359	0.622	0.360	0.191	0.419
	F1-score	0.410	0.303	**0.552**	0.493	0.336	**0.528**	0.403	0.250	**0.456**
Negative opinion	Precision	0.740	0.536	0.688	0.441	0.340	0.409	0.439	0.500	0.425
	Recall	0.281	0.333	0.514	0.508	0.500	0.578	0.388	0.173	0.210
	F1-score	0.368	0.366	**0.558**	0.446	0.378	**0.460**	**0.382**	0.242	0.257
Other	Precision	0.671	0.615	0.767	0.676	0.562	0.694	0.682	0.584	0.689
	Recall	0.752	0.707	0.819	0.670	0.640	0.693	0.693	0.740	0.765
	F1-score	0.705	0.652	**0.787**	0.669	0.590	**0.689**	0.681	0.648	**0.718**

As can be seen from the table, our features outperform bag-of-words for the *positive, negative* and *other* classes, for all studied classifiers. Note that the number of our features is much smaller compared with the bag-of-words size (e.g., 19 vs. 3437, respectively). Although bag-of-words exceeds our approach for the *advertising* and *informational* classes, the combination of our features with bag-of-words performs best for all categories, regardless of the classifier used. For example, the combination of features used as input to the SVM classifier has the highest performance for all classes. Precisely, it improves substantially, reaching almost a doubled performance compared with bag-of-words on the *positive* and *negative* classes. We conclude that each feature type from the combination captures some aspect of a tweet and hence, is important for the overall classification.

Comparison of SentiStrength with our Approach. We computed the results obtained by SentiStrength and found that our approach performs better in terms of F1-score (i.e., SentiStrength achieves 0.251 for the *positive* class and 0.232 for the *negative* class). SentiStrength has better recall (i.e., 0.580 for *positive*; 0.666 for *negative*), but it achieves a low precision (lower than 20%, i.e., 0.160 for *positive*; 0.140 for *negative*), while our approach obtains a precision higher than 60% for both *positive* and *negative* classes. These results can be justified by the fact that SentiStrength does not follow sentiments towards specific entities, focusing mainly on the overall sentiment of a tweet. We conclude that our proposed features are fairly good indicators of sentiments toward e-cigs.

Classifiers' Performance after Adding Different Categories of Features. Table 4 shows the performance achieved after we incrementally add each feature category from our approach, starting with traditional sentiment features. The reported results are computed employing 10 folds cross-validation and SVM.

Table 4. F1-scores obtained by sequentially adding the categories of features

FEATURES	Informational	Advertising	Positive	Negative	Other
SENTIMENT FEATURES					
TRADITIONAL FEATURES	0.000	0.484	0.208	0.080	0.258
+NEWLY DESIGNED	0.041	0.447	0.367	0.324	0.231
+USER INFORMATION	0.055	0.377	0.376	0.324	0.517
+TWEET STRUCTURE	0.589	0.634	0.380	0.372	0.710

Our features are grouped in the following categories: *sentiment features* comprised of traditional features (*noOfPositiveWords, noOfNegativeWords, noOfPositiveEmoticons, noOfNegativeEmoticons*) and new features tightened to e-cigs (*personalECigSenti, checkIfHasECigSenti*); features extracted from *user information* (*userHasKeyword, noOfRetweetsOverAVG*) and *tweet structure* (*hasQuestion, noOfWords, noOfKeywords, hasRepeatingCharacters, hasNumbersAndQuantities, hasLink, oneSentenceAndLink, hasSlangWords, hasHashtag*).

As can be seen in the table, the traditional sentiment features provide relevant knowledge for *advertising, positive* and *other* classes. Combined with traditional features, newly designed features perform very well, significantly raising the opinion classes' performance. Specifically, after adding newly designed features (*checkIfhasECigSenti, personalECigSenti*), the performance increased for the positive class with more than 0.1 and for the negative class with more than 0.3. Adding user information shows better results for almost all classes, over the setting that does not use this information. Features from the tweet structure result in the highest increase in performance over the previous setting, mainly for the *informational, advertising* and *other* classes. More precisely, after combining this feature category with those previously used, the performance increased with almost 0.5 for the *informational* class, 0.3 for *advertising* and 0.2 for *other*. This feature type brings also a slight boost in performance for the *opinion* classes.

Twitter Data Characterization. We automatically labeled the entire set of tweets employing the combination of our features, SentiStrength and bag-of-words and the SVM classifier trained on the labeled dataset. Our dataset contains tweets that are not entirely written in English, e.g., "*vaping* aja atuh beroh..." and " 『【最短でお届け‼】 *FUMI E-JUICE* ブルをる[天]." A closer analysis of the predicted labels for non-English tweets showed that they were assigned to the *other* category, although they may express sentiments. In future, it would be interesting to process them using machine translation. We computed statistics from the predicted labels and found that the majority of tweets are spread with *informational* purpose (almost 33% of tweets). Since *e-cigs* are relatively new products, online users post many informational tweets or links to pages that contain information about e-cigs, making it a trending subject. The second larger category (almost 28%) comprises the tweets that do not express sentiments, information or advertising (i.e., the *other* category), followed by the *advertising* category that represents almost 26% of the collected data. The tweets that express an opinion represent a small fraction of data. We found that users are more likely to share positive opinions/experiences (11%) than negative (3%).

Further, we detected the influential spreaders related to e-cigs from our data. To this end, we built a network which leverages tweets' relationships. Specifically, a node represents a tweet and an edge links two tweets if one is a retweet for the other. Each node is represented giving its importance: the bigger the node (i.e., its degree), the more important the corresponding tweet is. We show the network in Figure 1.

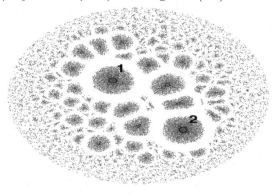

Fig. 1. Information spread network

As can be seen from the figure, there are two important nodes in the network (marked with bigger circles), which implies that there are two highly re-tweeted tweets and many other that are not so important, although they still have a fair amount of re-tweets. We identified the two most important tweets and the users who posted them originally. The first user was a regular user who posted substantial information about e-cigs. Specifically, the highest re-tweeted tweet (marked with "1" in figure) in the network provided a link to reviews. Because e-cigs are relatively new products, people are mainly interested in others' experiences, opinions or concerns. Not only they read the information, but they also share it further. The second highly re-tweeted tweet (marked with "2" in figure) was posted by a company for promotion. The tweet contains a link to information about company's products. An analysis of all tweets that receive a high number of re-tweets in our data show that highly shared tweets inside the network belong to our predominant categories (informational and advertising).

6 Discussion and Conclusion

In this paper, we proposed a supervised approach to identifying sentiments and information dissemination concerning e-cigs from Twitter data. Based on the results obtained using only a small portion of data (1200 labeled tweets), we see that our best setting (the combination of our features with bag-of-words, used as input to an SVM classifier) offers a clearer perspective on the e-cigs domain than other traditional sentiment analysis methods (SentiStrength and bag-of-words). That is, our approach identifies ≈80% of *advertising, informational* and *other* tweets, whereas the *opinion* tweets can be identified in a proportion of 55%.

We expanded our experiments to a more general case (i.e., all the collected dataset) and found that the majority of Twitter users share information concerning e-cigs or spread advertising tweets. Because e-cigarettes are relatively new products, users are mainly interested in sharing/finding meaningful information, while the producer companies are interested in promotion. Although opinions are shared in a small proportion, the general sentiments related to e-cigs tend to be positive. We also found that user information and the way a tweet is structured can be effectively used to automatically discover a tweet's purpose.

This study proposed an effective way of leveraging information posted in online social media to study public opinions and information dissemination related to e-cigarettes. Our method can facilitate the identification of trending behaviors concerning e-cigs, being able to use both current and past information from social networking sites. This approach can be used by various agencies to improve features of e-cigs or marketing strategy, based on public opinion. It is also a general-enough method, which can be easily adapted to study other entities. As future work, it would be interesting to study the type of information posted with respect to *e-cigs*, that is, if the posted information is in support for using e-cigs, or, quite on the contrary, this refers to the information that suggest the negative effects on human health. We further plan to extend our models, to analyze other entities that are legal, but potentially dangerous, such as energy drinks.

Acknowledgments. The authors would like to thank Kishore Neppalli for helping with the collection of the dataset.

References

1. U.S. Department of Health and Human Services. The health consequences of smoking 50 years of progress: A report of the surgeon general. Atlanta, GA: US Department of Health and Human Services, Centers for Disease Control and Prevention, National Center for Chronic Disease Prevention and Health Promotion, Office on Smoking and Health 17 (2014)
2. U.S. Department of Health and Human Services. How Tobacco Smoke Causes Disease: What It Means to You. Atlanta: Centers for Disease Control and Prevention, National Center for Chronic Disease Prevention and Health Promotion, Office on Smoking and Health (2010)
3. Centers for Disease Control and Prevention. QuickStats: Number of Deaths from 10 Leading Causes National Vital Statistics System, United States (2010), Morbidity and Mortality Weekly Report 2013:62(08);155
4. Grana, R., Benowitz, N., Glantz, S.A.: E-cigarettes: A scientific review. Circulation 129, 1972–1986 (2014)
5. Callahan-Lyon, P.: Electronic cigarettes: human health effects. Tobacco Control 23(suppl. 2), ii36–ii40 (2014)
6. World Health Organization, http://www.who.int/tobacco/publications/gender en_tfi_gender_women_addiction_nicotine.pdf
7. Kapoor, D., Jones, T.H.: Smoking and hormones in health and endocrine disorders. Eur. J. Endocrinol. 152, 491–499 (2005)
8. Hu, M., Liu, B.: Mining and summarizing customer reviews. In: The Tenth ACM SIGKDD International Conference on Knowledge Discovery and Data Mining (2004)
9. Ding, X., Liu, B., Yu, P.S.: A holistic lexicon-based approach to opinion mining. In: International Conference on Web Search and Data Mining. ACM (2008)

10. Pang, B., Lee, L., Vaithyanathan, S.: Thumbs up? Sentiment classification using machine learning techniques. In: ACL 2002 Conference on Empirical Methods in Natural Language Processing, pp. 79–86. Association for Computational Linguistics (2002)
11. Meng, X., Wei, F., Liu, X., Zhou, M., Li, S., Wang, H.: Entity-centric topic-oriented opinion summarization in twitter. In: The 18th ACM SIGKDD International Conference on Knowledge Discovery and Data Mining, pp. 379–387. ACM (2002)
12. Biyani, P., Caragea, C., Mitra, P., Zhou, C., Yen, J., Greer, G.E., Portier, K.: Co-training over Domain-independent and Domain-dependent Features for Sentiment Analysis of an Online Cancer Support Community. In: ASONAM (2013)
13. Bullen, C., Howe, C., Laugesen, M., McRobbie, H., Parag, V., Williman, J., Walker, N.: Electronic cigarettes for smoking cessation: a randomised controlled trial. The Lancet 382(9905), 1629–1637 (2003)
14. Popova, L., Ling, P.M.: Alternative Tobacco Product Use and Smoking Cessation: A National Study. Am. J. Public Health 103(5), 923–930 (2013)
15. Mysln, M., Zhu, S.H., Chapman, W., Conway, M.: Using Twitter to examine smoking behavior and perceptions of emerging tobacco products. Journal of Medical Internet Research 15(8) (2013)
16. De Marneffe, M.-C., MacCartney, B., Manning, C.D.: Generating typed dependency parses from phrase structure parses. In: LREC, vol. 6, pp. 449–454 (2006)
17. Thelwall, M., Buckley, K., Paltoglou, G.: Sentiment strength detection for the social web. J. Am. Soc. Inf. Sci. Technol., 163–173 (2012)

Determining User Similarity in Healthcare Social Media Using Content Similarity and Structural Similarity

Ling Jiang [✉] and Christopher C. Yang

College of Computing and Informatics, Drexel University, Philadelphia, USA
l.jenny.jiang@gmail.com, chris.yang@drexel.edu

Abstract. More and more health consumers discuss healthcare topics with peers in online health social websites. These health social websites empower consumers to actively participate in their own healthcare and promotes communication between people. However, it is difficult for consumers to find information efficiently from hundreds of thousands of discussion threads. Finding similar users for consumers enables them to see what their peers are doing or experiencing thus enables automated selection of "relevant" information. In this work, we proposed two different methods for computing user similarity in healthcare social media using content and structural information respectively. Experiment results showed that the method using structural information from a heterogeneous healthcare information network performed better than content similarity in finding active similar users. However, when the users are not as active or contributing relatively fewer messages in social media, content similarity performed better in identifying these users.

1 Introduction

Numerous studies showed that the Internet has become a significant source of health information for many people [1]. The increasing demands for healthcare information have boosted the emergence of online health social websites. Health consumers discuss medical conditions and treatments with peer consumers on these websites. More importantly, they share personal experiences and provide social support for others.

Although the Internet provides easily accessible sources of health information, consumers still find it difficult to search relevant health information [2]. Consumers usually cannot fully understand their conditions, or use different language frommedial terminologies [3]. These problems lead to poor query formation, and hinder effective information searching. In order to help consumers to improve the health information searching experience, many researchers studied consumers' health-searching behavior [3, 4], and provided possible solutions such as recommending queries to consumers [5] and designing specialized search engine for medical information [6].

Finding similar users in health social websites could be a solution. A primary impact of social networking on healthcare is that it enables consumers to see what their peers are doing or experiencing, thus enables automated selection of "relevant" information [7]. If we find similar users and recommend them to consumers, we could help to accelerate this selection process. In addition, finding similar users for health consumers can facilitate their connection with peers who are interested in common

© Springer International Publishing Switzerland 2015
J.H. Holmes et al. (Eds.): AIME 2015, LNAI 9105, pp. 216–226, 2015.
DOI: 10.1007/978-3-319-19551-3_28

healthcare topics, thus encourage social networking activities. Unfortunately, measuring similarity between users from healthcare social media is not a trivial task.

Content similarity is the most common approach of measuring similarity. It could be used to calculate two users' similarity based on their threads. However, there are still some challenges. On one hand, many users participated in very few discussion threads. Even though these users may provide useful information for a target user, it could be difficult to find them out of thousands of users. On the other hand, some active users contribute much more content and their discussions are in-depth and cover multiple aspects of the concerned healthcare topics. But the complex concerns of these users cannot be easily represented by simple keyword vectors.

Structural similarity is another approach. A health social website can be considered as a huge health information network, and the similarity problem can be treated as measuring the similarity of two ego-centered networks. Most existing studies assume information networks to be homogeneous, where nodes are objects of the same entity type and links are relationships from the same relation type. However, most real-world networks are heterogeneous, where nodes and links are of different types [8]. Healthcare information network is one typical heterogeneous network. A heterogeneous information network contains massive nodes and links carrying much richer information than homogeneous network does. Finding similar pairs of objects from heterogeneous networks may uncover underlying patterns from different perspective.

In this paper, we introduced two approaches for measuring user similarity in healthcare social media using content and structural information respectively. We also described the process of constructing a heterogeneous health information network.

2   Related Works

Many studies have been reported for measuring user similarity using different methods for different purposes. Generally, methods for similarity analysis fall into two categories: content-based approaches and structural analysis approaches.

Content-based similarity has its roots in Information Retrieval (IR). Extensive studies of similarity of documents have been done [9]. Many recommendation systems utilize the similarity between users to predict users' ratings of items. User-based collaborative filtering algorithm [10] usually first finds similar uses for a target user, then uses the ratings of the similar users to estimate the target user's interests for certain items. A common method is calculating similarity of users' profiles, which could be item ratings, browsing logs, clicks, queries and so on. Cosine similarity and Pearson's correlation are popular similarity measures in collaborative filtering [10-12].

Structural similarity is exploited frequently in information network studies. The problem can be considered as the proximity between any two nodes in a network. Some approaches adopted local similarity measures, based on the idea that two nodes are likely to be similar if they share a large number of neighbors in the network. The Friend-of-Friend algorithm, which is adopted by many popular online social websites such as Facebook.com, is based on the intuition that "if many of my friends consider Alice a friend, perhaps Alice could be my friend too" [13]. The most basic implementation of this idea is to compute the number of common neighbors [14]. Jaccard's coefficient and Adamic/Adar index are alternative similar measures based on common neighbors [15]. The structural features of a node can be represented by its ego-centered network and the similarity problem can be also viewed as calculating the similarity of two ego-centered networks. Xiang et al. proposed a metric of similarity between two subgraphs in a network. The idea is that two subgraphs having more connections or being simultaneously closely connected to other subgraphs are likely to have higher proximity to each other [16]. Hsu et al used the structural features of each user   to recommend users with common interests in a social network [17]. Most existing similarity measures are explored in homogeneous networks. However, most information networks in real world are heterogeneous rather than homogeneous.

3   Method

3.1   Content-Based Similarity

In our study, we are concerned with similar consumers who are interested in common health-related topics. In an online health social website, users participate in discussions on topics of interest. Therefore, the messages authored by a user can best represent his/her interests. Thus the problem of user similarity can be transformed into the problem of text similarity. Cosine similarity is a popular measurement for document similarity. A given document can be represented by a term vector that contains all the terms appear in the document. Cosine similarity measures the similarity of two documents by calculating the cosine of the angle between their word vectors. In this study, for each user, the messages authored by this user can be characterized by a term vector, and the value of each dimension in this vector corresponds to the frequency of each term in the messages. By calculating the cosine of two term vectors, we can measure how similar two set of messages are. The problem is formulated as follow.

Given a set of users $U = \{u_1, u_2, ..., u_n\}$ and a collection of messages $M = \{m_1, m_2, ..., m_n\}$, user u_i is the author of the messages m_i. Each user u_i can be represented by a term vector $\vec{t_i} = \{t_{i1}, t_{i2}, ..., t_{im}\}$, which are all terms in m_i . t_{i1} is the TF-IDF value of the term in M. In order to measure the similarity of u_i and u_j, we adopt the cosine similarity to calculate the similarity between vector $\vec{t_i}$ and $\vec{t_j}$:

$$S(u_i, u_j) = \frac{\vec{t_i} \cdot \vec{t_j}}{\| \vec{t_i} \| \| \vec{t_j} \|}$$

Nevertheless, content similarity has some shortcomings. Since content-based approach measures the similarity using textual content, the quality of the content is critical. However, consumer-contributed content from online social websites are mainly composed of noisy narrative content, and the poor quality of the content may impact the performance. Another challenge is that active users' interests cannot be easily represented by simple term vectors. Unlike traditional documents that are usually focused on a specific topic, an active user's messages could cover diverse topics. In that case, simple term vectors would not be able to best represent the user's complex interests. Therefore, we propose another approach based on structural information.

3.2 Structural Similarity (Profile Similarity)

An online health social community can be abstracted as a heterogeneous network. The nodes contain users, named entities appearing in threads such as drugs, diseases, and ADRs. The edges consist of user-interact with-user, drug-treat-disease, drug-cause-ADR, and so on. The structure information of the network could be utilized for calculating the similarity of nodes. Here we first give a definition of information network.

An *Information Network* is an un-directed graph $G = (\mathcal{V}, E; T, R)$ with an entity type mapping: $\varphi: \mathcal{V} \to T$ and a link type mapping: $\emptyset: E \to \mathcal{R}$. Vertex $v \in \mathcal{V}$ is an entity, while edge $e = \langle v, u \rangle \in E$ represents a relationship between v and u, where $v, u \in \mathcal{V}$. Type $t_i \in T = \{t_1, t_2, \ldots, t_n\}$ is an entity type, and $\varphi(v) \in T$. All vertexes $\mathcal{V} = \{V_1 \cup V_2 \ldots \cup V_n\}$ can be partitioned into n mutually exclusive subsets. Relation $r_j \in R = \{r_1, r_2, \ldots, r_m\}$ is a type of relationship, and $\emptyset(e) \in R$. All es $E = \{E_1 \cup E_2 \ldots \cup E_m\}$ can be partitioned into m mutually exclusive subsets. In a weighted network, $w(e)$ denotes the weights of $e = \langle v, u \rangle \in E$.

Most current studies consider information networks as homogeneous, that is, $n = 1$ for $T = \{t_1, t_2, \ldots, t_n\}$ and $m = 1$ for $E = \{E_1 \cup E_2 \ldots \cup E_m\}$. However, most information networks are heterogeneous in real world. A Heterogeneous Information Network is a specific type of Information Network, and it contains n $(n > 1)$ types of entities and m $(m > 1)$ types of relationships.

Given the above definition, we propose a Profile similarity approach to measure similarity between consumers in a heterogeneous healthcare information network. The Profile P_v^d of a user node v is defined as a vector of weights between v and its neighbor nodes within distance d:

$$P_v^d = \{ \overrightarrow{W_{r_1}}, \overrightarrow{W_{r_2}}, \ldots, \overrightarrow{W_{r_n}} \}$$

where

$$\overrightarrow{W_{r_i}} = \left(w(e_{vu_1}), w(e_{vu_2}), \ldots, w(e_{vu_m}) \right),$$

Where $r_i \in \{r_1, r_2, \ldots, r_m\}$ denotes different types of relationships in the network, and $w\left(e_{vu_j}\right)$ is the weight of the edge between node v and node u_j. In this study, we consider all links equally important, so we let $w\left(e_{vu_j}\right) = 1$ if there is a link between the two nodes, otherwise, we let $w\left(e_{vu_j}\right) = 0$. If two consumers talked about same entities in threads, it would be likely that they have very similar profile. Based on the Profile definition, the similarity of two users can be measured as follows:

$$S(v, u) = \sum_{i=1}^{m} \frac{\alpha_{r_i} \cdot P_v^d(\overrightarrow{W_{r_i}}) \cdot P_u^d(\overrightarrow{W_{r_i}})}{\left\| P_v^d(\overrightarrow{W_{r_i}}) \right\| \cdot \left\| P_u^d(\overrightarrow{W_{r_i}}) \right\|}$$

where α_{r_i} is the weight assigned to the type r_i. Since different types of links convey different semantic meanings, the profile is organized into several separate vectors based on the relationship types. Two consumers may have similar profiles because they talked about the same drug, or because they are interested in the same disease. In another word, consumers can be similar in different ways. By taking into account the heterogeneity of the network, we could provide personalized recommendation to consumers. For example, if consumers prefer to find similar users that are interested in same drugs, then we could set a higher weight for the user-interested in-drug relation.

Fig. 1 shows a toy example of two users' profiles in distance 1. There are four types of nodes in the network: user, drug, disease, and ADR. For a user, there could be three types of relationships: user-drug, user-disease, and user-ADR. According to the Profile algorithm, if we assign the same weight to the three types of relationships, then the similarity between user1 and user2 should be (0.5+1+0)/3=0.5.

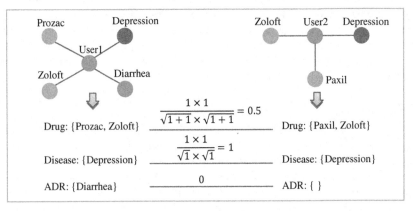

Fig. 1. Example of Profile Similarity

4   Experiment

4.1   Dataset

We collected the dataset from a popular online health social website MedHelp[1]. In MedHelp, there are hundreds of Medical Support Communities, each of which focuses on a specific type of medical condition. We collected all threads from 8 communities, including heart disease, depression, lung cancer, breast cancer, skin cancer, gastric cancer, stomach cancer, and dental health. Then we randomly extract 200 threads with more than one participant from each community and combine them into a dataset. The dataset contains a total of 1327 threads, because some communities do not contain as many as 200 threads with more than on participant. Each thread contains several messages. There are a total of 6654 messages in the dataset. Then we construct a heterogeneous health information network from the dataset.

---

[1] http://www.medhelp.org/

4.2   Heterogeneous Information Network

Nodes

In our study, we are interested in extracting consumers, drugs, diseases, and ADRs (Adverse Drug Reactions). We adopted external dictionaries to identify these entities. Recognizing consumers, namely healthcare social website users, is straightforward. However, we need to rely on dictionaries to identify drugs, diseases and ADRs.

For drugs, we used DrugBank[2] to build dictionary. DrugBank is a comprehensive online database containing 7685 drug entries [18]. For disease, we extracted all concepts with related string names under the semantic type "Disease or Syndrome" from UMLS[3] Metathesaurus to build a dictionary for diseases. For ADRs, we extracted dictionary from SIDER (Side Effect Resource)[4], which contains information of recorded adverse drug reactions of marketed medicines [19]. However, the situation for ADRs is more complicated. Consumers usually reach a consensus of names for drugs or diseases. Nevertheless, consumers often use a variety of expressions for ADRs. For instance, if a consumer experienced hair loss after taking a drug, he/she might describe it as "hair loss", "hair falling", or "baldness". On the other hand, because of the language gap between consumers and health professionals, there is a mismatch between expressions used by consumers and professional vocabularies. Take "hair loss" as example, the professional vocabulary for "hair loss" is "alopecia" in SIDER, which it is too professional for most consumers that they may not even know it. They are more likely to use "hair loss" instead of "alopecia". Therefore, we propose to use Consumer Health Vocabulary (CHV) to address this problem. Zeng et al. developed the open access and collaborative (OAC) CHV [20]. It was developed by identifying Consumer-Friendly Display (CFD) names and map CFD names to professional vocabulary. Compared with professional terms, the CHV terms are more likely to be used by consumers, and these terms can be used for expanding the professional terms.

Links

Co-occurrence analysis is the most direct way for extracting relations. The basic idea is that if two entities co-occur with each other, it implies an underlying relationship between them. An online thread could contain more than one message, and we propose to use message as analysis unit to extract entities as nodes and relations as links to construct the network. The reason we chose message over a whole thread is that topic digression usually occurs in thread. Especially in a long thread with tens of messages, messages posted by different users might be about totally different diseases or drugs. Under this circumstance, using co-occurrence analysis for relation extraction from the whole thread would generate a large number of false links. A message is usually focused on a single topic, so the entities in one message are more likely to be related to each other. For node frequency and link frequency, multiple appearances in one message only accounted for one occurrence. Notice that the relations extracted in non-directed. Table 1 gives some general information of the constructed network.

---

[2] http://www.drugbank.ca/
[3] http://www.nlm.nih.gov/research/umls/
[4] http://sideeffects.embl.de/

As we can see, the network is quite sparse. We then applied the proposed similarity analysis methods to this network.

Table 1. Network Information

# Nodes	# Links	Avg. Degree	Density	Diameter
5130	69487	13.564	0.005	10

4.3   Ground Truth

Our study is motivated to find similar users from online health social websites. Some consumers with similar interests might have already interacted with each other, while some others have never talked to each other and they might not even know the existence of each other. We should be able to measure not only the explicit similarity between consumers, but more importantly, the implicit similarity. In order to set up the ground truth, two human annotators were recruited to go through all the messages and determine whether a given pair of consumers is similar to each other.

In the dataset, a large portion of users only posted one message. For these users, we could not obtain enough textual content or network structural content for the similarity analysis. So, we pruned the network and only retain user nodes with frequency higher than 5. The pruned network contains a total of 153 user nodes, and the user node frequency falls in $[5, 191]$. Intuitively, the more messages a user posted, the more content would be available for the content-based similarity. In addition, the user would also have more connections to other nodes in the network. Based on this idea, we could speculate that similarity analysis methods might have different performance for active user and inactive users. Therefore, we put all 153 users into three groups with node frequency $freq < 10$, $10 \leq freq \geq 50$, and $freq > 50$ respectively. Then we randomly selected 5 users from each group and we got 15 users in total. For each of the 15 users, we randomly select 25 users from the other 152 users, and we have 375 pairs of users. The two human annotators then read through the 375 pairs of users' messages independently, and determine if each pair has similar interests.

We used the weighted Kappa [21] measure to compute the inter-rater agreement. Weighted Kappa measure is a statistical measure for computing the agreement between two annotators. It has a maximum value of 1 which indicates a perfect agreement and a value of 0 when the agreement is not better than by chance. In general, a weighted kappa measure value larger than 0.8 is considered to be a very good agreement. In our experiment, the weighted Kappa measure was 0.95, which means that the two annotators reached a very good agreement and the ground truth was reliable.

4.4   Evaluation Measurement

In this experiment, we use F1 score to measure the performance. For each target user of the 15 users, similarity analysis algorithms were used to calculate the similarity scores between the target user and the randomly selected 25 users. Then we got a list of users ranking in a descending order of the similarity scores. We consider the Top k ($1 \leq k \leq 25$) users are similar to the target user and use them for recommendation.

If one user in Top k is considered as similar to the target user by the ground truth, then we have a True Positive (TP). On the other hand, if one user is determined as dissimilar with the target user but is included in Top k, then we have a False Positive (FP). If one user is considered as dissimilar with the target user and is not in the Top k, then it is a True Negative (TN). Finally, if one user is considered as similar user to the target user but it is not ranked in Top k, then we have a False Negative (FN). Based on the definition, we can calculate the following:

$$precision = \frac{TP}{TP+FP} \qquad recall = \frac{TP}{TP+FN} \qquad F1 = \frac{2 \times precision \times recall}{precision + recall}$$

4.5 Results and Discussion

For each target user of the 15 users, 25 users were randomly selected to set up the ground truth. According to the ground truth, an average of 5.27 out of 25 users is similar to a target user. Therefore, we set k=1, 2, 3, 4, 5 for Top k and calculate the average F1 score from Top 1 to Top 5 for each proposed algorithm. There were three groups of users, and each group contained 5 users. We used the average F1 score of users in each group for evaluation. Table 2 gives the detailed average F1 score for each group of users. We compared the performance of content-based method and the structural-based algorithms. In this experiment, we tested the performance of Profile algorithm within distance $d = 1,2,3$.

Table 2. F1 Score

User Frequency	Top K	Content-based	Profile ($d = 1$)	Profile ($d = 2$)	Profile ($d = 3$)
<10	1	0.34	0.26	0.34	0.00
	2	0.57	0.43	0.40	0.00
	3	0.74	0.45	0.47	0.07
	4	0.78	0.44	0.55	0.18
	5	0.73	0.45	0.62	0.19
	Avg.	0.63	0.41	0.48	0.09
10-50	1	0.32	0.19	0.19	0.19
	2	0.44	0.39	0.39	0.27
	3	0.49	0.48	0.48	0.28
	4	0.55	0.65	0.47	0.29
	5	0.53	0.66	0.50	0.29
	Avg.	0.47	0.47	0.40	0.26
>50	1	0.07	0.28	0.04	0.04
	2	0.14	0.39	0.16	0.14
	3	0.20	0.48	0.29	0.17
	4	0.31	0.56	0.35	0.16
	5	0.44	0.62	0.31	0.19
	Avg.	0.23	0.46	0.23	0.14

The first noticeable pattern in the results is that when the distance d increases, the performance of Profile algorithm reduces except for users with less than 10 messages. The Profile algorithm measures similarity based on users' neighbors. Theoretically, when the distance d increases, more nodes would be considered as the central node's neighbors. Therefore, more noise could be added into the calculation. However, for users who posted less than 10 messages, there might be only a very small set of neighbors, which makes it hard to find similar users. In this case, increasing d could be likely to bring in relevant nodes rather than noisy ones. But as d increases and exceeds certain threshold, more noise could be brought in. In this experiment, $d = 2$ performed better for inactive users, and $d = 1$ performed better for active users.

Another interesting trend could be observed between the two methods in different user groups. Content-based method achieve an average F1 score higher than 0.6 when users participate in a very small set of threads. As users get more active, content-based approach's ability in identifying similar users reduces. The F1 score of content-based method for users who posted more than 50 messages is as low as 0.23. Contrarily, the performance of Profile algorithm ($d = 1$) increases as users get more active.

The trend can be explained by the different underlying basic idea of each method. Content-based method calculates similarity between two users based on the threads authored by each user. Active users usually participate in a great number of threads, and theses threads could be about a diversity of topics. On the contrary, inactive users who only posted a few threads are likely to be interested in only one or two topics. Therefore, inactive users have more focused interests, while active users' interests are diluted by being spread over a large number of threads. In this case, content-based similarity could yield better results for inactive users. On the other hand, structural approach measures similarity based on users' structural context such as users' neighbors. Active users are connected to much more entities than inactive users. Thus, the sub-graph of an active user bears richer structural information than that of an inactive user. Therefore, structural approach performs better for active users.

From practical perspective, recommending active users to a target consumer could be more meaningful than recommending inactive users. Because our ultimate goal is to help consumers find similar users so as to stimulate information propagation and social networking, recommending active users would serve the goal better. If we made a recommendation to a consumer and he/she found that the suggested similar user just posted one message and never showed up again, this recommendation would hardly make sense. The results showed that the proposed Profile algorithm with $d = 1$, which is only considering a user's direct neighbors, performed the best for finding active similar users.

5   Conclusions

In this paper, we proposed methods of measuring similarity based on both content and structural information. For the structural similarity, we consider an information network as heterogeneous. Experiments were conducted to compare the performance of different similarity analysis methods, the results showed that structural-based approaches performed better than content-based method in finding active similar users for health consumers. For future study, we may focus on developing new methods for structural similarity in heterogeneous information networks.

References

1. Fox, S.: The social life of health information, Pew Internet & American Life Project (2011),
   `http://alexa.pewinternet.com/~/media/Files/Reports/2011/PIP_Social_Life_of_Health_Info.pdf` (cited December 2014)
2. Arora, N.K., et al.: Frustrated and confused: the American public rates its cancer-related information-seeking experiences. Journal of General Internal Medicine 23(3), 223–228 (2008)
3. Zhang, Y., et al.: Health information searching behavior in MedlinePlus and the impact of tasks. In: Proceedings of the 2nd ACM SIGHIT International Health Informatics Symposium. ACM (2012)
4. Eysenbach, G., Köhler, C.: How do consumers search for and appraise health information on the world wide web? Qualitative study using focus groups, usability tests, and in-depth interviews. Bmj 324(7337), 573–577 (2002)
5. Zeng, Q.T., et al.: Assisting consumer health information retrieval with query recommendations. Journal of the American Medical Informatics Association 13(1), 80–90 (2006)
6. Luo, G., et al.: MedSearch: a specialized search engine for medical information retrieval. In: Proceedings of the 17th ACM Conference on Information and Knowledge Management. ACM (2008)
7. Eysenbach, G.: Medicine 2.0: social networking, collaboration, participation, apomediation, and openness. Journal of Medical Internet Research 10(3) (2008)
8. Sun, Y., Han, J.: Mining heterogeneous information networks: principles and methodologies. Synthesis Lectures on Data Mining and Knowledge Discovery 3(2), 1–159 (2012)
9. Baeza-Yates, R., Ribeiro-Neto, B.: Modern information retrieval, vol. 463. ACM Press, New York (1999)
10. Herlocker, J.L., et al.: An algorithmic framework for performing collaborative filtering. In: Proceedings of the 22nd Annual International ACM SIGIR Conference on Research and Development in Information Retrieval. ACM (1999)
11. Breese, J.S., Heckerman, D., Kadie, C.: Empirical analysis of predictive algorithms for collaborative filtering. In: Proceedings of the Fourteenth Conference on Uncertainty in Artificial Intelligence. Morgan Kaufmann Publishers Inc. (1998)
12. Wang, J., De Vries, A.P., Reinders, M.J.: Unifying user-based and item-based collaborative filtering approaches by similarity fusion. In: Proceedings of the 29th Annual International ACM SIGIR Conference on Research and Development in Information Retrieval. ACM (2006)
13. Chen, J., et al.: Make new friends, but keep the old: recommending people on social networking sites. In: Proceedings of the SIGCHI Conference on Human Factors in Computing Systems. ACM (2009)
14. Newman, M.E.: Clustering and preferential attachment in growing networks. Physical Review E 64(2), 025102 (2001)
15. Liben-Nowell, D., Kleinberg, J.: The link-prediction problem for social networks. Journal of the American Society for Information Science and Technology 58(7), 1019–1031 (2007)
16. Xiang, B., Chen, E.-H., Zhou, T.: Finding community structure based on subgraph similarity. In: Fortunato, S., Mangioni, G., Menezes, R., Nicosia, V. (eds.) Complex Networks 2009. SCI, vol. 207, pp. 73–81. Springer, Heidelberg (2009)

17. Hsu, W.H., et al.: Collaborative and Structural Recommendation of Friends using Weblog-based Social Network Analysis. In: AAAI Spring Symposium: Computational Approaches to Analyzing Weblogs (2006)
18. DrugBank. About DrugBank, http://www.drugbank.ca/about (cited December 2014)
19. Kuhn, M., et al.: A side effect resource to capture phenotypic effects of drugs. Molecular Systems Biology 6(1) (2010)
20. Zeng, Q.T., Tse, T.: Exploring and developing consumer health vocabularies. Journal of the American Medical Informatics Association 13(1), 24–29 (2006)
21. Cohen, J.: Weighted kappa: Nominal scale agreement provision for scaled disagreement or partial credit. Psychological Bulletin 70(4), 213 (1968)

Biomedical Concepts Extraction Based on Possibilistic Network and Vector Space Model

Wiem Chebil[1,2], Lina Fatima Soualmia[1,3(✉)], Mohamed Nazih Omri[2], and Stéfan Jacques Darmoni[1,3]

[1] LITIS-TIBS EA 4108, Normandie University,
Rouen University and Hospital, Rouen, France
wiem.chebil@yahoo.fr
[2] Research unit MARS, Monastir University, Monastir, Tunisia
Mohamednazih.omri@fsm.rnu.tn
[3] French National Institute for Health, INSERM, LIMICS UMR 1142, Paris, France
{Lina.Soualmia,Stefan.Darmoni}@chu-rouen.fr

Abstract. This paper proposes a new approach for indexing biomedical documents based on the combination of a Possibilistic Network and a Vector Space Model. This later carries out partial matching between documents and biomedical vocabularies. The main contribution of the proposed approach is to combine the cosine similarity and the two measures of possibility and necessity to enhance the estimation of the similarity between a document and a given concept. The possibility estimates the extent to which a document is not similar to the concept. The necessity allows the confirmation that the document is similar to the concept. Experiments were carried out on the OSHUMED corpora and showed encouraging results.

Keywords: Indexing · Biomedical documents · Possibilistic network · Vector space model · Partial matching

1 Introduction

In order to improve the performance of an information retrieval system, it is essential to develop an automatic indexing system that is able to have as output the most representative index of a document. To improve estimation of the similarity between a document and a given concept, a new approach for indexing biomedical documents is proposed in this paper. The proposed approach combines a Possibilistic Network (PN) and a Vector Space Model (VSM) [1] and exploits controlled vocabularies. These later are the Medical Subject Headings thesaurus (MeSH) [2] and the Systematized Nomenclature of Medicine Clinical Terms (SNOMED CT). Each concept of the controlled vocabularies is related to a set of terms and each term is composed of one or several words. The advantages of combining a PN and a VSM are: (i) the VSM exploits the weight of a word in the controlled resource, which improves the estimation of the relevance of the concepts [3, 4]. In fact, if the weights of the words of a term in the document are similar to their weights in the controlled resource, then it

© Springer International Publishing Switzerland 2015
J.H. Holmes et al. (Eds.): AIME 2015, LNAI 9105, pp. 227–231, 2015.
DOI: 10.1007/978-3-319-19551-3_29

improves the similarity between the term and the document; (ii) the VSM allows to reduce the relevance of a term that has not all its words occurring in the document and finally (iii) the PN allows the use of two measures (the possibility and the necessity) to estimate the relevance of a concept. These two measures improve the ranking of relevant concepts as in [5]. In fact, the Possibility Theory [6] is a powerful method for dealing with imprecision and uncertainty and has been efficiently applied in different fields including the measure of similarity [7] and information retrieval [8]. The encouraging results obtained in [8] motivated us to propose an approach based on a PN that outperformed several proposed approaches in the field of concept extraction from biomedical documents.

The paper is organized as follows: Section 2 describes the steps of the proposed model. Section 3, details the experiments, the obtained results and the discussion. Finally, Section 4 concludes the paper and presents some future work.

2   Indexing Approach

This section describes our approach which is composed of 4 steps: (1) Pre-treatment: this step is the same as in [5], (2) Concept extraction, (3) Filtering and (4) Final ranking.

2.1   Concepts Extraction

The concepts extraction step begins with the extraction of the terms related to concepts by using a Possibilistic Network and a Vector Space Model.

Extracting Terms Using a Possibilistic Network. Terms are extracted using a Possibilistic Network. The architecture of this later is as follows: T_j: is a term of a concept belonging to controlled vocabularies. W_k: is a word belonging to the document to be indexed or to a term. D_i: is the document to be indexed. The evaluation of a term is carried out through the propagation of the information given by the term in the network when it is instantiated. The links are activated by this instantiation from the term to the document and evaluated through two measures. The first is the possibility of the document being indexed given a term (Equation 1). The second is the necessity of the document given a term (Equation 2). Terms are then ranked according the sum of Equation 1 and Equation 2. The sorted terms are considered as the *Set 1*. One can find more details about the architecture of the PN and computing (1) and (2) in [5].

$$S1(T_j, D_i) = \Pi(d_i | T_j) = \frac{\Pi(T_j \wedge d_i)}{\Pi(T_j)} \tag{1}$$

$$S2(T_j, D_i) = N(d_i | T_j) = 1 - \Pi(\overline{d_i} | T_j) \tag{2}$$

Extracting Terms Using a Vector Space Model. The score of a term corresponds to the similarity between a document D_i and a term T_j, which is computed using the cosine similarity (Equation 3). To do that, two weights are computed: (1) Weight of Word in the Document (*WWDoc*) and (2) Weight of Word in a Term (*WWT*). These two weights are detailed in [4]. Terms are ranked according Equation 3.The sorted terms are considered as the *Set 2*. To compute Equation 3 we consider that T_j is a set of p words.

$$S3(T_j, D_i) = Sim(T_j, D_i) = \frac{\sum_{y=1}^{p} WWT_y \times WWDoc_y}{\sqrt{\sum_{y=1}^{p} (WWT_y)^2 \times (WWDoc_y)^2}} \tag{3}$$

The score of a concept. The ranked *Set 1* is merged with the ranked *Set 2* by deleting the doubloons. A new score *SF* (Equation 4) is computed for candidates terms. The score of a concept is the maximum score of its terms (Equation 5). The term having the maximum score is the Representative Term.

$$SF(Tj) = (S1(Tj) + S2(Tj) + S3(Tj)) \times a \tag{4}$$

$$Score(C_f) = \max_{T_j \in T(C_f)} (SF(T_j)) \tag{5}$$

$T(C_f)$ represents the set of terms of a concept C_f and a is a coefficient and its value belongs to]0,1]. We consider that $a=1$ if the words of terms are in the same phrase at least once, and $a<1$ if not (a is experimentally tuned).

2.2 Filtering and Final Ranking

The aim of this step is to keep only relevant concepts among those with their Representative Terms having a subset of their words not occurring in the document. In fact, we classified the non-extraction of these relevant concepts as a category of indexing errors in a previous work [9]. This step exploits the semantic relations and co-occurencies between concepts provided by the UMLS and performed such as in [5]. The details of the method can be found in [5]. The output of this step is a set of concepts. These later are re-ranked according to the score of the Equation 5 to obtain the final index.

3   Experimental Evaluations and Results

To test our approach a subset of the OHSUMED collection[1] selected randomly and composed of 120,000 MEDLINE citations was used. Each selected citation is composed by a title and an abstract. In all the experiments, only the first fifteen concepts

---

[1]http://trec.nist.gov/data/t9_filtering.html

were kept in the final index. In fact, the average number of concepts in the manual indexes in OSHUMED is 15 [3].

To highlight the effectiveness of our indexing approach, the performance of this later was compared to the performance of other approaches (Table 1) by computing the Main Average Precision (MAP), the F-score (Fs) and the precision at rank 5 (P@5), at rank 10 (P@10) and at rank 15 (P@15). MaxMatcher+ [10] was considered as the baseline against which the tested approaches were compared. The choice of MaxMatcher+ as a baseline is based on the fact that it is among the most recent tools developed for extracting concepts from biomedical documents. In addition, to show the statistically significant improvements, the paired-sample T-tests was computed between means of each ranking obtained by each experimented approach and the baseline. The difference between two given rankings is significant if $p<0.05$ (noted*), very significant if $p<0.01$ (noted**) and extremely significant if $p<0.001$ (noted***).

Table 1. Comparison of the combination of PN and VSM (PN & VSM) with other approaches

	MAP ($\pm\Delta\%$)	Fs ($\pm\Delta\%$)	P@5 ($\pm\Delta\%$)	P@10 ($\pm\Delta\%$)	P@15 ($\pm\Delta\%$)
MaMatcher+ [10]	0.455	0.585	0.771	0.651	0.459
AMTex [11]	0.393 (-13.62)	0.502 (-14.18)	0.691 (-10.37)	0.551 (-15.36)	0.407 (-11.32)
PoNeDI [5]	0.575 (+26.37)*	0.693 (+18.46)	0.965 (+25.16)	0.809 (+24.27)*	0.565 (+23.09)*
PN &VSM	0.688 (+51.12)***	0.803 (+36.75)	0.985 (+27.75)	0.945 (+45.16)**	0.673 (+46.62)**

When analysing Table 1, one can deduce that the combination of PN and VSM (PN &VSM) outperforms all the tested approaches. In addition, only our approach is extremely statistically significant compared to the baseline (p=2.44 $\times 10^{-6}$, df=64.75, t=6.08, M=3.20). These results confirm what was expected. In fact, using the possibility modelled by the necessity degree and the cosine similarity contributes to improve the extraction and the ranking of relevant concepts. The significant results achieved by our approach can be explained by two reasons: the first is the effectiveness of the contribution and the second is the limitations of the other existing approaches. In fact, as it is mentioned in the introduction, the advantages of using VSM for extracting terms don't characterise the PN, which allowed to out perform PoNeDI. In addition, MaxMatcher+ performs a partial matching between documents and a controlled vocabulary without a filtering step. Thus, irrelevant concepts having a subset of their words in the document may be extracted which decreases precision. All improvement rates of AMTex are negatives. In fact, AMTex exploits the C/NC-value, which is based on learning linguistic rules that depend on the corpus and the controlled vocabulary. This leads to decrease the performance of the indexing system when another corpus or/and several controlled vocabularies are used. The C/NC-value is also based on an exact matching that allows extracting only terms that are present in the document. The supervised approaches for controlled indexing were not tested. This is explained by the fact that these approaches are not suitable for controlled indexing due to the complexity of training a system for huge numbers of classes (around 24,000 classes with MeSH) [3]. The results of our approach depend also on parameters such as the parameter a that must be well-tuned to allow good results.

4   Conclusion

In this paper, a new approach for indexing biomedical documents was proposed. The main contribution is to combine the Possibilistic Network and the Vector Space Model to extract concepts, which improves estimation of the similarity between a document and a given concept. The experiments clearly showed the interest of our indexing approach, which may be extended by a step of disambiguation of indexing terms having more than one concept. The performance of an information retrieval system that integrates the proposed approach may also be evaluated and compared to other existing systems.

References

1. Singhal, A.: Modern information retrieval: A brief overview. IEEE Data Engineering Bulletin 24(4), 35–43 (2009)
2. Nelson, S.J., Johnson, W.D., Humphreys, B.L.: Relationships in Medical Subject Heading. In: Relationships in the Organization of Knowledge, pp. 171–184 (2001)
3. Ruch, P.: Automatic assignment of biomedical categories: towards a generic approach. Bioinformatics Journal 22(6), 658–664 (2006)
4. Chebil, W., Soualmia, L.F., Darmoni, S.J.: BioDI: A new approach to improve biomedical documents indexing. In: Decker, H., Lhotská, L., Link, S., Basl, J., Tjoa, A.M. (eds.) DEXA 2013, Part I. LNCS, vol. 8055, pp. 78–87. Springer, Heidelberg (2013)
5. Chebil, W., Soualmia, L.F., Omri, M.N., Darmoni, S.J.: Indexing biomedical documents with a possibilistic network. Journal of the Association for Information Science and Technology (in press, 2015), doi: 10.1002/asi.23435
6. Dubois, D., Prade, H.: Possibility Theory. Plenum (1988)
7. Omri, M.N., Chouigui, N.: Measure of similarity between fuzzy concepts for identification of fuzzy user's requests in fuzzy semantic networks. International Journal of Uncertainty, Fuzziness and Knowledge-Based Systems (IJUFKS) 9(6), 743–748 (2001)
8. Boughanem, M., Brini, A., Dubois, D.: Possibilistic networks for information retrieval. International Journal of Approximate Reasoning 50, 957–968 (2009)
9. Chebil, W., Soualmia, L.F., Dahamna, B., Darmoni, S.J.: Indexation automatique de documents en santé: évaluation et analyse de sources d'erreurs. BioMedical Engineering and Research 33(5-6), 129–136 (2012)
10. Dinh, D., Tamine, L.: Towards a context sensitive approach to searching information based on domain specific knowledge sources. Web Semantics: Science, Services and Agents on the World Wide Web 12-13, 41–52 (2012)
11. Hliaoutakis, A., Zervanou, K., Petrakis, E.G.M.: The AMTEx approach in the medical document indexing and retrieval application. Data Knowledge Engineering 68(3), 380–392 (2009)

Answering PICO Clinical Questions:
A Semantic Graph-Based Approach

Eya Znaidi[1(✉)], Lynda Tamine[1], and Chiraz Latiri[2]

[1] IRIT, University Paul Sabatier of Toulouse, Toulouse, France
eya.znaidi@irit.fr
[2] Computer Sciences Department, Faculty of Sciences of Tunis, Tunis, Tunisia

Abstract. In this paper, we tackle the issue related to the retrieval of the best evidence that fits with a PICO (Population, Intervention, Comparison and Outcome) question. We propose a new document ranking algorithm that relies on semantic based query expansion bounded by the local search context to better discard irrelevant documents. Experiments using a standard dataset including 423 PICO questions and more than 1, 2 million of documents, show that our aproach is promising.

Keywords: Evidence-based-medicine · PICO clinical queries · Medical information retrieval · Semantic query expansion

1 Introduction

Evidence-Based Medicine (EBM) has been defined as the conscientious, explicit and appropriate use of systematic research findings, in consultation with the patient, with the aim of optimizing the healthcare decision-making process of medical professionals [8]. One major issue faced by the professionals during the daily practice of EBM is the complexity of expressing precise, context-specific clinical queries that better facilitate the identification of the relevant evidence. These works rely heavily on a prior automatic annotation of PICO facets in both queries and documents. Unlikely, our approach (1) relaxes the condition of PICO facet identification in the documents, and (2) abstracts the word-based question formulation by highlighting the overall semantic picture of each question facet. Moreover, each question facet is separately expanded using concepts extracted from top ranked documents issued from the initial retrieval.

The remainder of the paper is structured as follows. In section 2, we first give an overview of related work. Section 3 details our aproah for PICO question elicitation and answering. In section 4, we describe the experimental setup and then present and discuss the results obtained using a standard clinical information retrieval dataset. Section 5 concludes the paper.

2 Related Work

While some previous work [1,4,11] tackled the issue of PICO element detection, as a prior stage before retrieving relevant documents, other studies, close to our

© Springer International Publishing Switzerland 2015
J.H. Holmes et al. (Eds.): AIME 2015, LNAI 9105, pp. 232–237, 2015.
DOI: 10.1007/978-3-319-19551-3_30

work [3,2,5] focused on the design of retrieval techniques and models that exploit the PICO facets in order to compute the relevance score of documents. To achieve this goal, Boudin et al. [3,2] automatically detected PICO elements in the documents and then revised the basic version of the IR language model [9]. More precisely, the authors revised the word-document weighting schema by taking into account both the distribution of PICO elements in the different passages of the documents and the distributions of the words in the different PICO parts. The experimental evaluation held on a collection of 1.5 million documents and 423 queries showed that the proposed model yields an improvement of 28% in mean average precision over state-of-the-art baselines. Demner-Fushman and Lin [5] also proposed an unified framework for both detecting and using the detected PICO elements in the relevance document scoring function S_{EBM}. The latter is based on the linear combination of partial relevance scores of the documents considering the three facets of EBM, namely, PICO (S_{PICO}), strenght of evidence (S_{SoE}) and task type (S_{task}). For instance, the PICO score relies on a linear combination of P, I, C and O facet scores considering the word overlap between the document and the question. Experiments carried out on 24 real-world clinical questions show that the approach outperforms a traditional PubMed search.

3   A Semantic Graph-based Approach for Answering PICO Questions

We describe in Figure 2 the general algorithm (main and function) for expanding the PICO query and ranking the best evidence to be returned as an answer to the clinician.

- *(Main) Steps 1-12*: Given a word-based PICO query Q, the related annotation Q_{PICO}, the subqueries Q_P, Q_{IC} and Q_O and the list of N_d top ranked documents D_N^* included in a document collection C, the algorithm builds first the semantic sub-graphs G_P, G_{IC} and G_O after (1) extracting, using our concept extraction method [6] build upon Metamap[1], the active concepts, respectively $Concepts(Q_P)$, $Concepts(Q_{IC})$ and $Concepts(Q_O)$; each active concept has an importance score $Score(c)$ that highlights the likelihood of similarity between the concept preferred entry and the query words, (2) building the associated graphs G_P, G_{IC} and G_O by appending to the active concepts the corresponding hypernyms through terminology function $HypG$ processed on medical terminology T until reaching the first common concept. Each returned active concept c is considered at relative level 0.

- *(Main) Steps 13-15*: for each sub-graph G_P, G_{IC} and G_O, we build the set of N_c concepts to be used for query expansion by applying function $Expand(G_x)$ considering $Maxlevel$ which denotes the maximum level used for query expansion beginning from level 0.

---

[1] http://metamap.nlm.nih.gov

1. Main: *Document ranking*

Input: $Q, Q_{PICO}, T, N_d, N_c, MaxLevel$
Output: G_P, G_{IC}, G_O, D_N^*
1: # Initial search
2: $D_N^* \leftarrow Top_D(Q, N_d, C)$;
3: # Query Graph Building
4: $Q_P \leftarrow Substr(Q, P)$;
5: $Q_{IC} \leftarrow Substr(Q, IC)$;
6: $Q_O \leftarrow Substr(Q, O)$;
7: $Concepts(Q_P) \leftarrow Extract(Q_P, T)$;
8: $G_P \leftarrow HypG(Concepts(Q_P), T)$;
9: $Concepts(Q_{IC}) \leftarrow Extract(Q_{IC}, T)$;
10: $G_{IC} \leftarrow HypG(Concepts(Q_{IC}), T)$;
11: $Concepts(Q_O) \leftarrow Extract(Q_O, T)$;
12: $G_O \leftarrow HypG(Concepts(Q_O), T)$;
13: $Q_P^e \leftarrow Expand(G_P)$;
14: $Q_{IC}^e \leftarrow Expand(G_{IC})$;
15: $Q_O^e \leftarrow Expand(G_O)$;
16: $Words(Q^e) \leftarrow Words(Q) \cup Entries(Q_P^e) \cup Entries(Q_{IC}^e) \cup Entries(Q_O^e)$;
17: # Final search
18: $D_N^* \leftarrow Top_D(Q^e, N_d, C)$;

2. Function: *Expand*

Input: G_x
Output: *Cexpand*
1: # Query expansion
2: # Process the top ranked documents
3: **for all** $d \in D_N^*$ **do**
4:     # Extraction of document concepts
5:     $Cexpand \leftarrow Extract(d, G_x)$;
6:     $level \leftarrow 0$;
7:     # Score Propagation
8:     **for all** $c \in Cexpand$ AND $level < Maxlevel$ **do**
9:         **for all** $csub \in Hypo(c, G_x)$ **do**
10:            $Score(csub) \leftarrow (Score(csub) + Lev(csub) * Score(c))$;
11:            $Score(csub) \leftarrow Normalized(Score(csub))$;
12:            $level \leftarrow level + 1$;
13:        **end for**
14:    **end for**
15: **end for**
16: $Cexpand \leftarrow Top_C(G_x, N_c)$;
17: **return** *Cexpand*;

Fig. 1. The document retrieval process

- *(Expand) Steps 1-17:* To build the set of candidate concepts *Cexpand*, we consider each document d in D_N^* and then (1) extract the set of common weighted concepts with G_x (where $x \in \{P, IC, O\}$) using the same concept extraction method [6]; (2) apply a score propagation algorithm that propagates the scores of the active concepts of each query sub-graph G_x from level 0 to level *Maxlevel* by iteratively summing the scores of the hyponym concepts through sub-graph G_x, $Hypo(c, G_x)$. The basic underlying idea is to leverage the importance and the specificity of the concepts by assigning the normalized scores $Normalized(Score(c))$ obtained step by step from less specific concepts to most specific ones, considering their level $Lev(c)$. The final score of a concept reflects its importance in the whole top ranked documents in terms of high specificity and matching degree with documents D_N^*. This fits with our intuition that favors the selection of most specific concepts that better match the search context gathered from the top ranked documents.

- *(Main) Steps 16-18:* The returned set of N_c top weighted concepts *Cexpand* extracted from each sub-graph G_x, are used to expand respectively the sub-queries Q_P, Q_{IC} and Q_O (resulting in Q_P^e, Q_{IC}^e and Q_O^e respectively) by adding to the intial word-based query Q the words belonging to their preferred entries ($Entries(Q_P^e)$, $Entries(Q_{IC}^e)$ and $Entries(Q_O^e)$ respectively) within terminology T. The final expanded query Q^e is processed and allows selecting the final list of documents D_N^* to be returned as an answer to the initial PICO query Q.

4   Experimental Evaluation

4.1   Experimental Setup

We used the CLIREC dataset which has been built with the specific aim of evaluating clinical information retrieval [3]. Some statistical characteristics of the collection are depicted in Table 1.We used the MeSH terminology which has been widely accepted as the main controlled vocabulary used to index biomedical citations [10]. Each node of the terminology represents a concept node referred to using a preferred entry.

Table 1. CLIREC test collection statistics

Number of documents	1.212.040 abstracts from PubMed
Average document length	246 words
Number of queries	423
Average number of query keywords	4.3 words
Average PICO query length	18.7 words
Average Number of relevant documents per query	19

For the purpose of evaluating and comparing retrieval effectiveness, we used under version 4.0 of the Terrier search engine[2]: 1) The Mean Average Precision (MAP) measure which is the mean of the AP measure over a set of queries; it is used to provide a single, overall measure of search performance. The performance measures have been computed using the standard TREC-eval tool[3]; 2) We used two state-of-the-art information retrieval models, namely the Okapi probabilistic model (BM25) [7] and the language model (LM) [9]. The Okapi model was parameterized as recommended in the literature: $k1 = 1.2$, $k3 = 7$ and $b = 0.75$. For the LM, the Dirichlet smoothing method with $\mu = 1000$ was used.

4.2   Results

We compared the retrieval effectiveness based on MAP of our semantic graph-based document ranking algorithm GQE with respect to the state-of-the-art ranking models $BM25$ and LM. Table 2 presents the obtained results in terms of the MAP measure and relevant retrieved documents as well as the corresponding pourcents of improvement and significance t values of the statistical t-test. We can see that our model (GQE) significantly overpasses word-based document

---

[2] http://www.terrier.org
[3] http//trec.nist.gov/trec_eval

Table 2. Comparison of the semantic graph-based query expansion impact on the retrieval effectiveness. $\%Chg$: Student test significance over the MAP measure *: $0.01 < t \leq 0.05$; **: $0.001 < t \leq 0.01$; ***: $t \leq 0.001$.

Model	MAP	%Change	t	Rel. Ret	% Change
$BM25$	0.1073	+25.44%	**	4783	+15.28%
LM	0.1052	+27.94%	**	4685	+17.69%
GQE	0.1346	-	-	5514	-

ranking approaches $(BM25, LM)$ from $25, 44\%$ to $27, 94\%$. From these results, we can highlight that our semantic approach allows achieving better results than state-of-the-art word-based IR models that do not specifically take into account the PICO framework; this yields a credit to our intuition behind question elicitation on the basis of the semantic hidden behind each question facet.

5   Conclusion

In this paper, we presented a novel approach to answer PICO clinical queries. The key underlying idea is to enhance each query facet with the most representative terminological concepts on the basis of a local search context. Moreover, we apply a score propagation algorithm that allows selecting the concepts with higher matching degree over the whole search context and across the different query facets. Experiments on a standard data set highlight that the proposed approach significantly overpasses state-of-the-art IR models. In future, we plan to integrate a weighting facet schema in the document ranking model in order to consider the differences in the importance of the question facets with respect to document relevance.

References

1. Boudin, F., Nie, J.-Y., Bartlett, J., Grad, R., Pluye, P., Dawes, M.: Combining classifiers for robust pico element detection. BMC Medical Informatics and Decision Making 10(1), 29 (2010)
2. Boudin, F., Nie, J.Y., Dawes, M.: Clinical information retrieval using document and PICO structure. In: NAACL HLT, pp. 822–830 (2010)
3. Boudin, F., Nie, J.-Y., Dawes, M.: Positional language models for clinical information retrieval. In: EMNLP, pp. 108–115 (2010)
4. Chung, G.Y.: Sentence retrieval for abstracts of randomized controlled trials. BMC Med. Inform. Decis. Mak. 9, 10 (2009)
5. Demner-Fushman, D., Lin, J.: Answering clinical questions with knowledge-based and statistical techniques. Comput. Linguist. 33(1), 63–103 (2007)
6. Dinh, D., Tamine, L.: Towards a context sensitive approach to searching information based on domain specific knowledge sources. Web Semantics: Science, Services and Agents on the World Wide Web 12 (2012)
7. Robertson, S., Jones, K.S.: Relevance weighting of search terms. Journal of the American Society on Informtion Science and Technology 27(3) (1976)

8. Sackett, D.L., Rosenberg, W.M.C., Gray, J.A.M., Haynes, R.B., Richardson, W.S.: Evidence based medicine: what it is and what it isn't. BMJ 312(7023), 71–72 (1996)
9. Song, F., Croft, W.B.: A general language model for information retrieval. In: ACM SIGIR, pp. 279–280 (1999)
10. Stokes, N., Cavedon, Y., Zobel, J.: Exploring criteria for succesful query expansion in the genomic domain. Information Retrieval 12, 17–50 (2009)
11. Zhao, J., Yen Kan, M., Procter, P.M., Zubaidah, S., Yip, W.K., Li, G.M.: Improving search for evidence-based practice using information extraction. BMC Medical Informatics and Decision Making 10(29) (2010)

Semantic Analysis and Automatic Corpus Construction for Entailment Recognition in Medical Texts

Asma Ben Abacha[✉], Duy Dinh, and Yassine Mrabet

Luxembourg Institute of Science and Technology (LIST), Luxembourg, Luxembourg
{asma.benabacha,duy.dinh,yassine.mrabet}@list.lu

Abstract. Textual Entailment Recognition (RTE) consists in detecting inference relationships between natural language sentences. It has a wide range of applications such as machine translation, question answering or text summarization. Significant interest has been brought to RTE with several challenges. However, most of current approaches are dedicated to open domains. The major challenge facing RTE in specialized domains is the lack of relevant training corpora and resources. In this paper we present an automatic corpus construction approach for RTE in the medical domain. We also quantify the impact of using (open-)domain RDF datasets on supervised learning based RTE. We evaluate the relevance of our corpus construction method by comparing the results obtained by an efficient memory based learning algorithm on PASCAL RTE corpora and on our automatically constructed corpus. The results show an accuracy increase of +6 to +28% and an improvement of +8 to +23% in terms of F-measure. We also found that semantic annotations from large open-domain datasets increased F1 score by 6%, while smaller medical RDF datasets actually decreased the overall performance. We discuss these findings and give some pointers to future investigations.

1 Background

Textual Entailment (TE) can be described as a directional relation expressing the fact that "the meaning of a text snippet is contained in the meaning of a second piece of text" [4]. The entailing and entailed texts are called *text* (T) and *hypothesis* (H). The first PASCAL Recognizing Textual Entailment Challenge (2004-2005) defined the task of Recognizing Textual Entailment (RTE) as deciding, given two text fragments, whether or not the meaning of one text (H) can be inferred (entailed) from the other one (T) [3].

RTE is an important component in Natural Language Understanding. It opens relevant tracks and perspectives for several applications such as Information Extraction, Machine Translation, Question Answering or Document Summarization. For instance, [5] argue that RTE can enable QA systems to identify correct answers with greater precision than keyword or pattern based methods. They showed that TE accuracy can be increased up to 20% overall when *filtering* or *ranking* the answers of a QA system.

While open-domain TE has been extensively addressed in the literature, RTE has been less addressed for more restricted and specialized fields such as the biomedical domain. [10] proposed a method to expand existing open-domain TE corpora. They extracted a large set of TE pairs from Wikipedia and used a semi-supervised machine learning method to make the extracted dataset homogeneous with the existing corpora.

© Springer International Publishing Switzerland 2015
J.H. Holmes et al. (Eds.): AIME 2015, LNAI 9105, pp. 238–242, 2015.
DOI: 10.1007/978-3-319-19551-3_31

Other efforts tackled the automatic generation of training corpora for a specific language. For instance, [7] proposed a method to create a Greek Textual Entailment Corpus that can be exploited for training or evaluating a system for RTE from Greek texts. As far as we know there are no training corpora for RTE in the medical domain.

Our first contribution is an automatic corpus construction method for RTE in the biomedical domain. In a second contribution, we analyze the impact of semantic annotations referring to (open-)domain RDF datasets on the RTE task. More precisely, we study the impact of annotations from DBpedia, SNOMED-CT and NCI. Our experiments showed the relevance of the automatically constructed corpus as the results were significantly better than those obtained with the training corpora from PASCAL RTE 1, 2 and 3. They also show the positive impact of semantic annotations with significant performance shifts when using large open-domain datasets and medical datasets.

The remainder of the paper is organized as follows: Section 2 presents the semantic features that we propose for the RTE task. In section 3 we present the supervised learning algorithm used in our experiments and the full set of features. Section 4 presents our methodology to automatically construct a learning corpus. Section 6 describes our experimental evaluation and a discussion of the obtained results. Finally, section 7 gives the conclusions and lines for future work.

2   Learning Algorithm and Baseline Features

In order to evaluate our corpus construction method and the semantic annotation features, we build a baseline approach based on the Tilburg memory-based learning classifier (TiMBL)[1]. TiMBL is a descendant of the k-nearest neighbour approach. It is based on analogical reasoning: the behaviour of new instances is predicted by extrapolating from the similarity between (old) stored representations and the new instances. Given that the training stage is done without abstraction but by simply storing training instances in memory, it is considerably faster than other machine learning algorithms.

In order to select the most relevant features, we first removed stop words and performed word stemming using the Porter algorithm for all (T, H) pairs. We then tested several knowledge-based and lexical features on 4 different Memory-based Learning algorithms implemented in Timbl, using the data from the RTE-3 challenge as learning data. These tests led to the selection of the following features for each (T, H) pair:

- **JC**: [6] combined both edge-counts as well as information content values using the WordNet 'is-a' hierarchy to compute the similarity between two words. The final similarity between T and H is the average of each couple of most similar words.
- **WO**: [8] defined the word overlap as the proportion of words that appear in both sentences normalized by the sentence's length. We compute the word overlap between T and H and normalize by the length of T.
- **NE**: NegEx has been proposed by [2] for finding terms used in negative senses. It relies on trigger terms, pseudo-trigger terms, and termination terms for identifying negation scope in either T and H respectively.
- **BS**: The best similarity between all tested similarity measures.

---

[1] http://ilk.uvt.nl/timbl/

Several Memory-based Learning algorithms are available in TIMBL. We used the above set of features and the train and test corpora from the PASCAL RTE-3 workshop to select the most efficient algorithm, which was IB1 [1] with an accuracy of 64.12%.

3 Semantic Annotations

Using semantic knowledge bases provides a semantic level of abstraction above the "words" level. We considered the annotation with both open-domain and medical ontologies represented in RDF, namely DBpedia, SNOMED-CT and NCI. SNOMED-CT is known as the most comprehensive clinical healthcare terminology. NCI is a recognized standard for biomedical coding. DBpedia is an knowledge base constructed from Wikipedia infoboxes. This is particularly suitable to text annotation as specialized ontologies do not represent general concepts (e.g. "challenge" has been annotated as <Histamine challenge> in NCI because it does not contain the general concept).

All semantic annotations were obtained automatically using *KODA*, an unsupervised ontology-based annotator which relies only on indexation and ontology-level co-occurrences to annotate the target texts [9]. Another interesting feature of *KODA* is that it can provide semantic interpretation of words according to the semantic context. For instance, in the sentence "To make a comprehensive evaluation of the efficiency of eradication therapy in patients with coronary heart disease (CHD) ..", the word "Eradication" has been annotated by the DBpedia entity <Eradication_of_infectious_diseases>.

The main features derived from these annotations are the number of common entities between the text T and the hypothesis H. Three features are defined to represent the number of common entities according to the point of view of each ontology (i.e. one feature per ontology). We will refer to these features as DBP, SCT, NCI, referring to the respective number of DBpedia/SnomedCT/NCI concepts in common between T and H. We study and discuss the impact of these features w.r.t. the baseline in section 6.

4 Automatic Corpus Construction

As shown by Google statistics on "search trends", the most searched diseases on Google (2004-to-present) are Heart diseases, Lyme disease and Celiac disease[2]. Following this observation, we collected 200 MEDLINE abstracts on heart diseases as the first part of our corpus. For the second part of the corpus we collect 200 MEDLINE abstracts on Depression. This last choice is motivated by the fact that articles about psychiatric diseases (e.g. symptoms of Depression) could include general terms that are not specific to the medical domain (e.g. Loss of interest in activities or hobbies, persistent sad or anxious feelings), which makes the comparison with open-domain corpora/systems more reliable. The 400 MEDLINE abstracts were obtained from a PubMed search with keywords relevant to each disease.

We created automatically 4 corpora of textual entailment (TE) examples by pairing the title (T), the first sentence of the abstract (I; for introduction) and the last sentence (C; for conclusion). We considered the following 4 hypotheses/scenarios:

---

[2] http://www.google.com/trends/explore#q=disease\&mpt=q

- **TI**: the title T implies the first sentence of the abstract I (T → I)
- **IT**: the first sentence of the abstract I implies the title T (I → T)
- **TC**: the title T implies the last sentence of the abstract C (T → C)
- **CT**: the last sentence of the abstract C implies the title T (C → T)

In order to test these hypotheses, we trained our classifier on the PASCAL-3-Dev corpus then tested it on the 4 candidate TE corpora. The best results were obtained with the IT pairs for both diseases (44.65% and 46.01% accuracy). From these empirical observations we selected the 400 IT pairs *(the first sentence of the abstract I implies the title T)* as positive examples. We extract negative examples from the same corpus of 400 MEDLINE abstracts. We collect two types of data: (i) pairs of consecutive sentences and (ii) pairs of sentences linked by contrast connectives such as *even though, in contrast*, etc. [5]. We selected also sentences linked by connectives such as: *besides, furthermore, moreover, in addition*. We do not consider all the available negative examples to guarantee a balanced number of negative and positive examples. We randomly selected 500 negative pairs. Finally we apply a semantic filter using DBpedia annotations. All positive pairs were annotated automatically with DBpedia using KODA. We then kept only the (T,H) pairs sharing at least one DBpedia concept. This process led to the selection of 175 positive pairs from the initial 400 pairs.

5 Evaluation

The goal of this investigation is (i) to evaluate our method for the automatic construction of a medical corpus for RTE, (ii) to test the benefits of domain-related corpora vs. open-domain corpora and (iii) test the impact of the semantic features. We constructed a test corpus from MEDLINE abstracts. We targeted two different diseases to test the portability of our method to other subfields of the medical domain: Lyme Disease and Celiac Disease (i.e. the second and third most "important" diseases according to Google's search trends). Starting from PubMed query results, we extracted automatically title/first sentence pairs and consecutive-sentence pairs, the ratio of each kinf of pairs is 50%. Finally, we selected manually 120 positive and negative pairs as a test benchmark. We calculate the *precision - P, recall - R, F-measure* and the *accuracy - A*.

Table 1. Results of the baseline classifier with the automatically-constructed medical corpus. MM1: Classification with only the baseline features. MM2: Classification with DBpedia annotations. MM3: Classification with SNOMED-CT. MM4: Classification with NCI.

	P	R	F	A
MM1	0.6400	0.8205	0.7191	0.7917
MM2	0.8400	0.7241	0.7778	0.8000
MM3	0.7800	0.6842	0.7290	0.7583
MM4	0.8200	0.7193	0.7664	0.7917

The baseline classifier and baseline features obtained 68% F-measure and 74% accuracy when trained with the Pascal RTE 3 corpus, 51% F-measure and 46% accuracy with Pascal RTE 2 and 44% F-measure and 65% accuracy with Pascal RTE 1. The same baseline classifier obtained the best performance of 77% F-measure and 80% accuracy with our automatically-built training corpus (resp. increase of 9% F1 and 6%

Acc. when compared to the best Pascal corpus), cf. table 1. This is a very positive result since no manual interventions were made to enhance our training corpus. Also, a higher performance could be reached with a better balance between the number of positive pairs and negative pairs (currently 175/400). Our results also show that DBpedia annotations outperformed both Snomed-CT and NCI. All knowledge bases had a positive impact on precision and a negative impact on recall. DBpedia annotations led to the best results (77% F-measure and 80% accuracy) due to their wide coverage for common terms.

6   Conclusion

We described an RTE approach dedicated to specialized domains for the construction of training RTE corpora and tested it on medical texts. The results confirm the relevance and enhanced performance of supervised learning approaches on domain-specific corpora instead of open-domain corpora. We also tested the impact of annotations referring to knowledge bases such as DBpedia, SNOMED CT and NCI. The ablation study showed that semantic features enhance significantly the F1 score and have a slight positive impact on accuracy. More particularly DBpedia led to significantly higher results than Snomed-CT and NCI. Perspectives of our work include the evaluation of semantic annotations with different supervised learning algorithms and additional corpora.

References

1. Aha, D.W., Kibler, D., Albert, M.K.: Instance-based learning algorithms. Mach. Learn. 6(1), 37–66 (1991)
2. Chapman, W.W., Bridewell, W., Hanbury, P., Cooper, G.F., Buchanan, B.G.: A Simple Algorithm for Identifying Negated Findings and Diseases in Discharge Summaries. Journal of Biomedical Informatics 34(5), 301–310 (2001)
3. Dagan, I., Oren et al.:Glickman. The pascal recognising textual entailment challenge. In: Proc. of PASCAL Challenges on Recognising Textual Entailment (2005)
4. Dagan, I., Roth, D., et al.: Recognizing Textual Entailment: Models and Applications. Synthesis Lectures on Human Language Technologies (2013)
5. Harabagiu, S., Hickl, A.: Methods for using textual entailment in open-domain question answering. In: Proc. of the 21st International Conference on Computational Linguistics, pp. 905–912. Association for Computational Linguistics (2006)
6. Jiang, J.J., Conrath, D.W.: Semantic similarity based on corpus statistics and lexical taxonomy. CoRR, cmp-lg/9709008 (1997)
7. Marzelou, E., Zourari, M., Giouli, V., Piperidis, S.: Building a Greek corpus of Textual Entailment. In: Proc. of the 6th Language Resources and Evaluation Conference, Marrakech, Morocco, pp. 1680–1686 (May 2008)
8. Metzler, D., Bernstein, Y., Croft, W.B., Moffat, A., Zobel, J.: Similarity measures for tracking information flow. In: Proc. of the 14th ACM International Conference on Information and Knowledge Management, pp. 517–524. ACM (2005)
9. Mrabet, Y., Gardent, C., Foulonneau, M., Simperl, E., Ras, E.: Towards Knowledge Driven Annotation. In: 29th AAAI Conference on Artificial Intelligence (2015)
10. Zanzotto, F.M., Pennacchiotti, M.: Expanding textual entailment corpora from wikipedia using co-training. In: In Proc of the 2nd Coling Workshop on The Peoples Web Meets NLP: Collaboratively Constructed Semantic Resources, pp. 28–36 (2010)

Automatic Computing of Global Emotional Polarity in French Health Forum Messages

Natalia Grabar and Loïc Dumonet[⊠]

CNRS UMR 8163 STL, Université Lille 3, 59653, Villeneuve d'Ascq, France
natalia.grabar@univ-lille3.fr, loicdumonet@yahoo.fr

Abstract. Social media provide the possibility for people to freely communicate. These discussion are rich with subjectivity and emotions, which is due to the anonymity of contributors. We propose to work on health fora in French and on subjective entities (*e.g.* emotions, feelings, uncertainties). Our specific interest is to study how the polarity of emotions is influenced by negation, uncertainty, modifiers and discoursive markers, and how the global polarity of sentences is constructed. We design a rule-based system and evaluate is against manually built reference data. Inter-annotator agreement is between 0.50 and 0.66. An evaluation of the automatic system shows between 40 and 56% precision.

1 Introduction

Social media dedicated to health topics provide the possibility for patients to freely communicate on their health conditions, drugs, procedures, medical doctors, etc. This communication is prone for expressing emotions, feelings [9], and more generally the subjectivity of patients, which is certainly due to their anonymity and to the topics discussed. Forum discussions may thus provide new insights on life and well being of patients. Health fora contain two main types of entities: conceptual (*e.g.* medical problems, drugs, procedures) and subjective (*e.g.* emotions, opinions, uncertainties). We propose to study the latter in order to observe how emotions interact among them, how they are influenced by negation and uncertainties, and how the global emotional polarity of sentences is constructed. Among the related studies, we can find those dedicated to the acquisition of emotion lexica in different languages [20,2]; to the emotion categorization [14,13,19]; to their relation with events and entities [3,18]; and to the exploitation of emotions in various NLP applications [4,5,15,11]. Besides, some NLP studies combine emotions with negation [17], while in logic studies researchers analyze logical impact of modifiers, uncertainty and negation [21,7].

2 Material and Material

Corpora. Two kinds of corpora in French are used: *QA* (993,383 occ.) and *Forum* (1,763,022 occ.) corpora. *QA* corpus is built from *MaSanteNet* website[1],

---

[1] www.masantenet.com

J.H. Holmes et al. (Eds.): AIME 2015, LNAI 9105, pp. 243–248, 2015.
DOI: 10.1007/978-3-319-19551-3_32

and contains questions submitted by patients and answers provided by medical professionals. *Forum* corpus also provides discussion threads, in which questions submitted by patients are usually answered by other patients with more personal experience. This corpus is built from *Doctissimo*[2] website.

Resources. Resources exploited for the detection of subjectivity and emotions cover different types of markers:

- Emotions (n=1,144) [2]. Lexicon entries are associated with over 30 emotions (*e.g. sadness, disgust, joy, shame*). Emotions are grouped in three categories: *sadness* is a negative emotion, *joy* is positive, *astonishment* is neutral.
- Uncertainty (n=101) is expressed with various linguistic units (*e.g. suppose, appear, suspect, possibility, hypothesis, likely, doubtful, maybe*), and indicates that given information is not fully certain and is to be taken with caution.
- Negation (n=20) can be expressed with various markers (*e.g. no, absence, negative, impossible, without*), and indicates that given information is absent.
- Modifiers or intensifiers (n=17) include markers such as *little, very little, extremely*, or *truly*. Two kinds of modifiers are distinguished: *modif-p* which increases the degree, and *modif-m* which decreases the degree.

Our work addresses the interaction between these various markers and discourse connectors, in order to compute the global emotion polarity of sentences.

Reference Data for the Evaluation of Global Polarity. Reference data are created by a manual annotation of sentences by two annotators (500 in *QA* and 80 in *Forum* corpora). The objective is to define the global emotion polarity of sentences. Possible categories are *positive, negative* and *neutral*.

2.1 Semantic Annotation of Corpora

Reaccenting the Corpora. Forum corpora often miss accented characters, which may have negative impact on the annotation. Hence, we generate reaccented version of corpora through a comparison with the reference lexicon.

Semantic Annotation. Semantic annotation consists of detection of various markers from the resources, and of non-lexical emotion marks: smileys or emoticons (=), ;-), :-/, XD), mark of laugh (*lol, mdr, haha, hihi*), emotional punctuation (*!!!??, !!!!!!!!!!*, words with duplicated letters (*maaaaaaal (paaaaaaain), noooooooon (nooooooooo)*)) These non-lexical emotion marks are also typed according to whether they denote positive (*e.g.,* =), *mdr, looool*), negative (*e.g.,* :-(, :-/) or neutral (*e.g., ???!!?, ohhhhh*) emotions.

2.2 Rule-Based System for Computing the Global Emotion Polarity

Context and Rules. Emotions are the processed units. These units are studied in windows of maximum seven words on the left and on the right [8]. The window size can be reduced when strong (*?, ., !*) or medium (*:, ;, (), []*) punctuation, or discourse connectors (*e.g. car (because), mais (but)*) are found. Within this

---

[2] forum.doctissimo.fr/sante/douleur-dos

window, we detect negation, uncertainty and modifier markers, and apply four rules that manage the scope of markers and their semantics:

1. *Negation.* If negation (*e.g. ne...pas (no), rien (nothing), aucun (any)*) is found, then the polarity of emotion is inversed (positive and neutral → negative, negative → positive). Maximal size of the negation window is five tokens.
2. *Modifiers.* If modifier is found, then the emotion polarity is amplified or attenuated according to modifiers. Modifiers can combine with negation and uncertainty. Maximal size of the modifier window is three tokens. When several modifiers are found, all of them influence the unity processed.
3. *Uncertainty.* If uncertainty is found within a maximal window of seven tokens, then the emotion polarity is attenuated.
4. *Connector.* If discoursive connector (*e.g. car (because), donc (hence), mais (but), cependant (however)*) is detected, then the emotion polarity is either amplified or attenuated according to connectors.

Combination of Markers. Different markers can co-occur within emotion contexts. Their combination requires specific principles and additional rules:

1. *negation + modif-p.* When negation is followed by *modif-p* modifier, this attenuates the polarity of negation.
2. *modif-p + modif-p.* When modifier *modif-p* is followed by modifier *modif-p*, this leads to a doubled increase of the emotion polarity.
3. *modif-p + modif-m.* When modifier *modif-p* is followed by *modif-m*, *modif-p* amplifies *modif-m*, which leads to a double attenuation of the polarity.

Occurrence of connectors within right or left context of emotions reduces the scope of other markers. Still, the impact of connectors varies according to their own scope and to the size of window they operate within [10]:

- *mais (but)* and *cependant (nevertheless/yet)* introduce separation between the text that precedes and the text follows the connector;
- *car (because)* strengthens preceding information by the following information;
- *et (and)* means enumeration of emotions;
- *donc (hence)* gives more importance to information that follows.

Computing the Global Emotion Polarity. Markers occurring in contexts of emotions modify their intensity and polarity. The starting point is the initial intensity associated with each emotion polarity [16,17]: +0.5 for positive emotions, -0.5 for negative emotions, and 0 for neutral emotions. Modifiers modify these initial values with +0.1 if they increase the intensity, -0.1 if they decrease the intensity, and -0.05 if they bring uncertainty. Negation inverses the polarity. If several polarities have the same score S, we apply the following principles:

- if $S_{pos} = S_{neg} \Rightarrow$ global polarity is neutral;
- if $S_{pos} = S_{neu} \Rightarrow$ global polarity is positive;
- if $S_{neg} = S_{neu} \Rightarrow$ global polarity is negative.

Table 1. Evaluation against the two annotators and the common dataset

Annotators	Corpus	BL	E1	E2	E3	E4
A1	QA	39.92	**42.07**	41.64	41.21	40.78
	Forum	41.08	**44.65**	41.08	40.00	40.00
A2	QA	49.79	**55.80**	55.80	54.94	54.51
	Forum	42.86	**42.86**	**42.86**	38.19	41.82
common	QA	44.06	**46.54**	46.04	46.04	45.55
	Forum	**45.10**	41.18	43.14	40.00	42.00

2.3   Evaluation

Evaluation of global emotion polarity is done against the reference data prepared by manual annotation. Evaluation is performed with the precision measure in order to assess the correctness of the output of the system.

3   Discussion of Results and Future Work

Inter-Annotator Agreement. Inter-annotator agreement between annotators is computed with the Cohen kappa [6]: 0.63 agreement in *QA* corpus, and 0.58 in *forum* corpus, which corresponds to good and moderate agreement, respectively [12]. We can observe that annotators show poorer agreement with neutral polarity, for which there is an hesitation to assign neutral polarity or to consider that there is no polarity to be assigned. The two other polarities are more consensual.

Evaluation of the Rule-Based System. Precision values of the rule-based system are indicated in Table 1. Several versions of the system are evaluated:

- *BL*: the baseline version corresponds to original annotations, on which the global emotion polarity is computed, but without the application of rules;
- *E1*: the proposed rules are applied and the global polarity is computed;
- *E2*: the corpus is reaccented on which the proposed rules are applied and the global polarity is computed;
- *E3*: the global polarity corresponds to the last emotion, which shows to be suitable for processing of emotions in Chinese sentences [10];
- *E4*: the global polarity corresponds to the last emotion and is computed on the reaccented corpus.

Automatically computed results are compared with the reference annotations provided by each annotator and with the *common* set containing common annotations. The best results (up to 56% precision) are obtained with the rule-based system we propose *E1*, which main advantage is to manage semantics of emotions, negation, modifiers, uncertainty and discourse connectors, and their interactions. These results are comparable with the published work [17,3]. With our system, we can gain up to 6% by comparison with our baseline. Besides, reaccenting of corpus is suitable for the task, while the last emotion uttered does not correspond to the global emotion polarity of sentences in French.

We have several direction for future work: producing larger reference set with consensual annotations; better adaptation of method and resources to forum discussions; exploitation of syntactic analysis for computing the scope of markers. The system can be applied to other fora and genres (*e.g.* novels, political texts). Besides, a fine-grained interaction between the operators used in our work can be defined [21,1,7]. These operators can also be transformed in order to be used by a supervised machine-learning system. Supervised approaches have shown to be efficient in the processing of this kind of material [14]. In this way, we expect to improve global performance of our system and to obtain more precise results.

References

1. Akdag, H., DeGlas, M., Pacholczyk, D.: A qualitative theory of uncertainty. Fundamenta Informaticae 17(4), 333–362 (1992)
2. Augustyn, M., Ben Hamou, S., Bloquet, G., Goossens, V., Loiseau, M., Rynck, F.: Constitution de ressources pédagogiques numériques: le lexique des affects, pp. 407–414. Presses Universitaires de Grenoble (2008)
3. Bakliwal, A., Foster, J., van der Puil, J., O'Brien, R., Tounsi, L., Hughes, M.: Sentiment analysis of political tweets: towards an accurate classifier (2013)
4. Battaïa, C.: L'analyse de lémotion dans les forums de santé. JEP-TALN-RECITAL, RECITAL pp. 267–280 (2012)
5. Chauveau-Thoumelin, P., Grabar, N.: La subjectivité dans le discours médical: sur les traces de l'incertitude et des émotions. In: EGC 2014, pp. 455–466 (2014)
6. Cohen, J.: A coefficient of agreement for nominal scales. Educational and Psychological Measurement 20(1), 37–46 (1960)
7. Cornelis, C., DeCock, M., Kerre, E.: Efficient Approximate Reasoning with Positive and Negative Information, pp. 779–785 (2004)
8. Feng, S., Zhang, L., Li, B., Wang, D., Yu, G., Wong, K.F.: Is twitter a better corpus for measuring sentiment similarity? In: EMNLP, pp. 897–902 (2013)
9. Gauducheau, N.: La communication des émotions dans les échanges médiatisés par ordinateur: bilan et perspectives. Bulletin de Psychologie 61(4), 389–404 (2008)
10. Huang, H., Yu, C., Lin, T., Chang, C., Chen, H.: Analyses of the association between discourse relation and sentiment polarity with a Chinese human-annotated corpus. LAW VII & ID, p. 70 (2013)
11. Huh, J., Yetisgen-Yildiz, M., Pratt, W.: Text classification for assisting moderators in online health communities. Journ. Biomed. Inform. 46(6), 998–1005 (2013)
12. Landis, J., Koch, G.: The measurement of observer agreement for categorical data. Biometrics 33, 159–174 (1977)
13. Li, S., Lee, S.Y.M., Chen, Y., Huang, C.R., Zhou, G.: Sentiment classification and polarity shifting. In: COLING, pp. 635–643 (2010)
14. Liu, Y., Yu, X., Liu, B., Chen, Z.: Sentence-level sentiment analysis in the presence of modalities. In: Gelbukh, A. (ed.) CICLing 2014, Part II. LNCS, vol. 8404, pp. 1–16. Springer, Heidelberg (2014)
15. Maurel, S., Curtoni, P., Dini, L.: L'analyse des sentiments dans les forums. Atelier Fouille des Données d'Opinion (2008)
16. Moreno-Ortiz, A., Pérez-Hernández, C., Del-Olmo, M., et al.: Managing multiword expressions in a lexicon-based sentiment analysis system for spanish. In: NAACL HLT 2013, vol. 13, p. 1 (2013)

17. Paroubek, P., Pak, A.: Le microblogage pour la microanalyse des sentiments et des opinions. TAL 51(3) (2010)
18. Ramteke, A., Malu, A., Bhattacharyya, P., Nath, J.S.: Detecting turnarounds in sentiment analysis: Thwarting. In: ACL, pp. 860–865 (2013)
19. Sayeed, A.B., Boyd-Graber, J.L., Rusk, B., Weinberg, A.: Grammatical structures for word-level sentiment detection. In: HLT-NAACL, pp. 667–676 (2012)
20. Tokuhisa, R., Inui, K., Matsumoto, Y.: Emotion classification using massive examples extracted from the web. In: COLING, pp. 881–888 (2008)
21. Zadeh, L.: A fuzzy-set-theoretic interpretation of linguistic hedges. Journal of Cybernetics 2(3), 4–34 (1972)

Automatic Symptom Extraction from Texts to Enhance Knowledge Discovery on Rare Diseases

Jean-Philippe Métivier[1], Laurie Serrano[2(✉)], Thierry Charnois[3],
Bertrand Cuissart[1], and Antoine Widlöcher[1]

[1] Laboratoire GREYC, Univ. de Caen B.-N., CNRS, UMR6072, Caen, France
{jean-philippe.metivier,bertrand.cuissart,antoine.widlocher}@unicaen.fr
[2] Laboratoire MoDyCo, Univ. Paris X, CNRS, UMR7114, Nanterre, France
laurie.serrano@u-paris10.fr
[3] Laboratoire LIPN, Univ. Paris-Nord, CNRS, UMR7030, Villetaneuse, France
thierry.charnois@lipn.univ-paris13.fr

Abstract. This paper reports ongoing researches on automatic symptom recognition towards diagnosis of rare diseases and knowledge acquisition on this subject. We describe a hybrid approach combining sequential pattern mining and natural language processing techniques in order to automate the discovery of symptoms from textual content. More precisely, our weakly supervised approach uses linguistic knowledge to enhance an incremental pattern mining process, in order to filter and make a relevant use of the discovered patterns.

Keywords: Biomedical knowledge acquisition · Symptoms and rare diseases · Text mining · Incremental sequential data mining · Biomedical natural language processing

1 Introduction

A disease which affects less than 1 over 2,000 people is called a rare disease (RD): RDs are often disabling and life-threatening and, for most of these, there is no available cure. The Orphanet initiative maintains a reference portal providing services for knowledge sharing among the RD community. The related database includes expert-authored and peer-reviewed syntheses describing current knowledge about each RD. These syntheses result from a manual and time-consuming monitoring of literature made by specialists of RDs.

The work introduced in this paper aims at automating the update of the Orphanet knowledge by automatically identifying new symptoms associated to RDs. Symptoms have been rarely studied for themselves within biomedical information extraction (IE) literature but are often included in more general categories such as "clinical concepts", "medical problems" or "phenotypic information". In this work, we use the term "symptoms" to refer indifferently to functional and clinical signs of a disease. A very few studies consider linguistic contexts of symptoms towards their

© Springer International Publishing Switzerland 2015
J.H. Holmes et al. (Eds.): AIME 2015, LNAI 9105, pp. 249–254, 2015.
DOI: 10.1007/978-3-319-19551-3_33

automatic recognition. Some tackled symptom recognition with manually developed annotation rules [4] whereas others like [8] used a statistical approach (CRFs) to process clinical records. More recently, [7] automatically identified phenotypic information using the HPO ontology in order to recognize already known symptoms and enhance online search facilities. Most of existing studies process clinical reports or narrative corpora [6], whereas our work aims at scientific monitoring and analyses abstracts from research articles.

The overview of literature put forward two main difficulties: first, few works have tackled the problem of mining symptoms from texts and therefore existing resources are limited and incomplete; second, a given symptom can be expressed by multiple and diverse textual expressions which makes its automatic extraction very complex [5]. The contribution of this paper is to address these problems, designing a hybrid approach that combines data mining and natural language processing (NLP). On the one hand, we use an incremental process of frequent sequential data mining in order to automatically discover regularities (patterns) over textual expression of symptoms. The extracted patterns are then used for symptom recognition, each step of the incremental process allowing to discover more numerous symptoms. On the other hand, NLP techniques are involved to enhance the mining process and select relevant patterns, dealing with the well-known limitation of pattern mining techniques which produce very large, and hard to use, sets of patterns. It is worth noting that our method is fully automated and weakly supervised: to boot the process, the corpora are automatically annotated using public resources and the patterns are not validated manually.

Section 2 presents our hybrid approach. In Section 3, we give some preliminary results with their analysis and some possible technical improvements. Finally, Section 4 summarizes our contributions and provides perspectives.

2   Discovery of New Symptoms through Data Mining and Natural Language Processing

The proposed method relies on an iterative process where each loop runs three steps (see Figure 1). A corpus of medical texts is required as input, and the output is an annotated version of these texts where symptoms are tagged. As a first step, the texts of the initial corpus are annotated with the current list of already known diseases and symptoms. Then the annotated texts are mined to extract frequent sequential patterns which contain at least one symptom. During the third step, the most relevant patterns are selected thanks to a quality measure. Selected patterns are applied to the corpus providing new potential symptoms which enhance the resources for the first step of the next iteration. Then, this allows new patterns to be discovered, and so on.

Tagging of the Corpus. Two existing resources are used to annotate abstracts during the preprocessing step:

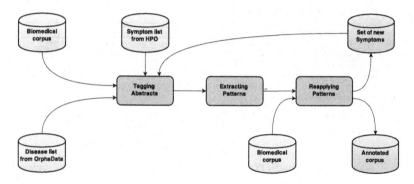

Fig. 1. Overall approach

1. OrphaData[1] provides a comprehensive, high-quality dataset related to rare diseases and orphan drugs. This resource allows to retrieve all the names of rare diseases and their aliases.
2. HPO[2] encapsulates a simple hierarchy of phenotypic anomalies. It does not provide a complete list of symptoms but this is a solid base to bootstrap the pattern mining phase.

These resources have been chosen for their specificity, rather than mostly used thesaurus (like UMLS *Unified Medical Language System* or MeSH *Medical Subject Headings*) that prove to be too large and generic for our objectives.

The corpus and the lists of terms coming from OrphaData and HPO are preprocessed using TreeTagger[3]: texts are tokenized, and each token is lemmatised and POS tagged. Each term (possibly composed of several tokens) coming from the external resources is matched against the corpus by comparing its tokens with those from the corpus. Terms coming from HPO are often generic (e.g. "weakness") and may be supplemented in medical texts with adjectives or object complements (e.g. "severe weakness of the tongue"). Thus, once a term matches, it can be expanded using the POS tags associated to surrounding terms.

Linguistic Pattern Mining. Sequential pattern mining was first introduced by [1] in the data mining field and was adapted to textual Information Extraction for instance by [2]. It is a matter of locating, in a set of sequences, sub-sequences (not necessarily contiguous) having a frequency above a given threshold. This mining process is applied to a base containing ordered sequences of itemsets where each sequence corresponds to a text unit (here sentences) and each itemset is a collection of features describing one word of a sequence. The goal is then to discover frequent sub-sequences of itemsets (called patterns).

---

[1] http://www.orphadata.org/

[2] http://www.human-phenotype-ontology.org/

[3] http://www.cis.uni-muenchen.de/~schmid/tools/TreeTagger/

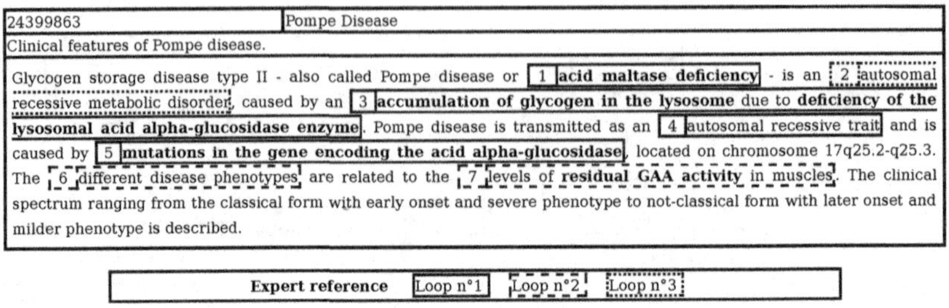

24399863	Pompe Disease
Clinical features of Pompe disease.	

Glycogen storage disease type II - also called Pompe disease or 1 acid maltase deficiency - is an 2 autosomal recessive metabolic disorder, caused by an 3 accumulation of glycogen in the lysosome due to deficiency of the lysosomal acid alpha-glucosidase enzyme . Pompe disease is transmitted as an 4 autosomal recessive trait and is caused by 5 mutations in the gene encoding the acid alpha-glucosidase, located on chromosome 17q25.2-q25.3. The 6 different disease phenotypes are related to the 7 levels of residual GAA activity in muscles. The clinical spectrum ranging from the classical form with early onset and severe phenotype to not-classical form with later onset and milder phenotype is described.

Expert reference   Loop n°1   Loop n°2   Loop n°3

Fig. 2. Three iterations applied on one abstract

In this work, we use the SDMC[4] extractor [2]: this tool provides several constraints (e.g. patterns length and gap between itemsets) to guide the search for useful patterns [3] and allows to get a condensed representation of the patterns without loss of information ("closed patterns"). Depending on the frequency threshold fixed, a very large number of sequential patterns may be extracted and it is necessary to filter them. To avoid a manual filtering, we use a quality measure relying on the following principle : if the number of occurrences of a pattern is by far larger than the number of occurrences from which it was discovered, this pattern probably involves too much noise.

Finding New Symptoms. Once the sequential patterns are extracted and filtered, these ones can be used to find new symptoms. Since they are recurrent structures announcing symptoms, they are matched against the corpus in order to detect symptoms (already known symptoms as well as new ones). New symptoms can improve the previous annotations and may allow to extract new sequential patterns, and so on.

3   Preliminary Results

Experimental Corpus and Parameters. The initial corpus is composed of 150 raw abstracts collected from PubMed[5]. Sentences are used as sequences for the pattern mining process, which is set as follows: a frequency threshold of $0,25\%$, at least one symptom annotation included in each sequential pattern, a minimal length of 3 itemsets, and a gap fixed to 0 (patterns of contiguous elements). To filter irrelevant patterns the quality threshold is set to 2 during the first loop. This threshold is decreased of 10% at each loop to avoid a snowball effect.

Abstract-Example and Qualitative Analysis by an Expert. Figure 2 depicts an example of an abstract processed using our method. Bold annotations correspond to symptoms manually asserted by an expert, and squared annotations to symptoms that have been automatically recognized (a different style

---

[4] http://sdmc.greyc.fr

[5] www.ncbi.nlm.nih.gov/pubmed

of square is used for each loop). Here, the expert marked five symptoms which were all recognized by our extractor, meaning that our method may have a good recall. Nevertheless, some annotations remain imperfect. Different kind of errors arise: firstly, the symptoms *accumulation of glycogen in the lysosome* and *deficiency of the lysosomal acid alpha-glucosidase enzyme* were tagged as a single annotation (3); secondly, two other annotations (2) (4) do not refer to symptoms but to inheritance expressions; thirdly, another false positive appears during the second loop (6).

On-Going Improvements. Most of the erroneous annotations could be resolved by inserting deeper linguistic knowledge at different stages of the method. The first problem (3) could be quite easily avoided by adding specific linguistic rules to detect causality expressions (e.g. *due to* or *leading to*). We also plan to develop similar rules to better annotate complex expressions of symptoms like enumerations. Furthermore, the integration of a syntactic analysis (particularly verbal and nominal groups segmentation) could fix wrong delimitations of entities (e.g. (7) compared to the expert choice). Finally, we noticed that many of the false positives annotated within the corpus were due to patterns having similar characteristics that can be classified and processed accordingly. For example, some errors come from too generic patterns like the ones containing only POS tags items and being quite short (a length of 3 itemsets).

4   Conclusions and Future Work

The outcomes of this research concern both the rare diseases and the IE domains: on one hand, we tackle automatic recognition of symptoms associated to RDs which is a problem poorly studied until now; on the other hand, our work explores a hybrid approach combining data mining and NLP techniques, following recent trends in the IE research community. It is worth noting that our system is weakly supervised, completely automatic and does not imply any manual operations from RD experts. The first experiments emphasize good results regarding the development cost and the (still basic) linguistic knowledge involved. The remaining extraction problems could be avoided by adding more sophisticated NLP techniques: a syntactic analysis of the corpus in order to better determine the symptoms' frontiers; the addition of linguistic constraints within the pattern mining process; the definition of linguistic rules to define and filter out categories of patterns that involve erroneous detections.

Acknowledgments. This research was supported by the Hybride project (ANR-11-BS02-002).

References

1. Agrawal, R., Srikant, R.: Mining sequential patterns. In: Proc. of the 11th International Conference on Data Engineering (1995)
2. Béchet, N., Cellier, P., Charnois, T., Crémilleux, B.: Discovering linguistic patterns using sequence mining. In: Proc. of the 13th International Conference on Computational Linguistics and Intelligent Text Processing (2012)
3. Dong, G., Pei, J.: Sequence Data Mining. Kluwer (2007)
4. Kokkinakis, D.: Developing resources for swedish bio-medical text mining. In: Proc. of the 2nd International Symposium on Semantic Mining in Biomedicine (2006)
5. Martin, L., Battistelli, D., Charnois, T.: Symptom extraction issue. In: Proc. of BioNLP 2014. Association for Computational Linguistics (2014)
6. Savova, G.K., Masanz, J.J., Ogren, P.V., Zheng, J., Sohn, S., Kipper-Schuler, K.C., Chute, C.G.: Mayo clinical text analysis and knowledge extraction system (ctakes): architecture, component evaluation and applications. Journal of the American Medical Informatics Association 17 (2010)
7. Taboada, M., Rodriguez, H., Martinez, D., Pardo, M., Sobrido, M.J.: Automated semantic annotation of rare disease cases: a case study. In: Database 2014 (2014)
8. Wang, Y., Liu, Y., Yu, Z., Chen, L., Jiang, Y.: A preliminary work on symptom name recognition from free-text clinical records of traditional chinese medicine using conditional random fields and reasonable features. In: Proc. of BioNLP (2012)

Prediction in Clinical Practice

A Composite Model for Classifying Parotid Shrinkage in Radiotherapy Patients Using Heterogeneous Data

Marco Pota[1(✉)], Elisa Scalco[2], Giuseppe Sanguineti[3], Maria Luisa Belli[4], Giovanni Mauro Cattaneo[4], Massimo Esposito[1] and Giovanna Rizzo[2]

[1] Institute for High Performance Computing and Networking (ICAR-CNR), Napoli, Italy
marco.pota@na.icar.cnr.it
[2] Institute of Molecular Bioimaging and Physiology (IBFM-CNR), Segrate MI, Italy
[3] Radiotherapy, Istituto Nazionale Tumori Regina Elena, Roma, Italy
[4] Medical Physics Department, San Raffaele Scientific Institute, Milano, Italy

Abstract. The identification of head-and-neck radiotherapy patients who will probably undergo the parotid gland shrinkage would help to plan adaptive therapy for them. The goal of this paper is to build predictive models to be included in a Decision Support System, able to operate with a wide set of heterogeneous data and classify parotid shrinkage. The main idea is to combine a set of models, each of them working distinctly with a group of features regarding clinical data, dosimetric data, or information extracted from Computed Tomography images, into one or more composite models using the most informative variables, in order to obtain more accurate and reliable decisions. Each of these models is built by using Likelihood-Fuzzy Analysis, which is based on both statistics and fuzzy logic, in order to grant semantic interpretability. This solution presents good accuracy, sensitivity and specificity, and compared with the well-known Fisher's Linear Discriminant Analysis results more effective in parotids classification, even in case of missing values. The best models operating with available features are achieved, and the advantages of acquiring data from different sources are outlined. Other interesting findings regard the confirmation of already known predictors, and the individuation of others still undisclosed.

Keywords: Fuzzy logic · Statistics · Parotid gland shrinkage · Radiotherapy

1 Introduction

Radiotherapy treatment (RT) in head-and-neck zone may induce the unpleasant effect of parotid gland shrinkage, with loss of salivary functionality, as widely evidenced [1]. Thus, before and during the RT, particular attention should be paid to the identification of patients who are susceptible to be concerned with parotid shrinkage, in order to program for them more specific cares as adaptive RT (ART) [2].

In this context, artificial intelligence was used with sundry results, by modelling data extracted from Computed Tomography (CT) images of patients, acquired during the treatment, in order to learn about the evolution of the shrinkage process. Classical works [2] studied the correlation between dosimetric features and parotid shrinkage, in order to find a model for volume decrease. More recent works were proposed for identifying patients at risk [3-7], by searching for predictors of parotid shrinkage,

© Springer International Publishing Switzerland 2015
J.H. Holmes et al. (Eds.): AIME 2015, LNAI 9105, pp. 257–266, 2015.
DOI: 10.1007/978-3-319-19551-3_34

among features extracted from CT images, as parotid volume [3,4], Jacobian index [5], and parotid mean density [3], or calculated from texture analysis [6,7].

The goal of this paper is to detect good sets of predictors, by building predictive models to be included in a Decision Support System (DSS), able to classify parotid shrinkage, by operating with a wider set of heterogeneous data. Interoperability issues of data coming from different sources are not examined here, while much concern is given to the construction of the best models employing sets of features coming from single or multiple sources, depending on their availability, a particular case being the model built with pre-treatment features only. In more detail, different sets of features will be used, consisting in general information pertaining the patient, dosimetric features set up by the therapist before the treatment start, anatomical information extracted from CT images taken before the treatment start, and the Jacobian index, extracted from CT images taken during the first two weeks of treatment.

The main idea is to first calculate the best model for each set of features by using the Likelihood-Fuzzy Analysis (LFA) [8,9], and then to build composite models by aggregating the simpler ones, thus considering different data sources at the same time, in order to obtain more accurate and reliable decisions. LFA is based on both statistics and fuzzy logic, and was chosen because it enables to handle data affected by uncertainty and including missing values, to build a classifier operating on the most informative among the available features, to present a confidence measure of results, and to grant semantic interpretability of the model, made of linguistic variables and *if-then* rules, which clearly and logically justify each prediction. The approach will be assessed in terms of accuracy, sensitivity and specificity in parotid classification, and compared with the well-known Fisher's Linear Discriminant Analysis (LDA).

The rest of the paper is structured as follows. In Section 2, the dataset is first presented. Then, the LFA approach for extracting simple predictive models as well as the method for composing them into a more complex one are described. Results are reported and discussed in Section 3, while Section 4 concludes the work.

2   Materials and Methods

2.1   Dataset

Available data regarding 40 parotid glands of 20 patients treated with intensity-modulated RT (IMRT) for nasopharyngeal cancer are pooled. For each patient, four sources of data are considered, whose features are specified as follows.

I) General Information. The age of the patient (*Age*) is extracted, since it was proved [2] to be a useful feature for the required model.

II) Dosimetric Information. The mean dose planned on parotid (*Dmean*), and the values of dose–volume histogram at planning (*V10*, *V15*, *V20*, *V30*, *V40*), corresponding to the percentage of parotid volume receiving at least 10, 15, 20, 30 or 40 Gy of dose, are used. Some instances are not available, thus, the dataset is incomplete.

III) Initial Clinical/Anatomical State. The following features are extracted from CT images acquired before the treatment (CT0): the planning target volume of high dose tumour (*PTVhd*), the absolute values of volume overlap between parotid gland and high dose tumour (*OVpghd*) and between the parotid gland and the lymph node chain (*OVpglc*), their respective relative values in percentage (*OVpghd%* and *OVpglc%*), and body thickness (*TH*) measured as the half-thickness at the level of vertebra C2.

IV) Evolution of Parotid Gland During the Early Phase of Treatment. The mean Jacobian index (*Jac*) is the determinant of the gradient matrix of the deformation field estimated from CT images acquired during the first and second week of treatment (CT1 and CT2). *Jac* quantifies the mean shrinkage or expansion of the single voxel, as global index to describe the early volume variation of the gland.

Parotid volume is measured from CT images taken before and after the treatment by using a dedicated algorithm [10]. The normalized relative difference between these values is assigned to a class, which can be significantly decreasing volume (*DV*) or approximately constant volume (*CV*). The method presented in [7] allows to divide samples into 30 belonging to the class *DV*, and 10 belonging to the class *CV*.

The sets of input variables corresponding to the features extracted from different sources are indicated with F_i, with $i=1,...,4$. Therefore, $F_1=\{Age\}$, $F_2=\{Dmean, V10, V15, V20, V30, V40\}$, $F_3=\{PTVhd, OVpghd, OVpglc, OVpghd\%, OVpglc\%, TH\}$, and $F_4=\{Jac\}$. The output class variable to predict is $Y\in\{DV, CV\}$.

2.2   Building a Fuzzy Model by Likelihood-Fuzzy Analysis

In this section, the procedure based on LFA and used to build a fuzzy model starting from a training dataset is explained.

The training dataset is constituted of N samples, each one corresponding to a pattern of values $\mathbf{x}_j=[x_j^{(1)},...,x_j^{(H)}]$, $j=1,...,N$, where H is the number of variables $X^{(h)}$ describing the features of the sample. A lack of knowledge about the data appears when some values $x_j^{(h)}$ are missing. Each sample is also associated to a class $y_j\in\{c_1,...,c_C\}$.

The knowledge extraction process consists in the fuzzy partition of each variable $X^{(h)}$ and in the construction of a rule base formulated according to the *if-then* structure.

The fuzzy partition of a variable X defines of a set of T membership functions (MFs) $\mu_t(x)$ of the fuzzy sets F_t, with $t\in\{1,...,T\}$ and $T>1$. Fuzzy sets are interpretable as terms of a linguistic variable if they satisfy some properties [11], i.e. normality, unimodality, continuity, distinguishability, coverage, and proper order. For this aim, $T-1$ sigmoid functions $S_t(x)=(1+\exp(a_tx+b_t))^{-1}$ are used with some constraints for a_t and b_t, to build the T MFs as follows, where $t\in\{2,...,T-1\}$ if $T>2$:

$$\mu_1(x)=1-S_1(x)\ ,\ ...,\ \mu_t(x)=S_{t-1}(x)-S_t(x)\ ,\ ...,\ \mu_T(x)=S_{T-1}(x)\ . \tag{1}$$

The fuzzy rule base is constituted by the complete set of rules $r_{\{t\_1,...,t\_H\}}$, with $\{t_1,...,t_H\}\in\{1,...,T_1\}\times...\times\{1,...,T_H\}$, made as follows:

$$\left(W_{\{t_1,...,t_H\}}\right)\ \textit{If } X^{(1)} \textit{ is } F_{t_1} \textit{ and ... and } X^{(H)} \textit{ is } F_{t_H} \textit{ then Y is } \begin{cases} \left(P_{\{t_1,...,t_H\}-1}\right)c_1 \\ ... \\ \left(P_{\{t_1,...,t_H\}-C}\right)c_C \end{cases} , \tag{2}$$

where the weight $W_{\{t\_1,...,t\_H\}}$ associated with the rule with respect to the others and the probability of the class k stated by the rule can be expressed as follows:

$$W_{\{t_1,...,t_H\}} = \frac{\sum\limits_{\kappa=1}^{C} w_{\{t_1,...,t_H\}-\kappa}}{\sum\limits_{\tau_1=1}^{T_1} \cdots \sum\limits_{\tau_H=1}^{T_H} \sum\limits_{\kappa=1}^{C} w_{\{\tau_1,...,\tau_H\}-\kappa}} \quad , \quad P_{\{t_1,...,t_H\}-k} = \frac{w_{\{t_1,...,t_H\}-k}}{\sum\limits_{\kappa=1}^{C} w_{\{t_1,...,t_H\}-\kappa}} \quad . \tag{3}$$

The number T of fuzzy sets as well as a_t and b_t, with $t \in \{1,...,T-1\}$ have to be found to define the fuzzy partition for each variable $X^{(h)}$, while the parameters $w_{\{t\_1,...,t\_H\}-k}$ have to be found to define the rule base.

In order to optimize all the parameters of the knowledge base, non-parametric likelihood functions, calculated from data even in case of some missing values, are approximated by a linear combination of membership functions:

$$p\left(c_k \mid x^{(h)}\right) \cong \sum_{t_h=1}^{T_h} \lambda_{t_h-k} \mu_{t_h}\left(x^{(h)}\right) . \tag{4}$$

In order to minimize the error of the approximation, a_{t_h} and b_{t_h}, with $t_h \in \{1,...,T_h-1\}$, λ_{t_h-k}, with $t_h \in \{1,...,T_h\}$ and $k \in \{1,...,C\}$, and the number of fuzzy sets T_h, are optimized all at once, separately for each variable $X^{(h)}$. Then, the fuzzy partitions (1) are defined by a_{t_h} and b_{t_h}, while the rule base (2) is defined by computing:

$$w_{\{t_1,...,t_H\}-k} = \frac{\lambda_{\tau_1-k} \cdot ... \cdot \lambda_{\tau_H-k}}{P(c_k)^{H-1}} . \tag{5}$$

The final model is made of the linguistically interpretable fuzzy partitions (1) and the transparent rule base (2), with the parameters optimized as shown above. When an unknown sample $\mathbf{x}=[x^{(1)},...,x^{(H)}]$ has to be classified, the firing strength of each rule is calculated by using the product T-norm of membership grades, the activation of the class k in this rule is computed by product implication, and the total activation of a class A_k is computed by weighted S-norm and Centre Of Area defuzzification. As demonstrated in [9], $A_k(\mathbf{x})$ approximates the probability of each class, given $\mathbf{x}$, $p(c_k|\mathbf{x})$.

In case of some missing value $x^{(h)}$ in the sample to be classified, it is not possible to calculate the corresponding value of the membership functions $\mu_{t\_h}(x^{(h)})$. Therefore, the value of the membership function is substituted with the value $P(c_k)/\lambda_{t\_h-k}$ of the constant *"don't care"* membership function $\mu_{dcth}(k)$. Doing this, the model results equivalent to that built without the missing variable, and $p(c_k|\mathbf{x})$ is still approximated.

2.3   Model Composition

The procedure for composing n different simple models M^1, ..., M^n, like (2), making use of n disjoint sets of variables, in a composite model $M^{Comp} := M^1 \otimes ... \otimes M^n$, comprising all the $H1+...+Hn$ variables, is described here. In detail, the number of rules of the combined model is obtained by multiplying the number of rules of simpler models. In other words, all combinations of one rule for each model are made, and for each combination, a rule $r^{Comp}_{\{t\_1,...,t\_(H1+...+Hn)\}}$ is obtained. The antecedent part is obtained by combining antecedent parts of different rules by using *and* connectives:

$$a^{Comp}_{\{t_1,...,t_{H1+...+Hn}\}} = a^1_{\{t_1,...,t_{H1}\}} \otimes^{ant} ... \otimes^{ant} a^n_{\{t_1,...,t_{Hn}\}} \,, \tag{6}$$

with $a \otimes^{ant} b := a$ *and* b, whereas the consequent part is calculated by combining different consequent weights as follows:

$$w^{Comp}_{\{t_1,...,t_{H1+...+Hn}\}-k} = w^1_{\{t_1,...,t_{H1}\}-k} \otimes^{cons-k} ... \otimes^{cons-k} w^n_{\{t_1,...,t_{Hn}\}-k} \,, \tag{7}$$

with $a \otimes^{cons-k} b := a \cdot b / P(c_k)$.

The combined model is equal to that extracted from data, using all the variables considered by the simpler models. Therefore, the class activation still approximates the class probabilities. However, the extraction of knowledge by LFA method, making use of combined models, allows to extract simple models from single variables or small groups of variables, and obtain the model comprising all the desired variables without extracting it again from the dataset.

3   Results and Discussion

The results reported and discussed here are obtained by applying the proposed approach for the construction of predictive models for parotid shrinkage. Different labelled datasets are considered, corresponding to the different sets of variables described in Section 2.1. LFA is applied by using a number of fuzzy sets $T_h=2$ for all variables, in order to avoid overfitting, since the dataset is made of a small number of samples. The leave-one-out cross-validation technique is applied to repetitively divide data into training set (39 samples) and test set (1 sample).

Different models are presented first in Section 3.1, each one considering no more than one source of data. Then, these models are merged, to fit the best models to be used when different data sources are available. It is straightforward to hypothesize that general information like age (F_1) is the first available. Moreover, the hypothesis is made here that if CT images during the therapy (F_4) are available, then also the CT images before the treatment (F_3) can be used. Therefore, in Section 3.2, the composite models built by using the following sets of variables are reported: $\{F_1+F_2\}$, $\{F_1+F_3\}$, and $\{F_1+F_2+F_3\}$, which refer to information that can be available before the treatment start, while those of Section 3.3, i.e. $\{F_1+F_3+F_4\}$ and $\{F_1+F_2+F_3+F_4\}$, comprise information available only after the treatment start. In Section 3.4, a discussion is given.

Fuzzy partitions of the most informative variables are reported in Fig. 1, while in Table 1, the performance values of all models considered in the following are reported in terms of accuracy, sensitivity and specificity. A comparison with the accuracy obtained by LDA approach is quoted as well.

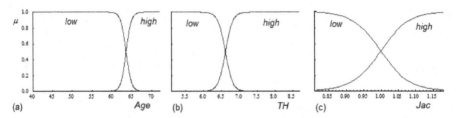

Fig. 1. Fuzzy partitions of the most informative variables: (a) *Age*, (b) *TH*, (c) *Jac*

Table 1. Classification results in accuracy (*acc*), sensitivity (*sens*) and specificity (*spec*) of the LFA and LDA with leave-one-out cross-validation. Each LFA model, indicated by the corresponding Equation, uses the most informative variables extracted from different data sources

Data source	Model variables	LFA model	LFA acc	LDA acc	LFA sens	LFA spec
$F_\emptyset$ or F_2	None	(8)	0.750	0.750	1.00	0.0
F_1 or $\{F_1+F_2\}$	$\{Age\}$	(9)	0.800	0.700	0.93	0.4
F_3	$\{TH\}$	(10)	0.800	0.750	0.90	0.5
F_4	$\{Jac\}$	(11)	0.800	0.800	0.90	0.5
$\{F_1+F_3\}$ or $\{F_1+F_2+F_3\}$	$\{Age, TH\}$	(9) $\otimes$ (10)	0.850	0.750	0.90	0.7
$\{F_1+F_3\}$ or $\{F_1+F_2+F_3\}$	$\{Age, TH, OVpghd\}$		0.875	0.725	0.93	0.7
$\{F_2+F_3\}$ or $\{F_1+F_2+F_3\}$	$\{V20, TH\}$		0.850	0.625*	0.97	0.5
$\{F_1+F_2+F_3\}$	$\{Age, TH, V15\}$		0.875	0.650*	0.97	0.6
$\{F_1+F_2+F_3\}$	$\{Age, TH, V20\}$		0.875	0.675*	0.97	0.6
$\{F_1+F_3+F_4\}$ or $\{F_1+F_2+F_3+F_4\}$	$\{Age, TH, Jac\}$	(9) $\otimes$ (10) $\otimes$ (11)	0.90	0.825	0.97	0.7

* 4 samples comprising missing values of dosimetric data are accounted as wrongly classified here.

3.1   Simple Models from Single Data Sources

$F_\emptyset$ **Model.** In case no information is available about the sample to be classified, the preferable model to use is the 0-rules one, considering only class prior probabilities:

$$Y \text{ is } \begin{cases} (0.75)\,DV \\ (0.25)\,CV \end{cases} \tag{8}$$

Its accuracy is equal to the greatest prior probability, therefore 0.75 in this case.

F_1 **Model.** In case only general information is available, the model built on F_1 makes use of only the variable *Age*. In Fig. 1(a), the fuzzy partition obtained for the variable *Age* is shown, and the simple rule base found is made of two rules as follows:

$$\textit{If Age is low then Y is } \begin{cases} (0.83)\,DV \\ (0.17)\,CV \end{cases}, \textit{If Age is high then Y is } \begin{cases} (0.29)\,DV \\ (0.71)\,CV \end{cases} \quad (9)$$

F_2 **Models.** In case only dosimetric information is available, all the models built with one or two variables of F_2 present an accuracy not higher than $F_\emptyset$ model. Therefore, no model is presented here, and (8) is the preferable model in this case.

F_3 **Models.** In case only CT images taken before the treatment are available, among the models built with one variable of F_3, the best one results that using the variable TH. All the other models, built with all couples of variables, present an accuracy not higher, therefore this is the preferable model with this set of features. In Fig. 1(b), the fuzzy partition obtained for the variable TH is represented, and the simple rule base found for this single variable is as follows:

$$\textit{If TH is low then Y is } \begin{cases} (0.13)\,DV \\ (0.87)\,CV \end{cases}, \textit{If TH is high then Y is } \begin{cases} (0.89)\,DV \\ (0.11)\,CV \end{cases} \quad (10)$$

F_4 **Model.** In case only CT images taken during the treatment are available, the model built on F_4 makes use of only the variable Jac. In Fig. 1(c), the fuzzy partition obtained for the variable Jac is represented, and the simple rule base found is as follows:

$$\textit{If Jac is low then Y is } DV, \textit{If Jac is high then Y is } \begin{cases} (0.19)\,DV \\ (0.81)\,CV \end{cases} \quad (11)$$

3.2   Composite Models from Heterogeneous Data Available Before Treatment

$\{F_1+F_2\}$ **Model.** In case general and dosimetric information is available, all the models built with one or two variables of F_1 and F_2 present an accuracy not higher than that of the model (9). Therefore, (9) is again the preferable model. It is worth noting that combining models (9) $\otimes$ (8), the result is (9) itself.

$\{F_1+F_3\}$ **Model.** In case general information and CT images taken before the treatment are available, the best model built with one or two variables of F_1 and F_3 corresponds to the combination of models (9) $\otimes$ (10), which uses Age and TH. A slight improvement of performances can be obtained by adding the variable $OVpghd$.

$\{F_1+F_2+F_3\}$ **Model.** In case general information, dosimetric information, and CT images taken before the treatment are available, one of the best models built with one or two variables of F_1, F_2 and F_3 corresponds to the combination of models (9) $\otimes$ (8) $\otimes$ (10), i.e. (9) $\otimes$ (10). The same performances can be obtained with the variables $\{V20,TH\}$, whereas a slight improvement can be achieved with some triplets of variables: $\{Age,TH,OVpghd\}$ (already found before), $\{Age,TH,V15\}$, and $\{Age,TH,V20\}$.

3.3   Composite Models from Heterogeneous Data Available During Treatment

$\{F_1+F_3+F_4\}$ **Model.** In case general information and CT images taken before and during the treatment are available, the best model built with one, two or three variables of F_1, F_3 and F_4 corresponds to the combination of models (9) $\otimes$ (10) $\otimes$ (11), which uses *Age*, *TH* and *Jac*.

{F_1+F_2+F_3+F_4} Model. In case general information, dosimetric information, and CT images taken before and during the treatment are available, the best model built with one, two or three variables of F_1, F_2, F_3 and F_4 corresponds to the combination of models (9) $\otimes$ (8) $\otimes$ (10) $\otimes$ (11), i.e. (9) $\otimes$ (10) $\otimes$ (11) already found above.

3.4   Discussion

In this section, some observations about the obtained results are given, going through those concerning performances, models, and predictors of parotid gland shrinkage.

The comparison between LFA and LDA performances shows that LFA overcomes LDA in most of the considered cases. A univariate paired t-test shows that the probability that these differences happened by chance is $1.1 \cdot 10^{-12}$, thus proving that LFA errors are significantly lower than LDA. Moreover, even if an unbalanced dataset is used, sensitivity and specificity of the best models result acceptable.

The models not reported and comprising variables as *V15* and *V20*, with missing values in the training dataset, are built using all available values of variables of interest. As shown in Section 2.3, samples with missing values can also be classified by all LFA models, whose accuracy results particularly higher than LDA in this case.

All of the extracted models result interpretable, and their complexity increases with the number of involved variables. It can also be seen that in models with only one variable, rule weights can be avoided. Therefore, in order to operate with heterogeneous data, the proposed DSS is structured by simple models, to be employed when single data sources are available, and to be composed when more sources are gathered. This allows to enhance readability of combined models, with respect to more complex ones using the whole set of available features and reaching similar accuracy.

Some predictors of parotid shrinkage can be individuated by analysing the best models listed above. In particular, among the features used in this work, those already individuated by previous works [2-4] as good predictors, which are the *Age* of the patient, body thickness (*TH*) and the mean Jacobian index of the deformation field (*Jac*), are confirmed here. Particular interest should be paid to *Age* and *TH*, and to the corresponding model (9) $\otimes$ (10), since they allow to well predict parotid shrinkage before the treatment start. Moreover, the interpretability of the models allows a simple qualitative description of the influence of features on shrinkage phenomenon. In particular, it can be deduced from simple models (9)-(11) and from Fig. 1, that the probability of class *DV* (significant shrinkage) increases for young patients (*Age* under 61/67 years), with high *TH* (over 6/7), and low *Jac* (under 1).

The reason why young patients are more susceptible of parotid shrinkage has been hypothesized before [2], while risk increase with initial body thickness *TH* can be explained by considering that risk increases with initial parotid volume *V* [7], and supposing a correlation between *TH* and *V*. *Jac* under 1 denotes an early decrease of voxels volume, therefore it is trivial to expect that it predicts final parotid shrinkage.

Some other features are individuated, however their predictive power should be confirmed by using a more numerous dataset. In particular, some features regarding the dose–volume histogram at planning (*V15* and *V20*), partially confirming previous results [12], and the overlapping between parotid gland and high-dose tumour (*OVpghd*), as could be expected, result useful in some measure. They seem not able to constitute an accurate model alone, but some of them can help improving performances of other models.

Different sources of information revealed respective advantages. General information (F_1) is the simplest to be obtained, and a good model can be constructed involving the variable *Age*. Dosimetric information (F_2) can also be obtained without invasive examination, however its usefulness cannot be confirmed by the analysis of this data set. Initial clinical and anatomical features extracted from CT0 (F_3), taking into account the difficulty of their acquisition, revealed their proficiency in improving the model accuracy before the treatment start. In particular, *TH* resulted a good predictor, however other features could be extracted from CT0 and their usefulness should be examined. Features extracted from CT1 and CT2 (F_4), taken during the early phase of treatment, surely can further improve the model, but these are available only after the therapy has begun. Here the usefulness of using only *Jac* is clear, however other predictors can be extracted as well [6,7].

Summarizing the results, the overall DSS should work as follows: if nothing is known, prior probabilities are assigned to possible classes as in (8), and the user is asked to insert first general information and then CT information. If the *Age* of the patient is known, then (9) can be used for class prediction. Before the treatment start, CT0 image information would increase accuracy by using *TH* and enabling to combine models (9) $\otimes$ (10). Integrating another variable like *OVpghd* (also extracted from CT0) or *V15* or *V20* (if dosimetric data are available), accuracy slightly increases, but also model complexity increases, therefore this can be avoided if interpretability is a main objective. Finally, if the treatment is started and information from CT images of the first weeks is available, the combined model (9) $\otimes$ (10) $\otimes$ (11) can be used, which ensures the highest accuracy.

4   Conclusion

In this work, a new approach based on fuzzy logic was applied to predict whether a parotid gland will be interested with significant shrinkage in patients under RT treatment. It essentially combines a set of interpretable models, built by using LFA and working distinctly with sets of features regarding clinical data, dosimetric data, or information extracted from CT images, into one or more composite models using the most informative variables, in order to obtain more accurate predictions, even in case of missing values. This approach was compared with LDA, resulting more effective in parotid classification, with good accuracy, sensitivity and specificity.

From a clinical perspective, the advantages of acquiring data from different sources were outlined, the best models operating with available sources are achieved (among them, the models operating before treatment), and some features (*Age*, *TH*, and *Jac*) were revealed as good predictors, according to previous works. The usefulness of other known predictors (*V15* and *V20*) and of another one individuated here (*OVpghd*) needs confirmation and expert discussion. However, some new and more significant findings are expected by applying the approach to a larger dataset, available in the next future, including more samples and more pre-treatment and CT-based features.

References

1. Hansen, E.K., Bucci, M.K., Quivey, J.M., Weinberg, V., Xia, P.: Repeat CT Imaging and Replanning During the Course of IMRT for Head-and-Neck Cancer. Int. J. Radiat. Oncol. 64, 355–362 (2006)
2. Broggi, S., Fiorino, C., Dell'Oca, I., Dinapoli, N., Paiusco, M., Muraglia, A., Maggiulli, E., Ricchetti, F., Valentini, V., Sanguineti, G.: A Two-Variable Linear Model of Parotid Shrinkage During IMRT for Head and Neck Cancer. Radiother. Oncol. 94, 206–212 (2010)
3. Fiorino, C., Rizzo, G., Scalco, E., Broggi, S., Belli, M.L., Dell'Oca, I., Dinapoli, N., Ricchetti, F., Rodriguez, A.M., Di Muzio, N.: Density Variation of Parotid Glands During IMRT for Head–Neck Cancer: Correlation with Treatment and Anatomical Parameters. Radiother. Oncol. 104, 224–229 (2012)
4. Fiorino, C., Maggiulli, E., Broggi, S., Liberini, S., Cattaneo, G.M., Dell'Oca, I., Faggiano, E., Di Muzio, N., Calandrino, R., Rizzo, G.: Introducing the Jacobian-Volume-Histogram of Deforming Organs: Application to Parotid Shrinkage Evaluation. Phys. Med. Biol. 56, 3301–3312 (2011)
5. Fiorentino, A., Caivano, R., Metallo, V., Chiumento, C., Cozzolino, M., Califano, G., Clemente, S., Pedicini, P., Fusco, V.: Parotid Gland Volumetric Changes During Intensity-Modulated Radiotherapy in Head and Neck Cancer. Brit. J. Radiol. 85, 1415–1419 (2012)
6. Scalco, E., Fiorino, C., Cattaneo, G.M., Sanguineti, G., Rizzo, G.: Texture Analysis for the Assessment of Structural Changes in Parotid Glands Induced by Radiotherapy. Radiother. Oncol. 109, 384–387 (2013)
7. Pota, M., Scalco, E., Belli, M.L., Sanguineti, G., Cattaneo, G.M., Esposito, M., Rizzo, G.: Likelihood-Fuzzy Analysis of Parotid Gland Shrinkage in Radiotherapy Patients. In: Graña, M., Toro, C., Howlett, R.J., Jain, L.C. (eds.) InMed 2014. Studies in Health Technology and Informatics, vol. 207, pp. 360–369. IOS press, Amsterdam (2014)
8. Pota, M., Esposito, M., De Pietro, G.: Combination of Interpretable Fuzzy Models and Probabilistic Inference in Medical DSSs. In: Skulimowski, A.M.J. (ed.) KICSS 2013. Advances in Decision Sciences and Future Studies, vol. 2, pp. 541–552. Progress & Business Publishers, Krakow (2013)
9. Pota, M., Esposito, M., De Pietro, G.: Best Fuzzy Partitions to Build Interpretable DSSs for Classification in Medicine. In: Pan, J.-S., Polycarpou, M.M., Woźniak, M., de Carvalho, A.C.P.L.F., Quintián, H., Corchado, E. (eds.) HAIS 2013. LNCS, vol. 8073, pp. 558–567. Springer, Heidelberg (2013)
10. Faggiano, E., Fiorino, C., Scalco, E., Broggi, S., Cattaneo, M., Maggiulli, E., Dell'Oca, I., Di Muzio, N., Calandrino, R., Rizzo, G.: An Automatic Contour Propagation Method to Follow Parotid Gland Deformation During Head-and-Neck Cancer Tomotherapy. Phys. Med. Biol. 56, 775–791 (2011)
11. Gacto, M.J., Alcalà, R., Herrera, F.: Interpretability of Linguistic Fuzzy Rule-Based Systems: An Overview of Interpretability Measures. Inform. Sciences 181, 4340–4360 (2011)
12. Broggi, S., Scalco, E., Fiorino, C., Belli, M.L., Sanguineti, G., Ricchetti, F., Dell'Oca, I., Dinapoli, N., Valentini, V., Di Muzio, N., Cattaneo, G.M., Rizzo, G.: The Shape of Parotid DVH Predicts the Entity of Gland Deformation During IMRT for Head and Neck Cancers. Technology in Cancer Research & Treatment (2014) (Epub ahead of print)

Feasibility of Spirography Features for Objective Assessment of Motor Symptoms in Parkinson's Disease

Aleksander Sadikov[1]([✉]), Jure Žabkar[1], Martin Možina[1], Vida Groznik[1], Dag Nyholm[2], and Mevludin Memedi[3]

[1] University of Ljubljana, Faculty of Computer and Information Science, Večna pot 113, Ljubljana, Slovenia
aleksander.sadikov@fri.uni-lj.si,
[2] Dept. of Neuroscience, Neurology, Uppsala University, Uppsala, Sweden
[3] Computer Engineering, Dalarna University, Borlänge, Sweden

Abstract. Parkinson's disease (PD) is currently incurable, however the proper treatment can ease the symptoms and significantly improve the quality of patient's life. Since PD is a chronic disease, its efficient monitoring and management is very important. The objective of this paper is to investigate the feasibility of using the features and methodology of a spirography device, originally designed to measure early Parkinson's disease (PD) symptoms, for assessing motor symptoms of advanced PD patients suffering from motor fluctuations. More specifically, the aim is to objectively assess motor symptoms related to bradykinesias (slowness of movements occurring as a result of under-medication) and dyskinesias (involuntary movements occurring as a result of over-medication). The work combines spirography data and clinical assessments from a longitudinal clinical study in Sweden with the features and pre-processing methodology of a Slovenian spirography application. The target outcome was to learn to predict the "cause" of upper limb motor dysfunctions as assessed by a clinician who observed animated spirals in a web interface. Using the machine learning methods with feature descriptions from the Slovenian application resulted in 86% classification accuracy and over 90% AUC, demonstrating the usefulness of this approach for objective monitoring of PD patients.

Keywords: Parkinson's disease · Movement disorder · Spirography · Spirography features · Objective monitoring

1 Introduction and Problem Statement

Parkinson's disease (PD) is a chronic neurological disorder associated with a number of motor and non-motor symptoms. Major motor symptoms include bradykinesia (slowness of movements), tremor and rigidity. While currently incurable, proper treatment can significantly ease the symptoms. As the disease progresses, however, patients start to experience motor fluctuations which adversely impact the quality of their life. Therefore, the treatment approaches

© Springer International Publishing Switzerland 2015
J.H. Holmes et al. (Eds.): AIME 2015, LNAI 9105, pp. 267–276, 2015.
DOI: 10.1007/978-3-319-19551-3_35

should be individualized in order to alleviate unwanted symptoms which occur as a result of insufficient levels of medication (Off state) and abrupt, involuntary movements (also known as dyskinesias) which occur as a result of excessive levels of medication. To this end, careful and objective monitoring of the disease, is of paramount importance. As the patients usually see the neurologist only few times per year (sometimes also just once per year), the neurologist often has only a very vague picture of their condition in-between the visits and has problems with prescribing the optimal drug dosage. Currently, patients monitor their long-term condition by keeping a simple diary. The entries in the diary, however, are subjective opinions of the patients and are not something measurable. Clinical scales like the Unified Parkinson's Disease Rating Scale (UPDRS) are not suitable for long-term and remote follow-up of the symptoms since they are relatively time-consuming [1], may need to be filled out at a clinical visit, require considerable clinical experience [2] and some of their items have poor inter-clinician reliability [3].

The digitalised spirography is a quantitative method for detection and evaluation of different types of tremors and other movement disorders. The system is usually composed of a computer with a specialised software, a graphic tablet or a touch-screen measurement device (e.g. a smartphone), and a stylus [14,4]. The patient is required to draw a spiral (or sometimes several spirals). The digitalised spirography enables us to store the exact timestamp of each point of the spiral in a two-dimensional area and thus provides an objective measurement. These systems allow extraction of detailed upper limb motor features from the spiral drawing tasks by analysing spatial and temporal artefacts of the spirals.

Our long-term goal is to develop a system for objective monitoring of PD patients that would also be able to automatically detect any significant changes in the patient's condition and report these changes to the neurologist. The spirals drawn have to be described mathematically by various features (some described in Table 3 later in the paper) for the machine learning algorithms to be able to analyse them automatically. This paper presents preliminary results and its main objective is to analyze whether the descriptive features and methodology developed for PARKINSONCHECK application for early detection of signs of Parkinsonian or Essential tremor [11,12] can be applied more generally. The specific application in this paper — which is different from PARKINSONCHECK's objective — is differentiation between states of bradykinesia (insufficient medication) and dyskinesia (overmedication) which is important for drug dosage adjustment, using spirography data collected in a Swedish study [5]. If this is the case, this would validate the PARKINSONCHECK's features for spiral description on a more general level as well as confirm the usefulness of spirography for this particular task.

The data and the differences with the data for which the features were originally constructed are described in the next section. Section 2 also describes the complete experimental setup, including used features and testing methodology. Section 3 presents the results, and Section 4 analyses and discusses the results. At the end we give some conclusions and ideas for further work.

2   Experimental Setup

2.1   Subjects

In this study, a retrospective analysis was conducted on spirography data of 65 patients with advanced idiopathic PD from eight different clinics in Sweden, recruited from January 2006 until August 2010 [6]. The patients were either treated with levodopa/carbidopa gel intestinal infusion or were candidates for receiving this treatment. There were 43 males and 22 females with median ($\pm$ inter-quartile range) age of 65 ± 11 years and total UPDRS of 49 ± 20.5. UPDRS is a widely used scale for clinical assessment of Parkinson's disease and consists of four parts: I: mentation, behaviour and mood, II: activities of daily living, III: motor examination, and IV: complications of therapy. All questions have five response options 0–normal, 1–slight, 2–mild, 3–moderate, and 4–severe. The sum over the answers to the questions gives the UPDRS rating of a patient. [16]

2.2   Spirography Data Collection

During the course of the clinical study, the patients used a touch screen telemetry device in their home environments [5]. On each test occasion, they were asked to trace a pre-drawn Archimedian spiral using the dominant hand. The pre-drawn spiral was shown on the screen of the device and the patients were instructed to use an ergonomic pen stylus to trace it from the center and out, as accurately and fast as possible, supporting neither hand nor arm. The patients were instructed to place the device on a table and to be seated in a chair. The raw data consisted of x-y coordinates and time-stamps of the pen tip, digitized at a sample rate of 10 Hz. In total, the database consisted of 10,272 test occasions having approximately 30,816 (3 * 10,272) spirals. Some example spiral drawings are shown in Figure 1.

2.3   Clinical Assessment of Motor Impairments

A clinician used a web interface that animated the spiral drawings, allowing him to observe different kinematic features during the drawing process and to rate task performance of the patients [7]. The interface initially retrieved spiral data from the database tables and then animated the drawing in real-time that is with the same speed as the patients initially drew the spirals. The interface randomly selected 3 test occasions per patient from the database and animated the 3 spirals that were drawn on that particular occasion. A number of motor features were assessed by the clinician including 'impairment' on a scale from 1 (normal) to 10 (extremely severe), 'speed', 'irregularity', and 'hesitation' on a scale from 0 (normal) to 4 (extremely severe). The motor features were considered specific for the type of upper limb motor movements found in patients with motor fluctuations. Finally, 'cause' of the said dysfunctions was marked on a 3-category scale including Tremor, Bradykinesia and Dyskinesia. In case the clinician could not decide which category of 'cause' to select, he had the option to skip the rating. There were 38 cases rated as bradykinesia, 119 as dyskinesia, 1 as tremor and 22 were skipped by the rater. Only the cases that were rated a bradykinesia and dyskinesia were included in the subsequent analysis.

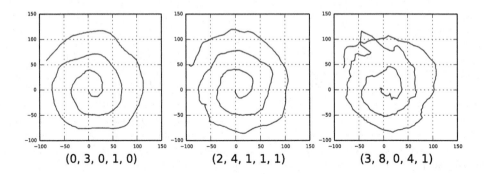

Fig. 1. Three example spiral drawings and ratings as given by the clinician. The values are for cause (0=none, 2=bradykinesia, 3=dyskinesia), impairment, speed, irregularity, and hesitation, respectively.

2.4   Differences with the Dataset from ParkinsonCheck

The two datasets, the PARKINSONCHECK and the Swedish one used in this study, were collected for a different purpose. PARKINSONCHECK is an application for *early* detection of signs of Parkinsonian or Essential tremor (ET, the most common differential diagnosis of PD) and for differentiation between these two types of tremor, while the Swedish data is collected during a longitudinal study aimed at monitoring the *advanced* PD patients.

As straightforward as spirography looks, the two datasets that is Swedish and Slovenian (PARKINSONCHECK) were collected with different data collections schemes. The following are the main discrepancies between the two schemes:

- A different equipment (smartphones or tablets vs specialized device) was used for drawing the spirals using a very different sampling rate (> 50 Hz vs 10 Hz);
- The spirals were drawn with a stylus instead of with fingers alone (different motoric skills involved);
- Different direction of drawing (counter-clockwise vs clockwise);
- Completely unsupervised data collection (patients were on their own) and without safeguards for detecting the center of the screen and direction of drawing;
- In the Swedish study, patients were asked to repeat the spiral test (tracing the pre-drawn spiral template on the screen) 3 times per test occasion using dominant hand, while PARKINSONCHECK data consists of four drawings with repetitions: with and without the template visible, both performed with both hands;

- The Swedish patients were specifically instructed to complete the spiral drawing test in approximately 10 seconds per drawing, while no such instruction was given for ParkinsonCheck data.

As the two datasets differ in so many aspects, it is interesting to investigate the extent of symptom information resolution of the previously developed features and symptom scoring methodology of ParkinsonCheck applied on the Swedish dataset.

2.5   Features and Pre-processing

The starting point of the data analysis phase was the raw data gathered with the Swedish telemetry device. A spiral drawn by a patient was described as a sequence of triples, (t, x, y), where t denotes the time (in ms) and x, y denote a Cartesian coordinate of a point of the spiral. We used raw data to calculate the features from the ParkinsonCheck application, also precisely matching all the pre-processing involved. The exact calculation including the pre-processing such as smoothing and normalisation are too extensive to describe here in any detail and are given in [10]. For each of the three spirals (repetitions), the constructed features included: root mean squared error (RMSE) between the patient's spiral and the optimal spiral, computed in polar coordinates, radial and tangential speed of drawing, the percentage of the spiral length when the patient is drawing towards the centre, and the parameters of oscillations. The meaning of the most important features is briefly described in the next section. These features were aggregated over the three repetitions using operators such as min, max, average and range over all three spirals.

Using these features, a learning example is composed of only aggregated features over all three repetitions, and a 'cause' class as appraised by the clinician. The learning situation was thus identical to that the neurologist had when initially classifying the examples. Only cases rated as bradykinesia or dyskinesia were included for the learning problem, giving the majority class of roughly 76%. Each case (learning example) represents a test occasion.

2.6   Machine Learning Methods

We tested four machine learning methods using Orange machine learning suite [15]: logistic regression (LR), naïve Bayes classification (NB), support vector machines (SVM), and random forests (RF). The first two are linear and their classification models are simple to understand, whereas the second two can extract also nonlinear patterns. All continuous attributes were first automatically discretized with the entropy-based discretization [13].

The methods were evaluated with a 10-times repeated tenfold cross-validation procedure with stratified sampling, for the following reasons: (a) using cross-validation will result in less biased estimates, (b) repeating cross-validation procedure on different splits will result in a smaller variance on an accuracy estimate, and (c) stratified sampling decreases the differences between class distributions in the learning and testing sets. To prevent overfitting, the discretization was first applied only on the learning data and then the same thresholds were used on the testing data. To compare the qualities of learned models, we used the following measures: classification accuracy (CA), area under the curve (AUC), and Brier score, which is the quadratic loss of the probability estimates.

3   Results

Table 1 summarizes the results for various machine learning algorithms for differentiating between the state of bradykinesia and the state of dyskinesia. There is no significant difference between the algorithms, they differentiate between the two states almost equally well. In the continuation, we will therefore focus on logistic regression (LR) as its model is relatively easy to understand as compared to other algorithms. Comprehensibility, while not being an unconditional requirement, is a welcome feature, especially so with new methodology still being validated. The confusion matrix for logistic regression model is given in Table 2.

Table 1. The results for logistic regression (LR), random forests (RF), support vector machines (SVM), and naïve Bayes classifier (NB)

	Majority	LR	RF	SVM	NB
CA	0.758	0.846	0.864	0.841	0.853
Brier	0.367	0.221	0.195	0.232	0.314
AUC	0.500	0.914	0.925	0.896	0.848

Table 2. The confusion matrix for logistic regression model. The results are averaged over all repetitions of 10-fold cross-validation.

	Bradykinesia (predicted)	Dyskinesia (predicted)
Bradykinesia (clinician)	23.2	14.8
Dyskinesia (clinician)	9.4	109.6

Table 3 contains ten most important features for the logistic regression model. The three most important features (avgP.min) all describe variability in speed (radial, tangential, and absolute) of drawing over the whole range of the spiral. The minimum over all three spiral drawings is taken. The features plrErrComCnt (avg and max) describe the level of curvature or smoothness of the spirals. The percentage of time the patient draws towards the centre is also quite important (percNeg feature) as well as the general misfit of the drawing as compared to the ideal spiral in polar coordinates (plrErrFit). The number of times the spiral crosses itself (rot.avgP) is also important — it is a good measure of severe fluctuations during drawing.

Table 3. The coefficients of the logistic regression with pre-discretization of attributes. Only ten most influential attributes (as measured by beta value range) are given.

Attribute	Importance	General description
radSp.avgP.min	1.13	radial speed variability
tangSp.avgP.min	1.02	tangential speed variability
absSp.avgP.min	0.78	absolute speed variability
plrErrComCnt.avg	0.70	level of curvature/smoothness of the spiral
radSp.percNeg005.min	0.69	percentage of time the patient drew towards the centre
plrErrComCnt.max	0.67	level of curvature/smoothness of the spiral
plrErrFit.avg	0.65	general misfit from the ideal spiral (template)
tangSp.avgP.rng	0.65	tangential speed variability
tangSp.avgP.max	0.63	tangential speed variability
rot.avgP.min	0.62	number of times the spiral crosses itself

4   Discussion

The main observation is that all the algorithms are clearly better than the majority classifier. This indicates that the features of the Slovenian PARKINSONCHECK application contain relevant symptom information for objective assessment of PD motor symptoms when applied to data collected by a telemetry device used in a three years Swedish clinical study. Even though the features were designed for early detection of PD and ET symptoms, the findings indicate that a set of them can be used for recognizing upper limb motor movements specific to Off episodes and peak-dose dyskinesias, which are prominent in advanced patients experiencing motor fluctuations.

In order to cover cases from all the patients involved in the Swedish study and to make it possible for the clinicians to rate the spirals, a sample of spirals from the whole database has been drawn by randomly selecting 3 test occasions per patient [7]. The results presented in this paper are preliminary since the web interface is currently being used by other clinicians.

However, we could not assess whether the features are useful for detecting tremor using the Swedish dataset. This is because the patients in the Swedish study did not have action tremor hence the rater identified 'cause' in only 1 out of 260 cases as tremor. The spatial and temporal characteristics of this case were different from those cases with 'cause' rated as bradykinesia and dyskinesia. Therefore, in the future it would be interesting to investigate the feasibility of the features for capturing the whole spectrum of Off symptoms including both bradykinesia and tremor as well as dyskinesias.

The results presented in this paper were obtained using only the aggregated features over all three spiral drawings. While experimenting, we also fitted models using the non-aggregated features, and the observed classification accuracies were up to 90% (with increases in other metrics as well). However, we decided to present the results only for aggregated features as we currently do not have a good explanation why any given spiral (first, second, or third attempt) would be more important than the others. It does indicate, though, that there is more information that can be extracted from this data. From the confusion matrix presented in Table 2, we can conclude that there were more misclassifications for bradykinesia class than dyskinesia. This can probably be because of the unbalanced data design where majority of the spirals (76%) were rated as dyskinesia. This is something that we are looking into while continuing this research. Moreover, it has to be noted that both possible misclassifications carry equal weight as both conditions are unpleasant for the patient and both need to be properly addressed.

In contrast to other technology-based symptom assessment strategies which are mainly based on the use of wearable sensors [8], spirography has been used mainly for assessing the severity of the symptoms. To our knowledge, only [9] have tackled the problem of assessing motor fluctuations using spirography tasks. However, they have mainly focused on quantifying the severity of dyskinesias only, by limiting data processing on frequency bands relevant to dyskinesias, and with no reference to Off symptoms. In contrast, our approach is designed to capture movement patterns exhibited by patients being in Off (bradykinesia) and dyskinesia motor states.

5   Conclusions and Future Work

The present study demonstrates that a lot of information about the PD patient's condition can be extracted from his or her spirographic data. The main conclusion is that it is feasible to apply PARKINSONCHECK's features and pre-processing methodology to quite a different set of spirographic data. The features can thus be thought of as quite general for the description of the spiral drawings.

In the long term this result suggests that spirography could be used as a valid method for objective monitoring of PD patients, especially combined with other tests that could detect those conditions that were currently misclassified. The latter could be improved with new features as well, however, we suspect that tests complementary to spirography will have a more significant impact.

The obvious future work is to look into the misclassified cases and try to either improve the model or get an understanding of why the misclassifications occurred. It would be interesting for a clinician to review the misclassified cases, perhaps changing his opinion or pointing the reasons for the misclassification. This could lead to potential new features for describing the spirals. Or it could hint at the lack of information in the spirals for this particular problem. Another helpful avenue of work is to visualise the most important characteristics of the spirals for each difficult case – this would make the clinicians' assessment much easier.

In the future, the plan is to collect more ratings on animated spirals from more clinicians. This would allow us to investigate the feasibility of time-space reconstruction of the spirals to clinicians and to investigate how the machine learning approach would adjust itself to individual ratings of multiple raters. The long-term plan is also to include multiple objective motor function measurements with different sensors including wearable sensors, eye tracking and upper limb touch screen tests (tapping and spirography) as well as video recording the patients while performing the tests and executing standardized motor tasks. This would allow us to investigate the relationship of the objective measures and blinded video ratings as well as their relationship to plasma levodopa concentration.

Acknowledgements. This work was partly supported by Swedish Knowledge Foundation, Nordforce Technology AB, Animech AB, and Dalarna University under PAULINA project and partly by Slovenian Research Agency (Artificial Intelligence and Intelligent Systems research programme), Slovenian Ministry of Education, Science and Sport, and European Regional Development Fund (PARKINSCHECK project). M. Memedi and D. Nyholm are shareholders in Jemardator AB, holder of IP of a test battery for collecting symptom data.

References

1. Martinez-Martin, P., Gil-Nagel, A., Gracia, L.M., Gomez, J.B., Martinez-Sarries, J., Bermejo, F.: Unified Parkinsons disease rating scale characteristics and structure. Movement Disorders 8, 76–83 (1994)
2. Taylor Tavares, A.L., Jefferis, G.S., Koop, M., Hill, B.C., Hastie, T., Heit, G., Bronte-Stewart, H.M.: Quantitative measurements of alternate finger tapping in Parkinsons disease correlate with UPDRS motor disability and reveal the improvement in fine motor control from medication and deep brain stimulation. Movement Disorders 20, 1286–1298 (2005)
3. Hagell, P., Whalley, D., McKenna, S.P., Lindvall, O.: Health status measurement in Parkinsons disease: Validity of the PDQ-39 and Nottingham health profile. Movement Disorders 18, 773–783 (2003)
4. Haubenberger, D., Kalowitz, D., Nahab, F.B., Toro, C., Ippolito, D., Luckenaugh, D.A., Wittevrongel, L., Hallett, M.: Validation of digital spiral analysis as outcome parameter for clinical trials in essential tremor. Movement Disorders 26, 2073–2080 (2011)
5. Westin, J., Dougherty, M., Nyholm, D., Groth, T.: A home environment test battery for status assessment in patients with advanced Parkinsons disease. Computer Methods and Programs in Biomedicine 98(1), 27–35 (2010)
6. Palhagen, S.E., Dizdar, N., Hauge, T., Holmberg, B., Jansson, R., Linder, J., Nyholm, D., Sydow, O., Wainwright, M., Widner, H., Johansson, A.: Interim analysis of long-term intraduodenal levodopa infusion in advanced Parkinson disease. Acta Neurologica Scandinavica 126, e29–e33 (2012)
7. Memedi, M., Bergqvist, U., Westin, J., Grenholm, P., Nyholm, D.: A web-based system for visualizing upper limb motor performance of Parkinsons disease patients. Movement Disorders 28, S112–S113 (2013)
8. Maetzler, W., Domingos, J., Srulijes, K., Ferreira, J.J., Bloem, B.R.: Quantitative wearable sensors for objective assessment of Parkinsons disease. Movement Disorders 28, 1628–2637 (2013)
9. Liu, X., Carroll, C.B., Wang, S.Y., Zajicek, J., Bain, P.G.: Quantifying drug-induced dyskinesia in the arms using digitised spiral-drawing tasks. Journal of Neuroscience Methods 144, 47–52 (2005)

10. Sadikov, A., Žabkar, J., Možina, M., Groznik, V., Georgiev, D., Bratko, I.: ParkinsonCheck: A decision support system for spirographic testing. Tech. Rep., University of Ljubljana, Faculty of Computer and Information Science (2014)
11. Sadikov, A., Groznik, V., Žabkar, J., Možina, M., Georgiev, D., Pirtošek, Z., Bratko, I.: ParkinsonCheck smart phone app. In: Proceedings of European Conference on Artificial Intelligence, pp. 1213–1214 (2014)
12. Groznik, V., Sadikov, A., Možina, M., Žabkar, J., Georgiev, D., Bratko, I.: Attribute Visualisation for Computer-Aided Diagnosis: A Case Study. In: Proceedings of the IEEE International Conference on Healthcare Informatics, pp. 294–299 (2014)
13. Fayyad, U.M., Irani, K.B.: Multi-interval discretization of continuous-valued attributes for classification learning. In: Proceedings of the 13th International Joint Conference on Artificial Intelligence, pp. 1022–1029 (1993)
14. Elble, R.J., Sinha, R., Higgins, C.: Quantification of tremor with a digitizing tablet. Journal of Neuroscience Methods 32, 193–198 (1990)
15. Demšar, J., Curk, T., Erjavec, A., Gorup, Č., Hočevar, T., Milutinović, M., Možina, M., Polajnar, M., Toplak, M., Starič, A., Štajdohar, M., Umek, L., Žagar, L., Žbontar, J., Žitnik, M., Zupan, B.: Orange: Data Mining Toolbox in Python. Journal of Machine Learning Research 14, 2349–2353 (2013)
16. Fahn, S., Elton, R.: UPDRS Development Committee: Unified Parkinsons disease rating scale. Recent Developments in Parkinson's Disease, 2, 153–163, 293–304 (1987)

Using Multivariate Sequential Patterns to Improve Survival Prediction in Intensive Care Burn Unit

Isidoro J. Casanova[1], Manuel Campos[1(✉)], Jose M. Juarez[1],
Antonio Fernandez-Fernandez-Arroyo[2,3], and Jose A. Lorente[2,3,4]

[1] Computer Science Faculty, University of Murcia, Murcia, Spain
manuelcampos@um.es
[2] University Hospital of Getafe, Madrid, Spain
[3] European University of Madrid, Madrid, Spain
[4] CIBER Enfermedades Respiratorias, Madrid, Spain

Abstract. Resuscitation and stabilization are key issues in Intensive Care Burn Units and early survival predictions help to decide the best clinical action during these phases. Current survival scores of burns focus on clinical variables such as age or the body surface area. However, the evolution of other parameters (e.g. diuresis or fluid balance) during the first days is also valuable knowledge. In this work we suggest a methodology and we propose a Temporal Data Mining algorithm to estimate the survival condition from the patient's evolution. Experiments conducted on 480 patients show the improvement of survival prediction.

1 Introduction

Intensive Care Burn Units (ICBU) are specialized units in which the main pathologies treated are inhalation injuries and severe burn injuries. Early mortality prediction after admission is essential before an aggressive or conservative therapy can be recommended. Severity scores are simple but useful tools for physicians when evaluating the state of the patient. Scoring systems aim to use the most predictive pre-morbid and injury factors to yield an expected likelihood of death for a given patient [14]. Baux and prognostic burn index (PBI) scores provide a mortality rate by summing age and percentage of total burn surface area (%TBSA) [2], while the abbreviated burns severity index (ABSI) also considers the gender and presence of inhalation injury [15].

Nevertheless, the evolution of other parameters during the resuscitation phase (first 2 days) and during the stabilization phase (3 following days) can also be important. The initial evaluation and resuscitation of patients with large burns that require inpatient care can only be loosely guided by formulas and rules. The inherent inaccuracy of formulas requires continuous re-evaluation and adjustment of infusions based on resuscitation targets. Incomings, diuresis, fluid balance, acid base balance (pH, bicarbonate, base excess) and others help to define objectives and to assess the evolution and treatment response.

© Springer International Publishing Switzerland 2015
J.H. Holmes et al. (Eds.): AIME 2015, LNAI 9105, pp. 277–286, 2015.
DOI: 10.1007/978-3-319-19551-3_36

In the ICBU, patient's evolution is registered but not considered in scores for mortality prediction. We believe this could be a relevant improvement for current knowledge. This knowledge can be discovered with Temporal Data Mining (TDM). TDM has the capability of mining activities, inferring associations of contextual and temporal proximity, some of which may also indicate a cause-effect association.

In this work, we face three main challenges: a) to provide the physicians with insight knowledge of the patient's evolution, b) to extract a manageable amount of knowledge, and c) to generate understandable models that could be interpreted by the expert. To this end, we have conducted different experiments within a 4-step knowledge discovery process.

The rest of the paper is organized as follows. Section 2 describes the methods for discovering sequential patterns and for classification. Section 3 describes the case study and the data preprocessing. Section 4 shows the results and discusses the methods. Finally, we provide the conclusions and future works.

2   Methods

2.1   Background Work

Some related work on the use of patterns as predictors can be found in the literature. There is a good experience in using association rules with algorithms such as CBA or CMAR [10], but these patterns do not consider the evolution of the variables. Other authors use temporal abstraction techniques [7], where the original data is abstracted into interval sequences and then association rules are discovered, or focus on measures for selecting patterns, such as the relative risk or a coverage measure [9]. In [19] sequences are used to classify good and bad plans in production systems. In [5], the authors propose an optimization technique to weight the patterns. In the clinical domain, univariate frequent episodes of SOFA subscores during the first days after admission were identified in [16]. Then, the authors selected a reduced number of patterns using Akaike's Information Criterion to build a logistic regression model for predicting the survivability of patients suffering from multiorganic failure. Later, in [17] the same authors showed that the use of univariate patterns as predictors is at least as effective as clinical scores.

Regarding the ICBU, few works have dealt with the problem of survival prediction using machine learning or intelligent data analysis [8]. As far as we know, none of them consider patient's evolution.

2.2   4-Step Knowledge Discovery Process

In order to build models for predicting mortality in ICBU, we define a 4-step knowledge discovery process. The first two steps focus on the pre-processing of the database and use a pattern discovery technique to show the patients' evolution. Then, we propose a post-processing of the patterns in order to reduce the

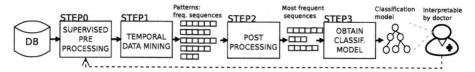

Fig. 1. 4-step knowledge discovery process

number of patterns discovered. Finally, in order to obtain interpretable models, the remaining patterns are used to build classification models in the form of rules and decision trees.

Step 0: Discretization of Temporal Attributes. The first step focuses on the discretization of all temporal attributes for three reasons: (1) we avoid the variability in splitting points of continuous attributes calculated in every branch of the decision tree, (2) the patterns are easy to interpret by the clinicians since they contains their usual language, and (3) we increase the legibility of the patterns due to the reduced number of variables.

In order to discretize, on the one hand, we can use a measurement like entropy, based on information gain with respect the class. On the other hand, an expert can provide a qualitative abstraction. The latter can introduce a bias, and even the predictive capacity of the variable may decrease. In our case, we adopted an expert driven discretization approach since the formulae for transforming the original data also allows us to normalize the data, and hence, to have a fairer pattern comparison regardless other patient's variables.

Step 1: Mining Multivariate Sequential Patterns. In this paper we focus on in the extraction of frequent sequences from a set of patient's sequences. In order to define the problem, we introduce the following concepts:

Definition 1. *Let $\Sigma = \{te_1, te_2, \ldots, te_n\}$ be a set of items and let $\mathcal{O}$ and $\mathcal{T}$ two attributes, where $dom(\mathcal{O})$ and $dom(\mathcal{T})$ denotes the domain of $\mathcal{O}$ and $\mathcal{T}$, respectively. A transactional dataset D is a set composed by r transactions, $D = \{D[0], D[1], \ldots, D[r]\}$, where $D[i]$ is a 3-tuple (o, t, E), with $o \in dom(\mathcal{O})$, $t \in dom(\mathcal{T})$, and $E \subseteq \Sigma$.*

The $\mathcal{O}$-attribute represents a real world entity. Each $o \in \mathcal{O}$ is a sequence of the dataset composed of a set of attributes. $\mathcal{T}$ describes the temporal context associated with the transactions. Table 2 shows an example of a dataset formed by 4 objects, where each object is associated with an enumeration of transactions.

Definition 2. *Let D be a set of transactional data formed by a set of r 3-tuple (o, t, E). If we assume that $|dom(\mathcal{O})| = n$, D can be divided into n disjoint subsets, each one associated with a particular object. Therefore, each o_i is associated with its corresponding subset denoted by D^{o_i} and formed by r_i tuples, $D^{o_i} = \{(t, E^{o_i})\}$, where $\sum_{i=0}^{n} r_i = r$. Each D^{o_i} corresponds to an input sequence formed by a set of events $S^{o_i} = \{e_1^{o_i}, e_2^{o_i}, \ldots, e_m^{o_i}\}$, where $e_j^{o_i} = (te, t) = (te_t)$. The union of the whole set of sequences generates the set of sequences D^S related to D.*

Seq. Id	Tr. time	Itemset
	10	C D
1	15	A B C
	20	A B F
	25	A C D F
2	15	A B F
	20	E
3	10	A B F
	10	D G H
4	20	B F
	25	A G H

1-Frequent Sequences
(A):4
(B):4
(D):2
(F):4

2-Frequent sequences
(A B):3
(A F):3
(B) (A):2
(B) (F):4
(D) (A):2
(D) (B):2
(D) (F):2
(F) (A):2

3-Frequent sequences
(A B F):3
(B F) (A):2
(D) (B) (A):2
(D) (B) (F):2
(D) (F) (A):2

4-Frequent sequences
(D) (B F) (A):2

Fig. 2. Ordered transactional dataset

Definition 3. *From the D^S set we can define the support of a sequence S_i as support$(S_i) = \frac{fr(S_i)}{|O|}$, where $fr(S_i)$ denotes the frequency of the sequence. A sequence S_i is frequent if and only if support$(S_i) > \sigma$, where σ is the minimum support defined by the expert of the domain.*

In the right part of Figure 2 we can see the set of sequences D^S associated with the set D with different sizes. For example, the 3-frequent sequence "(B F) (A):2" means that the items "(B F)" are found together twice before the itemset that only contains "(A)".

Regarding the algorithms for mining sequential patterns, there are three pioneer proposals: GSP algorithm with the Apriori strategy [1], SPADE algorithm with the Equivalence Classes strategy [18], and PrefixSpan with Pattern Growth strategy [12]. A number of algorithms based on the three above-mentioned proposals have focused on improving the efficiency by using different search strategies or data structures.

In this article we use the FasPIP algorithm[6]. FaSPIP is based on the Equivalence Classes Strategy and it is able to mine both points and intervals. Besides, FaSPIP uses a novel candidate generation algorithm based on boundary points and efficient methods to avoid the generation of useless candidates and to check their frequency.

Step 2: Post-processing. The pattern explosion phenomenon is one important drawback of using patterns as predictors for classifiers. If the support is low, the number of frequent patterns increases sharply. This problem becomes extremely limiting when we work with large databases. One interesting approach used to solve this problem consists of searching for patterns with specific properties such as closed patterns [11] or maximal patterns [3].

Definition 4. *A frequent sequence S_i is a closed sequence if there is no another frequent supersequence with the same support.*

Definition 5. *A frequent sequence S_i is a maximal sequence if there is no another frequent supersequence of it.*

Clearly, the collection of frequent closed sequences is smaller than the collection of all frequent sequences. And the collection of frequent maximal sequences is smaller than the collection of closed sequences. The search of closed patterns provides two benefits at the same time: a reduction in the number of candidates, and a more compact output while maintaining the maximum amount of information [11]. However, with the maximal sequences we lose some information and we are not able to rebuild the original database since some supports are missing.

In this article we explore the use of closed and maximal patterns instead of the frequent ones as predictors in order to increase the discriminative capacity.

Step 3: Classification Algorithms with Interpretable Models. In the knowledge discovery process we chose a model easy to interpret by the physician. We opted for using two different algorithms to cover possible differences in the database structure: one that generates a general model and one that is able to find local models.

On the one hand, we chose a decision tree [13]. Some of the advantages of decision trees are: they are easy to understand, they are easily converted to a set of production rules, and they can classify both categorical and numerical data.

On the other hand, we chose a sequential covering algorithm, such a Repeated Incremental Pruning to Produce Error Reduction, RIPPER [4]. In this case, rules are learned one at a time, and each time a rule is learned, the tuples covered by the rule are removed. This process is repeated until there are no more training examples or if the quality of a rule obtained is below a user-specified threshold.

3   Case Study

The database has 480 patients registries recorded between 1992 and 2002. From the database, we have removed all patients with missing data on the variables selected for this study. Although it was not necessary for mining sequential patterns, we removed them to be able to compare the results with the burn severity scores. After this cleansing, 379 patients remain, where 79.95% (303/76) of them survived, 69.39% (263/116) are male, and 47.23% (179/200) of them have inhalation injuries. Table 1 depicts a summary of the static attributes of the database.

One of the objectives of the resuscitation phase is to restore the fluids. Incomings (INC) were originally given in cc, we decided to make them uniform to the weight of the patient and to the %TBSA according to the Parkland's formula for resuscitation (the most used one). We have used quartiles to make four intervals: $[<, 2.3), [2.3, 3.66), [3.66, 5.78), [5.78, >]$. The usual unit with meaning for diuresis (DIU) is cc/kg/h, so we have divided all values between weight and 24 (every value is daily register with cumulated 24 hours). Clinical terms usually used in adults for diuresis are oliguria under 0.5 cc/kg/h, normal diuresis within

Table 1. Attribute summary

Attribute	Min	Max	Mean	Std. Dev
Age (years)	9	95	46.57	20.75
Weight (kg)	25	120	71.1	10.76
Length of stay (days)	5	163	26.11	25.31
Total burn surface area (%)	1	90	31.78	20.61
Deep burn surface area (%)	0	90	17.67	18.16
SAPS	6	58	20.76	9.57

0.5 and 1 cc/kg/h, and augmented diuresis over 1 cc/kg/h. Values above 1 mean a normal functioning, but we have used the third quartile to differentiate augmented from high values. Intervals defined are [0, 0.5), [0.5, 1), [1, 1.9), [1.9, >]. The fluid balance (BAL) measures the difference between the incomings and the total fluid output (not only diuresis). A desired value would be slightly positive balance. In this case, the therapeutic goal is fulfilled every day, and we have used the median of the consecutive days as a way of improvement. We defined the intervals [<, -2), [-2, 10.5), [10.5, 20.4), [20.4, 52.22), [52.22, >], being 10.5, 20.4 and 52.22 the medians of the forth, third and second day respectively.

For pH, bicarbonate and base excess, there is no standard criterion for qualitative discretization. A possible abstraction is the distinction of pH values in severe acidosis [<,7.20), moderate acidosis [7.20,7.30), mild acidosis [7.30,7.35), normal [7.35,7.45), mild alkalosis [7.45,7.50), moderate alkalosis [7.50,7.60), and severe alkalosis [7.6, >).

The qualitative abstraction of base excess (BE) is done with respect pH and maintaining pCO2 in 40 mmHg. Normal values of BE are between -2 and 2 mEq/L. We have used 4 intervals for different level of acidosis and alkalosis: [<,-4), [-4,-2), [-2,2), [2,4), [4,>].

Normal levels of bicarbonate (BIC) are within [21,25] mmol/L, and we have defined the following intervals using the interquartile difference Q3-Q1 to create a reference around normal values: [<, 17), [17,21), [21,25), [25,29), [29, >].

4   Experiments and Discussion

We have run several experiments that mine patterns and use them as predictors in the classifiers. In the first place, we consider only patterns as extracted from the database with FasPIP with different supports. Then, we have explored the number of closed patterns and maximal patterns as well as their main features. Table 2 shows the number of patterns discovered with different support values, the maximum length of the patterns in days, and the maximum number of events in the patterns. If we use a high support, only very common and short patterns are found; these patterns have less discriminative value since they appear in both survivors and non survivors with similar support. We did not use supports below 5% since the longest pattern at 10% already span to the 5 days.

The set of closed patterns is smaller than the original one, and the set of maximal patterns is the smallest one. In general, long patterns should be more prone to overfitting, but if we consider the monotonicity property, a closed pattern summarizes all its subpatterns without losing information (the support). When we chose only maximal patterns, we get the essential evolution, but we lose information about the support. Usually, a set of long patterns (containing more than 5 elements in our case) would have a common prefix and differ only in a few elements, with similar discriminative capacity than their superpatterns.

Since we wanted to extract rules on both survivors and non survivors, we also run a second experiment that extracts patterns from the subset of survivors and from the subset of non-survivors in order to remove common behaviour or patient's evolution that is not discriminative. In order to get more robust rules, we included patterns with a small degree of overlap in both classes (patterns that are found in survivors and at most in 2% of non survivors). In Tables 2 and 3 they are called *contrast patterns* and *robust contrast patterns* respectively. For example, with support at 15% we found 42 closed contrast patterns and 81 robust contrast patterns. As expected, the number of patterns (predictors) is clearly reduced using the same support.

Table 2. Number of patterns and maximum length in each test

Support	Type	All	Closed	Maximal	days/events
40%	Full	311	289	227	3 / 4
20%	Full	4295	4269	3137	4 / 6
15%	Full	11525	11498	8424	4 / 7
10%	Full	43193	43151	31236	5 / 8
5%	Full	373051	372013	261560	5 / 9
15%	Contrast	43	42	41	4 / 6
10%	Contrast	16115	14828	13526	5 / 9
15%	Robust	82	81	77	4 / 6
10%	Robust	16154	14867	13546	5 / 9
10%	Class pattern	24878	24873	18123	4 / 7

We carried out a third experiment to try to keep more discriminative patterns. To that end, we included the class as a new transaction in day 6 in every patient sequence. After mining the patterns, we discarded the frequent patterns that did not contain the class as last item. Then, we remove the class and check again the patients whose sequence contains the pattern (regardless they survive or not). We name them *class patterns* in Tables 2 and 3. Contrary to what we thought, we found even more patterns of this kind using the same support because the class is very frequent in the database and it is found in many patterns.

In Table 3 we compare the classifiers built with static knowledge and those built using patterns as predictors with the three previous experiments. For the predictors, we used the patterns obtained with 10% support in order to avoid overfitting with too specific patterns (experiments with higher support values provided worse results, but we omitted them due to space reasons). In both cases, we configured the classifiers with the same minimum number of elements in each leaf or rule to 2% of the instances. In the database with static attributes, we did not use the LOS attribute since it contains information that extends over

Table 3. Results of the experiments with RIPPER algorithm

	Sensitivity	Specificity	Accuracy	AUC
Static attributes	91.9%	38.16%	80.47%	0.6681
Full Patterns	88.78%	19.74%	74.93%	0.54
Full Patterns (Closed)	91.09%	31.58%	79.16%	0.606
Full Patterns (Maximal)	94.06%	19.74%	79.16%	0.574
Contrast Patterns (Closed)	100%	80.26%	96.04%	0.899
Robust Contrast Patterns (Maximal)	100%	78.95%	95.78%	0.87
Class Patterns (Full)	94.72%	25%	80.74%	0.6031

the five first days after admission. The accuracy, sensitivity, specificity and AUC
are calculated with a 10-fold cross validation.

As expected, the sensitivity is very high in all the experiments, since the
proportion of survivors is about 80% in the database. The low specificity in
experiments that do not use contrast patterns may be caused by the high number
of sequential patterns and the low number of patients in the database. In general,
closed patterns keep more information than maximal ones.

The use of contrast patterns improved the specificity given by the classifier
with static data. This is due to the fact that the models are able to include rules
for a better prediction of the deceased. In the case of robust contrast patterns, the
models do not show significant difference in neither accuracy nor AUC. The use
of non-partial patterns did not improve the classifiers. This may be because the
class variable is very common and the patterns obtained were not discriminative.
RIPPER generated only 2 rules for normal, closed and maximal patterns.

In this database, a high number of redundant patterns is generated since some
of the variables are closely related, e.g. fluid balance is related to incomings and
diuresis. However, the meaning of these variables is different since incomings
are a sign related to the treatments, while diuresis is a sign of how the kidney
behaves. Although the algorithms do not include correlated patterns in the same
model, it would be interesting to do the same experiment using fewer variables.

```
RULE 1:
IF (BIC_LOW => BAL_VERY_HIGH => EB_NORMAL) AND NOT (EB_NORMAL => PH_NORMAL)
        AND NOT (BAL_POSITIVE => (BIC_NORMAL+PH_NORMAL)) THEN NOT SURVIVE
RULE 2:
IF (EB_VERY_LOW => (DIU_AUGMENTED + EB_VERY_LOW))
        AND NOT (INC_HIGH + BIC_NORMAL) => DIU_AUGMENTED)
        AND NOT (INC_HIGH => PH_NORMAL => DIU_AUGMENTED)
        AND NOT (BAL_VERY_POSITIVE => (INC_LOW + BAL_POSITIVE)) THEN NOT SURVIVE
RULE 3: ELSE SURVIVE
```

Fig. 3. A RIPPER model using multivariate sequential patterns

Finally, we also drew our attention to the size of the models. We found that the
RIPPER models are smaller than the decision trees. The rules usually contain
only few patterns (from 3 up to 11), and they can be easily understood and
interpreted by the expert. As an example, Figure 3 depicts a model that shows
a default rule for survivors and several for deceased. The rules usually contain

a pattern with an evolution, and several patterns negated (see "and not") that contains events that are not observed in the patient.

In order to compare our classifier with clinical scores, we have calculated the Brier Score for the Baux (0.12), R-Baux (0.12), and ABSI (0.14) scores of burn patients, for SAPSII (0.14) score, and for our classifier (0.04). Our classifier clearly outperforms the clinical scores for mortality prediction.

5   Conclusions and Future Work

In this article we propose a 4-step knowledge discovery process to build a model for predicting mortality of patients in a database of an ICBU with 480 patients.

First, a physician-driven pre-processing was done based on temporal data discretization. The second step consisted of the discovery of multivariate sequential patterns that describe the evolution of six variables during the first five days after the admission of patients in an ICBU. We used the novel FasPIP algorithm, an efficient algorithm based on boundary items to mine the patterns.

The third step focused on reducing the amount of patterns to deal with the pattern explosion problem. A novel contribution of this paper is the exploration of the support property for pattern selection. We have shown the results with closed and maximal multivariate sequential patterns.

As regards to classification, we chose models that make it easy for the physician to interpret the survival prediction rationale. We opted to use a sequential covering algorithm and a decision tree. We have compared the accuracy, sensitivity, specificity and AUC of these models with other state-of-art classifiers to show their performance.

To the best of our knowledge, this is the first paper where multivariate sequential patterns are used as mortality predictors in ICBU or ICU.

The results of the classification tests show that our approach is comparable to the burn severity scores used currently by physicians. Unlike these scores, based on data at admission time, our proposal is based on data of the first five days. We highlight the interest of physicians in this kind of patterns since they can provide insights about the possible evolution of the variables of the patient (and hence, the response to the treatment).

For further research we plan to include temporal information in the patterns. In this sense, we can abstract the patterns into intervals or to include metric information in the patterns with the relative distance between the variables.

Acknowledgment. We thank Francisco Palacios, M.D,PhD, for his valuable comments on this work. This work was partially funded by the Spanish Ministry of Economy and Competitiveness under project TIN2013-45491-R, and by European Fund for Regional Development (EFRD), and Instituto de Salud Carlos III (Ref: FIS PI 12/2898).

References

1. Agrawal, R., Srikant, R.: Mining sequential patterns: generalisations and performance improvements. In: Apers, P.M.G., Bouzeghoub, M., Gardarin, G. (eds.) EDBT 1996. LNCS, vol. 1057, pp. 3–17. Springer, Heidelberg (1996)
2. Baux, S.: Contribution a létude du traitement local des brulures thermiques etendues. PhD thesis, Paris (1962)
3. Bayardo Jr., R.J.: Efficiently mining long patterns from databases. In: Procs of the 1998 ACM SIGMOD Int. Conf. on Management of Data, SIGMOD 1998, pp. 85–93. ACM, New York (1998)
4. Cohen, W.W.: Fast effective rule induction. In: Procs of the 20th Int. Conf on Machine Learning, pp. 115–123. Morgan Kaufmann (1995)
5. Exarchos, T.P., Tsipouras, M.G., Papaloukas, C., Fotiadis, D.I.: A two-stage methodology for sequence classification based on sequential pattern mining and optimization. Data and Knowledge Engineering 66(3), 467–487 (2008)
6. Gomariz, A.: Techniques for the Discovery of Temporal Patterns. PhD thesis, University of Murcia (March 2014)
7. Ho, T.B., Nguyen, T.D., Kawasaki, S., Le, S.Q., Nguyen, D.D., Yokoi, H., Takabayashi, K.: Mining hepatitis data with temporal abstraction. In: Proc. of the 9th ACM SIGKDD Int. Conf. on Knowledge Discovery and Data Mining, pp. 369–377. ACM, New York (2003)
8. Jimenez, F., Sanchez, G., Juarez, J.M.: Multi-objective evolutionary algorithms for fuzzy classification in survival prediction. Artificial Intelligence in Medicine 60(3), 197–219 (2014)
9. Li, I., Huang, J., Liao, I., Lin, J.: A sequence classification model based on pattern coverage rate. In: Park, J.J(J.H.), Arabnia, H.R., Kim, C., Shi, W., Gil, J.-M. (eds.) GPC 2013. LNCS, vol. 7861, pp. 737–745. Springer, Heidelberg (2013)
10. Li, W., Han, J., Pei, J.: CMAR: accurate and efficient classification based on multiple class-association rules. In: Proceedings IEEE International Conference on Data Mining, ICDM 2001, pp. 369–376 (2001)
11. Pasquier, N., Bastide, Y., Taouil, R., Lakhal, L.: Discovering frequent closed itemsets for association rules. In: Beeri, C., Bruneman, P. (eds.) ICDT 1999. LNCS, vol. 1540, pp. 398–416. Springer, Heidelberg (1998)
12. Pei, J., Han, J., Mortazavi-Asl, B., Wang, J., Pinto, H., Chen, Q., Dayal, U., Hsu, M.: Mining sequential patterns by pattern-growth: The prefixspan approach. IEEE Transactions on Knowledge and Data Engineering 16(11), 1424–1440 (2004)
13. Quinlan, J.R.: Induction of decision trees. Machine Learning 1(1), 81–106 (1986)
14. Sheppard, N.N., Hemington-Gorse, S., Shelley, O.P., Philp, B., Dziewulski, P.: Prognostic scoring systems in burns: A review. Burns 37(8), 1288–1295 (2011)
15. Tobiasen, J., Hiebert, J.M., Edlich, R.F.: The abbreviated burn severity index. Annals of Emergency Medicine 11(5), 260–262 (1982)
16. Toma, T., Abu-Hanna, A., Bosman, R.J.: Discovery and integration of univariate patterns from daily individual organ-failure scores for intensive care mortality prediction. Artificial Intelligence in Medicine 43(1), 47–60 (2008)
17. Toma, T., Bosman, R.J., Siebes, A., Peek, N., Abu-Hanna, A.: Learning predictive models that use pattern discovery-a bootstrap evaluative approach applied in organ functioning sequences. Journal of Biomedical Informatics 43(4), 578–586 (2010)
18. Zaki, M.J.: SPADE: An efficient algorithm for mining frequent sequences. Machine Learning 42(1/2), 31–60 (2001)
19. Zaki, M.J., Leshand, N., Ogihara, M.: Planmine: Predicting plan failures using sequence mining. Artif. Intell. Rev. 14(6), 421–446 (2000)

A Heterogeneous Multi-Task Learning for Predicting RBC Transfusion and Perioperative Outcomes

Che Ngufor[✉], Sudhindra Upadhyaya, Dennis Murphree, Nageswar Madde, Daryl Kor, and Jyotishman Pathak

Division of Biomedical Statistics and Informatics, Mayo Clinic, Rochester, MN, USA
Ngufor.Che@mayo.edu

Abstract. It would be desirable before a surgical procedure to have a prediction rule that could accurately estimate the probability of a patient bleeding, need for blood transfusion, and other important outcomes. Such a prediction rule would allow optimal planning, more efficient use of blood bank resources, and identification of high-risk patient cohort for specific perioperative interventions. The goal of this study is to develop an efficient and accurate algorithm that could estimate the risk of multiple outcomes simultaneously. Specifically, a heterogeneous multi-task learning method is proposed for learning outcomes such as perioperative bleeding, intraoperative RBC transfusion, ICU care, and ICU length of stay. Additional outcomes not normally predicted are incorporated in the model for transfer learning and help improve the performance of relevant outcomes. Results for predicting perioperative bleeding and need for blood transfusion for patients undergoing non-cardiac operations from an institutional transfusion datamart show that the proposed method significantly increases AUC and G-Mean by more than 6% and 5% respectively over standard single-task learning methods.

Keywords: Multi-task Learning · Machine learning · Blood transfusion · Health care · Regression · Classification

1 Introduction

Bleeding in patients undergoing surgical procedures is a serious and relatively common complication that has been found to be associated with significant morbidity and increased mortality [1]. Excessive bleeding, re-operation for bleeding and intraoperative red blood cell (RBC) transfusion are common both during and shortly after major surgical procedures. In spinal surgery for example, between 30% and 60% of patients require allogeneic blood transfusion [2]. Re-operation for bleeding and administration of blood products are associated with postoperative complications including transfusion associated lung injury (TRALI) and transfusion-associated circulatory overload (TACO) [3]. Despite the increased risk of postoperative complications and mortality, various studies have shown large variability in the number of units of blood products transfused among

© Springer International Publishing Switzerland 2015
J.H. Holmes et al. (Eds.): AIME 2015, LNAI 9105, pp. 287–297, 2015.
DOI: 10.1007/978-3-319-19551-3_37

different centers in the US. According to the national blood collection and utilization survey [4], the number of RBC units transfused annually is about 14 million. At an estimated cost of $761 per unit of RBC, this amounts to $10.5 billion in health care expenditures [4]. Methods are therefore needed to more accurately estimate the risk of bleeding and the need for blood products during surgical procedures.

Many studies have derived scores to assess the risk of bleeding during surgical procedures [5,6], however, most of these methods are based on standard statistical regression techniques. These models require assumptions regarding the functional form of the prediction function and the distribution of variables. If any of these assumptions are incorrect, derived relationships may be misleading. Machine learning (ML) methods on the other-hand can estimate complex relationships between the outcome and predictors with reasonable accuracy, thus producing robust and consistent risk scores.

However, it is not sufficient to simply apply standard ML methods and hope to improve prediction accuracy. The traditional learning in ML, where single tasks are learned one at a time, may be counterproductive in some applications. In particular, single task learning (STL) ignores potential sources of information that may be available in some related tasks. Instead, the multiple tasks can be learned simultaneously, sharing what each task learns to improve prediction accuracy. This type of learning is known as multi-task learning (MTL) [7]. Specifically, MTL deals with the problem of learning multiple prediction tasks (such as regression or classification) jointly such that information can be shared efficiently among the tasks. A major advantage of MTL over conventional STL is that it can achieve significantly better generalization performance, especially when the number of labeled examples per task is very small.

MTL has gained a lot of research interest in the past decade and many methods have been proposed [8,9,10]. The method has been advantageously applied in many areas including sentiment classification, document categorization, image retrieval, predicting future stock returns, etc. [11]. However, very few applications of MTL can be found in healthcare. This study proposes a new regularization-based MTL for predicting important surgical outcomes such as perioperative bleeding (PB), intra-operative RBC transfusion (Intra-RBC), Re-operation for bleeding (Re-OP), need for ICU care, need for post-operative mechanical ventilation (Post-MV), ICU length of stay (ICU-LOS), and hospital length of stay (LOS). In addition to predicting these relevant outcomes, an important feature of the proposed method is that some Pre-, Intra-, and Post-operative measurements such as fresh frozen plasma (FFP) and platelet transfusions that are often of interest to clinicians are incorporated as additional tasks. These additional outcomes which will be called *nuisance tasks* are outcomes that one would not normally predict, or are outcomes that only become available after predictions of some relevant outcomes must be made. For example predicting preoperative plasma transfusion may not be of interest for a population with international normalization ratio (INR) greater than 1.5, but information on whether a patient was administered FFP or not might help in predicting PB or Intra-RBC. The nuisance tasks are usually available in the training set and can be used in MTL to donate information and help the performance of predicting the relevant tasks.

Application of the proposed heterogeneous MTL to predict perioperative outcomes for patients undergoing non-cardiac operations show that the method can improve overall predictive accuracy over STL. Specifically, using 50 Monte Carlo experiments, the AUC and G-Mean for predicting PB were significantly increased (p-value $< 10^{-16}$) by 6.10% and 6.84% respectively while the corresponding values for Intra-RBC were 6.02% and 5.33%.

2 Methods

This section briefly reviews two learning tasks commonly employed in multi-task learning: regression and classification. Regularized kernel least squares regression is considered for regression tasks while extreme logistic regression [12] is considered for classification tasks because of its speed and scalability properties. Different from previous studies, the considered regression and classification tasks are represented in a unified heterogeneous multi-task framework for learning continuous and discrete outputs from a common set of input variables simultaneously.

2.1 Regularized Least Squares Regression

The goal of nonparametric regression is to predict the value of a scalar response variable $y_i = f(x_i) \in \mathbb{Y}$ corresponding to an input vector $x = (x_1, \ldots, x_d) \in \mathbb{X}$ under the assumption that the joint distribution of $(\mathbb{X}, \mathbb{Y})$ or the function f is possibly unknown.

In kernel based regression, the input data is mapped onto a higher dimensional feature space through a map function ϕ such that $\phi : x \to \phi(x) \in \mathbb{R}^{d_f}$. In the higher dimensional feature space, which can be infinite, linear functions can be constructed that represents non-linear functions in the input space. Specifically, given a set of i.i.d training examples $\mathcal{D} = \{(x_i, y_i), i = 1, \ldots n\}$, the regularized kernel least squares regression (RKLS) method finds estimates of the parameters β that solves the optimization problem:

$$\min_{\beta, \varepsilon} L(\beta, \varepsilon) = \frac{1}{2}\|\beta\|^2 + \frac{\gamma}{2}\sum_{i=1}^{n} \varepsilon_i^2$$

$$\text{subject to}: \quad z_i = \beta^\mathsf{T}\phi(x_i) + \varepsilon_i, \quad \forall \ i = 1, \ldots n \ , \tag{1}$$

where $\|\cdot\|$ is the L^2-norm, ε_i is the error on example x_i and $z_i = y_i$. The solution to the optimization problem can be solved using Lagrange multipliers. However, the map function $\phi(\cdot)$ is usually not known. In [12], this problem is addressed by explicitly mapping $\phi : x \to \phi(x) \in \mathbb{R}^p(x)$ into a finite randomize feature space. This significantly reduces the cost of computing the corresponding kernel matrix.

2.2 Extreme Logistic Regression

Extreme logistic regression (ELR) is a recent algorithm introduced in [12] that extends the extreme learning machine (ELM) theory [13] to kernel logistic regression (KLR) by replacing the square error loss of ELM with the logistic loss function.

As in ELM, ELR replaces the expensive kernel computation of KLR with a cheap randomized feature space kernel to obtain a simple, fast and minimally tuned algorithm with comparative generalization performance to support vector machines (SVM) and KLR. In addition to its good generalization performance, a major benefit of ELR compared to ELM and SVM is that it produces class posterior probability outcomes, whereas SVM and ELM outputs class decisions. The constrained optimization problem of ELR as derived in [12] is given by

$$\min_{\boldsymbol{\beta},\boldsymbol{\varepsilon}} L(\boldsymbol{\beta},\boldsymbol{\varepsilon}) = \frac{1}{2}\|\boldsymbol{\beta}\|^2 + \frac{\gamma}{2}\sum_{i=1}^{n} w_i \varepsilon_i^2$$

$$\text{subject to}: \quad z_i = \boldsymbol{\beta}^{\mathsf{T}}\boldsymbol{\phi}(x_i) + \varepsilon_i, \quad \forall \ i = 1,\ldots n, \tag{2}$$

where $\boldsymbol{\beta} = (\beta_1,\ldots,\beta_p)^{\mathsf{T}}$ are model parameters, $\boldsymbol{\phi}$ is the output function that maps the input data to a p dimensional randomized feature space $\boldsymbol{\phi}(x) \in \mathbb{R}^p$, and $w_i = \pi(x_i)(1 - \pi(x_i))$ are weights for each example with $\pi(x_i) = 1/(1 + \exp(-\boldsymbol{\beta}^{\mathsf{T}}\boldsymbol{\phi}(x_i)))$ the class conditional probability for each example. z_i represents a modified outcome variable given by $z_i = \boldsymbol{\beta}^{\mathsf{T}}\boldsymbol{\phi}(x_i) + \frac{1}{w_i}(y_i - \pi(x_i))$.

Observe that except for the weights w_i, the form of the optimization problem for RKLS in (1) is exactly the same as that for ELR. This representation provides a simple and unified framework for simultaneously learning of both regression and classification tasks, i.e. heterogeneous multi-task learning.

3 Multi-Task Learning

Multi-task learning (MTL) is an approach where knowledge is transfered or shared among related tasks. By transferring knowledge, the learned model can generalize better on unseen data compared to learning the tasks independently. MTL can be especially beneficial in situations where the number of training examples per task is very small.

The goal of MTL is to find T prediction functions $\mathcal{F}_T = \{f_1,\ldots,f_T\}$ such that $f_t(x_t) \approx y_t$ in a joint manner with information shared among the tasks. This is in contrast to traditional learning where each f_t is estimated separately. Various learning algorithms have been proposed for MTL. In neural network methods [7], the networks share their first hidden layer, while all the remaining layers are specific to each task. Bayesian methods [8] enforces task similarity through a common prior probability distribution on task parameters. Recently, much attention has been focused on the regularization-based multi-task learning strategy [9,10], which is also the approach pursued in this work.

This paper considers the set-up where there are T related regression or classification tasks, each associated with its own list of n_t training examples $\mathcal{D}_t = \{(x_{it}, y_{it})\} \in \mathbb{X}^t \times \mathbb{Y}^t$. For simplicity, it is assumed that all tasks have the same input space, i.e $\mathbb{X}^1,\ldots,\mathbb{X}^T = \mathbb{X}$ $(n_t = n)$ and each $x_i \in \mathbb{X} = \mathbb{R}^d$ is a d-dimensional column vector of feature variables and $y_{it} \in \mathbb{R}$ for regression tasks while $y_{it} \in \{0,1\}$ for classification tasks.

3.1   Regularized Multi-Task Learning with RKLS and ELR

The multi-task formulation in this study is based on the regularized multi-task learning proposed in [9]. In this approach, all similar tasks are forced to share a common mean, i.e. the tasks specific parameter vector is taken as $\beta_t = \beta_0 + \mathbf{v}_t$. If $\mathbf{v}_t$ is small, then the task are "close" or similar to each other. The goal then is to estimate all $\mathbf{v}_t$ as well as the common mean β_0 simultaneously. Based on the approach in [9], the optimization problem for the proposed MTL method formulated for RKLS and ELR is given by

$$\min_{\beta_0, \mathbf{v}, \varepsilon} L(\beta_0, \mathbf{v}, \varepsilon) = \sum_{t=1}^{T} \sum_{i=1}^{n} w_i^{\delta_{it}} \varepsilon_{it}^2 + \frac{\lambda_1}{T} \sum_{t=1}^{T} \|\mathbf{v}_t\|^2 + \lambda_2 \|\beta_0\|^2$$

$$\text{subject to}: \quad z_{it} = \beta_t^{\mathsf{T}} \phi(x_i) + \varepsilon_{it} \; \forall \; i = 1, \ldots n, \; t = 1, \ldots, T, \tag{3}$$

where λ_1, λ_2 are positive regularization parameters controlling task similarity and $\delta_{it} = 1$ if task t is classification and 0 otherwise.

Let β_0^* and $\mathbf{v}_t^*$ be the optimal solution of problem (3), then applying the Lagrange method it can be shown that $\beta_0^* = \frac{\lambda_1}{T\lambda_2} \sum_{t=1}^{T} \mathbf{v}_t^*$. This relation suggests that β_0 can be replaced with an expression of $\mathbf{v}_t$ in (3) to produce a heterogeneous MTL problem that depends only on the $\mathbf{v}_t$'s.

3.2   Dual Solution to Heterogeneous MTL Optimization Problem

By using a similar feature map as in [9], the dual of problem (3) is linked to the dual of RKLS or ELR which allows easy optimization of the Lagrangian function. Specifically, a feature map function $\Phi : \mathbb{X} \times \{1, \ldots, T\} \to \mathbb{R}$ is defined to connect the prediction functions $f_t(x)$ by $f_t(x_i) = \beta^{\mathsf{T}} \Phi(x_i; t)$ where

$$\Phi(x_i; t) = \left(\frac{\phi(x_i)^{\mathsf{T}}}{\sqrt{\mu}}, \underbrace{\mathbf{0}, \ldots, \mathbf{0}}_{t-1}, \phi(x_i)^{\mathsf{T}}, \underbrace{\mathbf{0}, \ldots, \mathbf{0}}_{T-t} \right)^{\mathsf{T}} \in \mathbb{R}^{pT' \times 1},$$

and $\beta = (\sqrt{\mu}\beta_0^{\mathsf{T}}, \mathbf{v}_1^{\mathsf{T}}, \ldots, \mathbf{v}_T^{\mathsf{T}})^{\mathsf{T}} \in \mathbb{R}^{pT' \times 1}$ and $T' = T+1$. $\mathbf{O}$ denotes a row vector of length p whose entries are all zero and $\mu = \frac{T\lambda_2}{\lambda_1}$.

With these transformations, the following theorem for heterogeneous MTL is similar to theorem 2.1 in [9].

Theorem 1. *Let* $\gamma = \frac{\lambda_1}{T}, \mu = \frac{T\lambda_2}{\lambda_1}$ *and define the randomize feature space kernel* $K_{ts}(x_i, x_j) = \Phi(x_i; t)^{\mathsf{T}} \Phi(x_j; s), t, s = 1, \ldots, T$. *Then the dual of problem* (3) *is given by*

$$\sum_{t=1}^{T} \sum_{j=1}^{n} \alpha_{js} K_{ts}(x_j, x_i) + \frac{1}{w_i^{\delta_{it}}} \frac{\alpha_{it}}{\gamma} = z_{it}, \quad i = 1, \ldots, n, \; t = 1, \ldots, T \tag{4}$$

If α_{it}^* *is a solution to the problem above, then the solution to problem* (3) *is given by*

$$f_t^*(x_i) = \sum_{s=1}^{T} \sum_{j=1}^{n} \alpha_{js}^* K_{ts}(x_j, x_i) \tag{5}$$

Proof. See the on-line supplementary material at
http://informatics.mayo.edu/CLIP/files/SupplementaryMaterialAIME2015.
pdf.   □
The parameter μ controls tasks similarity where small values indicates tasks are
related.

Let

$$\phi(\mathbf{X}) = \text{a } n \times p \text{ matrix containing } \phi(x_i)^{\mathsf{T}} \text{ on its } i\text{-th row}, \tag{6}$$

$$\boldsymbol{\Phi} = \boldsymbol{\Phi}(\mathbf{X}; T) = \begin{pmatrix} \frac{1}{\mu}\phi(\mathbf{X}) & \phi(\mathbf{X}) & \mathbf{O} & \cdots \cdots & \mathbf{O} \\ \frac{1}{\mu}\phi(\mathbf{X}) & \mathbf{O} & \phi(\mathbf{X}) & \cdots & \mathbf{O} \\ \vdots & \vdots & & \ddots & \vdots \\ \frac{1}{\mu}\phi(\mathbf{X}) & \mathbf{O} & \cdots & \cdots & \phi(\mathbf{X}) \end{pmatrix} \in \mathbb{R}^{nT \times pT'},$$

$$\boldsymbol{\alpha} = (\alpha_{11}, \ldots, \alpha_{n1}, \ldots, \alpha_{12}, \ldots, \alpha_{n2}, \ldots, \alpha_{1T}, \ldots, \alpha_{nT})^{\mathsf{T}} \in \mathbb{R}^{nT \times 1},$$

$$\mathbf{Y} = (y_{11}, \ldots, y_{n1}, \ldots, y_{12}, \ldots, y_{n2}, \ldots, y_{1T}, \ldots, y_{nT})^{\mathsf{T}},$$

$$\boldsymbol{\pi} = (\pi_{11}, \ldots, \pi_{n1}, \ldots, \pi_{12}, \ldots, \pi_{n2}, \ldots, \pi_{1T}, \ldots, \pi_{nT})^{\mathsf{T}},$$

$$\mathbf{W} = \mathbf{diag}(w_i^{\delta_{it}}, i = 1, \ldots, n, t = 1, \ldots, T) \text{ a diagonal weight matrix,}$$

$$\boldsymbol{\delta} = \mathbf{diag}(\delta_{it}, i = 1, \ldots, n, t = 1, \ldots, T),$$

then the expression in (4) can be written in matrix form as:

$$\left(\boldsymbol{\Phi}\boldsymbol{\Phi}^{\mathsf{T}} + \frac{1}{\gamma}\mathbf{W}^{-1}\right)\boldsymbol{\alpha} = \mathbf{z} \tag{7}$$

where

$$\mathbf{z} = \boldsymbol{\delta}\boldsymbol{\Phi}\boldsymbol{\Phi}^{\mathsf{T}}\boldsymbol{\alpha} + \mathbf{W}^{-1}(\mathbf{Y} - \boldsymbol{\delta}\boldsymbol{\pi}) \tag{8}$$

Equations (7) and (8) represents the standard iterative reweighted least squares
(IRLS) problem whose solution proceeds iteratively by updating $\boldsymbol{\alpha}$ in (7) and
$\mathbf{z}$ in (8). This recursive solution is applicable only for classification tasks. Since
$\mathbf{z} = \mathbf{Y}$ for regression, (7) is a simple linear system that can be solved directly.

Predictions. Given the training set $\mathbf{X}$ and a test example x^*, the predicted re-
sponse for a regression task is given by $y_t^* = \boldsymbol{\Phi}(x^*; t)^{\mathsf{T}}\boldsymbol{\Phi}(\mathbf{X}; t)^{\mathsf{T}}\boldsymbol{\alpha}_t$, while
the class probability for a classification task is given by $\pi_t^* = 1/(1 + \exp(-\boldsymbol{\Phi}(x^*; t)^{\mathsf{T}}$
$\boldsymbol{\Phi}(\mathbf{X}; t)^{\mathsf{T}}\boldsymbol{\alpha}_t))$.

This solution in $\boldsymbol{\alpha}$ can be computationally very expensive since the complete
training set has to be stored for prediction. The next section presents some
efficient strategies to mitigate this problem among others.

3.3   Approximate Multi-Task Learning with RKLS and ELR

The recursive training of classification tasks can be expensive for large data sets.
Each iteration involves the inversion of a $nT \times nT$ matrix which has a $\mathcal{O}(n^3T^3)$
computational cost. Strategies to reduce this cost have been described elsewhere
[14,15] and only the results of applying these methods are presented here.

For the case where $n \gg p$, [15] transformed (7) into a much smaller $pT' \times pT'$ system by writing $\boldsymbol{\alpha}$ in terms of $\boldsymbol{\beta}$. Likewise, [14] proposed a simple approximation of the logistic function which transformed the IRLS problem into a least squares problem. Applying these transformations, a simple and fast heterogeneous MTL algorithm is obtained and given by

$$\left(\boldsymbol{\Phi}^\mathsf{T}\boldsymbol{\Phi} + \frac{1}{\gamma}\widetilde{\mathbf{W}} \right) \beta = \boldsymbol{\Phi}^\mathsf{T}\widetilde{\mathbf{z}} \tag{9}$$

where for each task t, $\widetilde{\mathbf{W}}_t = 4^{\delta_t}\mathbf{I}_{pT'}$, and $\widetilde{\mathbf{z}}_t = 4^{\delta_t}(\mathbf{Y}_t - \frac{\delta_t}{2})$. $\mathbf{I}_{pT'}$ is a $pT' \times pT'$ identity matrix.

Given a test example x^*, the predicted response for a regression task is computed as $y_t^* = \boldsymbol{\beta}^\mathsf{T}\boldsymbol{\Phi}(x^*; t)$ while class probability for a classification task is given by $\pi_t^* = 1/\left(1 + \exp\left(-\boldsymbol{\beta}^\mathsf{T}\boldsymbol{\Phi}(x^*; t)\right)\right)$

4   Multi-Task Learning of Perioperative Outcomes

In transfusion studies, there are often many outcomes of interest such as PB, Intra-RBC, Re-OP, need for ICU care, LOS, and mortality. Some of these outcomes are very related (e.g ICU care, ICU-LOS, Post-MV and LOS, massive PB and Intra-RBC) such that in principle knowledge can be borrowed or shared between models for each of these outcomes. In addition there is often not enough labeled examples for some of these outcomes to learn a good model independently. Under such circumstances, it is advantageous to share information across models for similar tasks. Tasks with sufficient training examples can provide information to help prediction for tasks with very few training examples.

Knowledge can also be borrowed from tasks that one is not specifically interested in or may consider irrelevant. In the perioperative environment, valuable measurements may become available only after predictions of an outcome of interest must be made. For example, FFP or platelets administered 24 hours after surgery when bleeding occurs during surgery. These measurements cannot be used as inputs for the bleeding model because they will not be available at prediction time. Equally, some measurements are available before predictions are to be made, but one will normally not need to use them as inputs or as outcomes.

In both cases and especially in the former, if training is performed off-line, then these measurements can be used as extra tasks in MTL to donate information and help improve performance of the relevant tasks. These extra tasks are referred to as nuisance tasks in this study because they are not of immediate interest but are needed to help boost the performance of the main tasks. The predictions made on the nuisance tasks are discarded when the MTL model is used.

4.1   Study Population

Screening for study participation was performed using an institutional perioperative datamart [16] that captures data for all patients admitted to acute care environments. To be considered for study participation, patients must have met the following criteria: age $\geq$ 18 years, noncardiac surgery, and an INR $\geq$ 1.5 in the 30 days preceding surgery. Between 2008 and 2011, a total of 1,234 patients were identified and comprised the study population.

The distributions of the main and nuisance outcomes for the entire population are shown in Table 1. All classification tasks are binary (Yes/No). With respect to bleeding, there was a significant difference (p-value $= 1 \times 10^{-8}$) in age between patients who bled (mean age $= 61$) and those who did not (mean age $= 67$). Males were more common in both groups but not statistically significant between groups. A total of 55 predictors were considered for inclusion in the analyses (see the on-line supplementary material).

Table 1. Distribution of Main and Nuisance Outcomes

	Classification	PB	Intra-RBC	Re-OP	ICU Care	Post-MV		
	No	811	910	1169	757	917		
	Yes	423	324	65	477	317		
Main Outcomes	Regression	ICU-LOS	LOS					
	mean (days)	3.38	13.25					
	Classification	Pre-FFP	Pre-Platelets	Intra-FFP	Intra-Platelets	Post-RBC	Post-FFP	Post-Platelets
Nuisance Outcomes	No	1095	1207	890	1058	974	1069	1123
	Yes	139	27	344	176	260	165	111

4.2 Results

To investigate the improvement in performance of MTL over STL, first independent regression or classification models are learned using RKLS or ELR described in Sections 2.1 and 2.2 respectively. Second, a MTL model is learned to predict each of the main outcomes: Main = { PB, Intra-RBC, Re-OP, ICU Care, Post-MV, ICU-LOS, LOS}. Finally, the nuisance outcomes are grouped into Pre-, Intra- and Post-operative outcomes and incorporated as extra tasks in the main MTL model. This step produces 4 models: Main + Pre = {Main, Pre-Plasma, Pre-Platelets}, Main + Intra = { Main, Intra-Plasma, Intra-Platelets}, Main + Post = {Main, Post-RBC, Post-Plasma, Post-Platelets} and All = {Main, Pre, Intra, Post}.

A five fold cross-validation training procedure was performed with $p = 300$ (number of random features) and $\gamma = 0.05$ for both STL and MTL. It should be noted that these pre-selected values are the default parameters for the ELR algorithm and may not be optimal. The task similarity parameter was also set to 0.1.

Table 2 presents average performance measures for predicting the main outcomes on the test sets. AUC and G-mean ($\sqrt{\text{sensitivity} + \text{specificity}}$) are reported for classification tasks while mean absolute error (MAE) and mean square error (MSE) are reported for regression tasks. The results show that MTL increases AUC and G-mean for PB and Intra-RBC by more than 5%. Student t-test from 50 Monte Carlo experiments confirmed that this increase was statistically significant at the 95% confidence level (p-value $< 10^{-16}$). Corresponding

Table 2. Performance of STL and MTL: $p = 300, \gamma = 0.05, \mu = 0.1$

	STL		MTL								
			Main		Main+Pre		Main+Intra		Main+Post		All	
Outcome												
Classification	AUC	G-mean	AUC	G-mean	AUC	G-mean	AUC	G-mean	AUC	G-mean	AUC	G-mean
PB	0.82	0.73	**0.87**	**0.78**	0.86	0.75	0.87	0.77	0.87	0.77	0.86	0.76
Intra-RBC	0.83	0.75	**0.88**	0.78	0.87	0.78	0.88	0.78	0.88	**0.79**	0.88	0.78
Re-OP	0.73	0.68	**0.74**	**0.72**	0.74	0.70	0.74	0.68	0.74	0.69	0.74	0.69
ICU Care	0.78	0.71	**0.81**	0.73	0.80	0.73	0.80	0.73	0.80	0.73	0.80	**0.74**
Post-MV	0.86	0.79	**0.87**	0.78	0.87	**0.80**	0.87	0.78	0.87	0.79	0.87	0.78
Regression	MAE	MSE	MAE	MSE	MAE	MSE	MAE	MSE	MAE	MSE	MAE	MSE
ICU-LOS	0.79	1.16	0.63	0.80	**0.62**	**0.76**	0.64	0.81	0.63	0.80	0.62	0.78

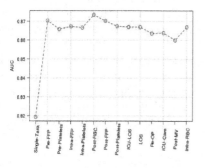 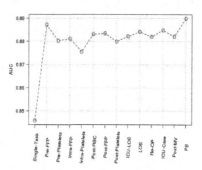

(a) Perioperative bleeding   (b) Intraoperative RBC transfusion

Fig. 1. Performance of STL and incremental addition of tasks in MTL

increase for ICU Care was also significant. Values for RE-OP and Post-MV increases as well but not significant (AUC p-values: 0.4 and 0.15, G-Mean p-values: 0.3 and 0.02 respectively). PB , Intra-RBC and ICU Care appeared to be more related while Re-Op and Post-MV appeared to be also related. These results suggest that the tasks do not equally learn from each other.

MTL also significantly reduced MAE and MSE for all regression tasks by large margins compared to STL (p-value $< 10^{-16}$) . Optimal performance was seen for the MTL model that includes main outcomes and pre-operative nuisance outcomes.

It is interesting to investigate the improvement in performance when tasks are added incrementally starting from a single task classifier. Figure 1 shows the AUC for PB and Intra-RBC as the nuisance tasks are added sequentially based on the order in the perioperative period when they become available. This is then followed by inclusion of the main tasks. The single addition of Pre-FFP increases AUC by more than 4%. Clearly, superior predictive performance for PB can be obtained through a MTL model that includes Pre, Intra and Post-RBC nuisance outcomes.

5 Conclusion and Future Work

A simple and accurate MTL algorithm is derived in this study based on RKLS and ELR algorithms and applied to predict perioperative outcomes. Different from previous regularized MTL methods in the literature, the proposed heterogeneous MTL approach seamlessly combines regression and classification tasks into a unified formula, thus facilitating knowledge transfer between tasks and allowing for easy implementation. Results for predicting perioperative outcomes in a blood transfusion study show that the method can improve predictive performance by large margins compared to learning the task independently. An interesting feature of the study is that, outcomes observed in the perioperative period that one will not normally predict are used as additional tasks. This was found to be particularly helpful in improving the performance of regression tasks. The results suggest that additional perioperative measurements which are usually considered irrelevant should be reported during data collection. The outcome of this study could facilitate optimal planning and utilization of hospital blood bank resources, and aid in identification of specific groups of patients most suitable for administration of blood products.

A limitation of the comparison results presented in this study is that the results may not be optimal for some methods as the tuning parameters were preselected, however, the same training condition was applied to all methods. The presented work can be extended in several possible directions. For example, as indicated by the results, knowledge is not transfered equally among tasks, thus extensions to include task clustering can investigated. Similarly, methods to select optimal tuning parameters, especially the task relatedness parameter, can be studied.

Acknowledgments. This work was funded in part by the Mayo Clinic Kern Center for the Science of Health Care Delivery.

References

1. Vivacqua, A., Koch, C.G., Yousuf, A.M., Nowicki, E.R., Houghtaling, P.L., Blackstone, E.H., Sabik III, J.F.: Morbidity of bleeding after cardiac surgery: is it blood transfusion, reoperation for bleeding, or both? The Annals of Thoracic Surgery 91(6), 1780–1790 (2011)
2. Zheng, F., Cammisa Jr., F.P., Sandhu, H.S., Girardi, F.P., Khan, S.N.: Factors predicting hospital stay, operative time, blood loss, and transfusion in patients undergoing revision posterior lumbar spine decompression, fusion, and segmental instrumentation. Spine 27(8), 818–824 (2002)
3. Kor, D.J., Stubbs, J.R., Gajic, O.: Perioperative coagulation management–fresh frozen plasma. Best Practice & Research Clinical Anaesthesiology 24(1), 51–64 (2010)
4. US Department of Health and Human Services and others: The 2009 national blood collection and utilization survey report. US Department of Health and Human Services, Office of the Assistant Secretary for Health, Washington, DC (2011)
5. Despotis, G., Avidan, M., Eby, C.: Prediction and management of bleeding in cardiac surgery. Journal of Thrombosis and Haemostasis 7(s1), 111–117 (2009)
6. Thomas, I.C., Sorrentino, M.J.: Bleeding risk prediction models in atrial fibrillation. Current Cardiology Reports 16(1), 1–8 (2014)
7. Caruana, R.: Multitask learning. Springer (1998)

8. Bakker, B., Heskes, T.: Task clustering and gating for bayesian multitask learning. The Journal of Machine Learning Research 4, 83–99 (2003)
9. Evgeniou, T., Pontil, M.: Regularized multi–task learning. In: Proceedings of the Tenth ACM SIGKDD International Conference on Knowledge Discovery and Data Mining, pp. 109–117. ACM (2004)
10. Gong, P., Ye, J., Zhang, C.: Robust multi-task feature learning. In: Proceedings of the 18th ACM SIGKDD International Conference on Knowledge Discovery and Data Mining, pp. 895–903. ACM (2012)
11. Pan, S.J., Yang, Q.: A survey on transfer learning. IEEE Transactions Knowledge and Data Engineering 22(10), 1345–1359 (2010)
12. Ngufor, C., Wojtusiak, J.: Extreme logistic regression. Advances in Data Analysis and Classification, 1–26 (2014)
13. Huang, G.B., Zhou, H., Ding, X., Zhang, R.: Extreme learning machine for regression and multiclass classification. IEEE Transactions on Systems, Man, and Cybernetics, Part B: Cybernetics 42(2), 513–529 (2012)
14. Ngufor, C., Wojtusiak, J.: Learning from large-scale distributed health data: an approximate logistic regression approach. In: Proc. ICML 2013: Role of Machine Learning in Transforming Healthcare (2013)
15. Ngufor, C., Wojtusiak, J., Hooker, A., Oz, T., Hadley, J.: Extreme logistic regression: A large scale learning algorithm with application to prostate cancer mortality prediction. In: The Twenty-Seventh International Flairs Conference (2014)
16. Herasevich, V., Kor, D., Li, M., Pickering, B.: Icu data mart: a non-it approach. a team of clinicians, researchers and informatics personnel at the mayo clinic have taken a homegrown approach to building an icu data mart. Healthcare Informatics: the Business Magazine for Information and Communication Systems 28(11), 42–44 (2011)

Comparison of Probabilistic versus Non-probabilistic Electronic Nose Classification Methods in an Animal Model

Camilla Colombo[1]([✉]), Jan Hendrik Leopold[2], Lieuwe D.J. Bos[2], Riccardo Bellazzi[1], and Ameen Abu-Hanna[2]

[1] University of Pavia, Pavia, Italy
`camilla.colombo02@ateneopv.it`
[2] Academic Medical Center, Amsterdam, The Netherlands

Abstract. An electronic nose (eNose) is a promising device for exhaled breath tests. Principal Component Analysis (PCA) is the most used technique for eNose sensor data analysis, and the use of probabilistic methods is scarce. In this paper, we developed probabilistic models based on the logistic regression framework and compared them to non-probabilistic classification methods in a case study of predicting Acute Liver Failure (ALF) in 16 rats in which ALF was surgically induced. Performance measures included accuracy, AUC and Brier score. Robustness was evaluated by randomly selecting subsets of repeatedly measured sensor values before calculating the model variables. Internal validation for both aspects was obtained by a leave-one-out scheme. The probabilistic methods achieved equally good performance and robustness results when appropriate feature extraction techniques were applied. Since probabilistic models allow employing sound methods for assessing calibration and uncertainty of predictions, they are a proper choice for decision making. Hence we recommend adopting probabilistic classifiers with their associated predictive performance in eNose data analysis.

Keywords: Electronic nose · Probabilistic classification · Internal validation · Calibration · Discrimination

1 Introduction

In recent years, there has been an increasing interest in exhaled breath analysis as a diagnostic tool due to its non-invasive nature and its versatility [1]. Analyzing the spectrum of volatile organic compounds (VOCs) present in breath can give insight into the physiological and pathological processes operative in the entire organism in different clinical conditions [2]. Electronic nose (eNose) technology has been proposed for real-time characterization of VOC patterns.

An eNose is a device composed of an array of gas sensors with partial specificity coupled with a pattern recognition software [3]. Each sensor reacts to different fractions of VOCs and the collective output of the array yields a unique

© Springer International Publishing Switzerland 2015
J.H. Holmes et al. (Eds.): AIME 2015, LNAI 9105, pp. 298–303, 2015.
DOI: 10.1007/978-3-319-19551-3_38

fingerprint of the gaseous mixture under study [4]. Appropriate data analysis techniques must be applied to extract the biological information of interest [5].

eNoses are mainly used for classification purposes after training with an appropriate algorithm [6]. The choice of data analysis method is crucial to the suitability and effectiveness of the instrument for specific detection applications. The most commonly used algorithms include Principal Component Analysis (PCA), Linear Discriminant Analysis (LDA) and cluster analysis [7]. More complex classifiers, like Neural Networks (NN) and Support Vector Machine (SVM) are also used [6]. However, the use of probabilistic classification methods is scarce.

Wlodzimirow et al. [8] first investigated exhaled breath analysis by eNose as a non-invasive test for Acute Liver Failure (ALF) in an animal model. They used an eNose to capture breath traces of 16 rats in which ALF was surgically induced. They developed and validated four non-probabilistic classifiers that use the first and second principal component from PCA of the eNose data to discriminate exhaled breath measurements during ALF from other conditions.

In this paper, we introduce four additional probabilistic classifiers and compare them to the current classifiers in terms of performance and robustness.

2   Methods

2.1   Experimental Setting

An established animal model of ALF in rats was studied in which each rat was its own control. In order to resemble clinical ALF, complete liver ischemia (LIS) was induced in 16 rats by means of a two-step procedure. In the first step, an end-to-side portacaval shunt was performed (PCS); the rats were then allowed to recover for 3 days. In the second step, complete ischemia of the liver was performed by ligation of the hepatic artery and common bile duct. To capture a potential confounding effect of PCS and LIS procedures, two sham operations were performed in 3 rats.

Breath samples were collected by means of an eNose. Each measurement lasted about 15 minutes. The eNose data consisted of the signals from its eight sensors, stored in the on-board database and then copied into an offline database.

Our design implied that measurements were divided into the following groups:

1. *healthy group*: measurements in healthy rats twice a day for 3-5 days.
2. *PCS group*: measurements in PCS rats twice a day for 3 days.
3. *LIS group*: measurements in LIS rats every hour until the rat was sacrificed.
4. *sham1 group*: measurements in three rats after the sham PCS procedure.
5. *sham2 group*: measurements in three rats after the sham LIS procedure.

Due to the limited amount of data, a combined control group was formed from the *healthy*, *PCS* and *sham* groups.

During the preprocessing phase, for each 15-minute measurement a delta value was calculated as the difference between the maximum and the minimum signal value for a sensor. For each rat, the median of the deltas in each of the two groups *(LIS* and *c-p-s)* was computed; these variables were named *pS1-pS8*. 11 rats had both a *c-p-s* and a *LIS* stage, while 2 rats which died early and 3 rats subjected to the sham operations only had measurements in the *c-p-s* group.

Data analysis was conducted in the statistical environment R 3.1.0.

2.2 Classification Methods

The signals from the eNose sensors were used as predictors in binary classification models to discriminate measurements in the *LIS* group from the *c-p-s* group.

Wlodzimirow at al. [8] had previously developed four standard non-probabilistic classifiers (described below). Only 14 rats were used to develop these methods, as the other two lacked a signal from an extra CO_2 sensor; since this sensor was not used in this paper, results were updated using all 16 rats.

- *PC1 threshold.* A new observation is classified based on whether its first principal component PC1 is above or below a fixed threshold. The threshold is chosen as the value minimizing the classification error on the training set.
- *Average distance.* A new observation is classified as belonging to the closest group in the sense that the average Euclidean distance in the PC1-PC2 space to each point of the group is less than to the other group.
- *k nearest neighbors (kNN).* Euclidean distances in the PC1-PC2 space are calculated and a new observation is classified as belonging to the majority group of its *k* nearest neighbors. Models are implemented for *k*=3, 5.

We introduced four additional probabilistic classifiers:

- *Logistic regression (LR).* A logistic regression model is developed using the median delta values *pS1-8* as predictors. Feature selection based on the Akaike Information Criterion is applied using a backward stepwise algorithm.
- *Principal Component Analysis and logistic regression.* PCA is performed on the median delta data *pS1-8*. The principal components are then used as predictors for a logistic regression model. The first PCs that explain at least 95% of the cumulative variance are included in the model. Additionally, a model using only the first principal component PC1 as predictor is developed.
- *Partial Least Squares (PLS) and logistic regression.* A PLS regression model is fitted using *pS1-8*. PLS components are selected choosing the number that minimizes the root mean square error of prediction (RMSEP). The selected PLS components are used as predictors for a logistic regression model.

For all the probabilistic classifiers, an optimal cutoff value for the predicted probabilities is found in order to obtain a predicted class for each observation. The value is chosen as the point on the receiver operating curve (ROC) closest to the top-left part of the plot with perfect sensitivity and specificity.

2.3 Validation

A leave-one-out strategy was used to evaluate the performances of all the classifiers. At each iteration, one rat was used as a test set, and the remaining rats formed the training set.

The following performance measures were adopted [9]: accuracy, Area under the Receiving Operator Characteristic curve (AUC), Brier score.

When the test rat had two observations (one in the *LIS* and one in the *c-p-s* stage), a mean value of the predicted probability and of the accuracy was used to account for the fact that those two predictions were obtained on the same rat. Therefore, each performance index calculated on each test rat within the leave-one-out procedure was assigned a 1 weight if the test rat had only a *c-p-s* stage, and a 0.5 weight if the rat had both a *c-p-s* and a *LIS* stage. The final global performance index was computed as a weighted mean for all the rats.

A sensitivity analysis to the preprocessing procedure was also performed. The performances of the classifiers on the original dataset were compared to the performances of the same classifiers on a dataset constructed by randomly sampling delta values for each stage in each rat (instead of computing the median).

An iterative procedure was developed. At each iteration, for each rat one measurement for the *c-p-s* stage and one for the *LIS* stage (if available) were randomly sampled; a new dataset was thus created. Each classifier was developed and validated on the new dataset. These steps were repeated 500 times.

The performances of all the classifiers were further compared to a reference random classifier which at each iteration assigned to the observations of the dataset a class obtained from the permutation of the true class values.

3 Results

Table 1. Classification results: performances (left) and sensitivity analysis (right)

method	acc	AUC	Brier	mean acc	sd acc
LR	0.69	0.68	0.31	0.7	0.1
PCA + LR	0.78	0.86	0.12	0.7	0.09
PC1 LR	0.91	0.87	0.1	0.72	0.09
PLS + LR	0.81	0.86	0.14	0.7	0.09
PC1 threshold	0.91	-	-	0.74	0.1
PCA + 3NN	0.91	-	-	0.71	0.1
PCA + 5NN	0.91	-	-	0.72	0.1
PCA + average	0.78	-	-	0.64	0.1

The performances of the classifiers are shown in the left side of Table 1. When comparing the two best probabilistic and non-probabilistic models (logistic regression based on PC1 and PC1 threshold method), they are found to yield the same class predictions in the leave-one-out validation process; significance testing would therefore not lead to identifying any differences. The right side of the table shows the mean and the standard deviation of the distributions of the accuracies obtained in the iterative procedure for the sensitivity analysis.

The percentage of cases within the iterative procedure in which each classifier had better accuracy performances than the permutation classifier was: 84.4% for logistic regression, 82.6% for PCA and logistic regression, 90% for logistic regression based on PC1, 83.4% for PLS and logistic regression, 94.2% for PC1 threshold method, 84% for PCA and 3 nearest neighbors, 85.4% for PCA and 5 nearest neighbors, 72.4% for PCA and average distance.

4 Discussion

The non-probabilistic classification methods developed by Wlodzimirow et al. [8] achieved very good results on the dataset. When appropriate feature extraction techniques such as PCA and PLS were employed, the probabilistic methods based on logistic regression performed equally well. In both cases models based on the first principal component PC1 alone yielded the best performances. It may be useful in further studies to apply additional evaluation approaches, such as bootstrapping and leave-two-out cross validation.

The sensitivity analysis showed that when models were trained on datasets where the two stages in the rats were assigned a randomly sampled measurement instead of the median value, the accuracy performances were worse, though still adequate. Both non-probabilistic and probabilistic models proved sufficiently robust to the preprocessing strategy. In particular, the two models based on PC1 which achieved the best results on the preprocessed dataset also performed best within the sensitivity analysis.

While not harming overall performance and robustness, relying on a probabilistic approach for the detection of ALF provided deeper insight in the inherent uncertainty associated to the prediction, thereby adhering to the Murphy's consistency principle [10]. Performance measures such as the Brier score and the AUC could be employed in tandem to evaluate calibration and discrimination of the models, which were overlooked by the other classifiers, in order to facilitate decision making about individual cases.

References

1. Cao, W., Duan, Y.: Current status of methods and techniques for breath analysis. Critical Reviews in Analytical Chemistry 37, 3–13 (2007)
2. Buszewski, B., Kęsy, M., Ligor, T., Amann, A.: Human exhaled air analytics: biomarkers of diseases. Biomedical Chromatography 21, 553–566 (2007)
3. Oh, E.H., Song, H.S., Park, T.H.: Recent advances in electronic and bioelectronic noses and their biomedical applications. Enzyme and Microbial Technology 48, 427–437 (2011)
4. Röck, F., Barsan, N., Weimar, U.: Electronic nose: current status and future trends. Chemical Reviews 108, 705–725 (2008)
5. Turner, A.P., Magan, N.: Electronic noses and disease diagnostics. Nature Reviews Microbiology 2(2), 161–166 (2004)
6. Di Natale, C., Paolesse, R., Martinelli, E., Capuano, R.: Solid state gas sensors for breath analysis: A review. Analytica Chimica Acta 824, 1–17 (2014)
7. Wilson, A.D., Baietto, M.: Applications and advances in electronic-nose technologies. Sensors 9, 5099–5148 (2009)

8. Wlodzimirow, K., Abu-Hanna, A., Schultz, M., et al.: Exhaled breath analysis with electronic. Biosensors and Bioelectronics 53, 129–134 (2014)

9. Medlock, S., Ravelli, A.C., Tamminga, P., Mol, B.W., Abu-Hanna, A.: Prediction of mortality in very premature infants: a systematic review of prediction models. PLoS One 6, e23441 (2011)

10. Murphy, A.H.: What is a good forecast? an essay on the nature of goodness in weather forecasting. Weather and Forecasting 8, 281–293 (1993)

Knowledge Representation
and Guidelines

Detecting New Evidence for Evidence-Based Guidelines Using a Semantic Distance Method

Qing Hu[1,2(✉)], Zhisheng Huang[1], Annette ten Teije[1], and Frank van Harmelen[1]

[1] Department of Computer Science, VU University Amsterdam,
Amsterdam, The Netherlands
{qhu400,huang,annette,Frank.van.Harmelen}@cs.vu.nl
[2] College of Computer Science and Technology,
Wuhan Univesity of Science and Technology, Wuhan, China

Abstract. To ensure timely use of new results from medical research in daily medical practice, evidence-based medical guidelines must be updated using the latest medical articles as evidences. Finding such new relevant medical evidence manually is time consuming and labor intensive. Traditional information retrieval methods can improve the efficiency of finding evidence from the medical literature, but they usually require a large training corpus for determining relevance. This means that both the manual approach and traditional IR approaches are not suitable for automatically finding new medical evidence in realtime. This paper propose the use of a semantic distance measure to automatically find relevant new evidence to support guideline updates. The advantage of using our semantic distance measure is that this relevance measure can be easily obtained from a search engine (e.g., PubMed), rather then gathering a large corpus for analysis. We have conducted several experiments that use our semantic distance measure to find new relevant evidence for guideline updates. We selected two versions of the Dutch Breast Cancer Guidelines (2004 and 2012), and we checked if the new evidence items in the 2012 version could be found by using our method. The experiment shows that our method can not only find at least some evidence for 10 out of the 16 guideline statements in our experiment (i.e. a reasonable recall), but it also returns reasonably small numbers of evidence candidates (i.e. a good precision) with an acceptable real-time performance (an average of approximately 10 minutes for each guideline statement).

1 Introduction

Based on the latest scientific research results, evidence-based medical guidelines[1] are developed to guide daily medical practice and to provide better medical practice. The scientific publications selected in the guideline are named as evidence to support the guideline conclusions. Ideally, a guideline should be updated immediately after new relevant evidence is published, so that the updated guideline can serve medical practice using latest medical research evidence[10]. However, the update of the guideline is often lagging behind medical scientific publications

---

[1] For brevity, we will simply speak of "guidelines"

© Springer International Publishing Switzerland 2015
J.H. Holmes et al. (Eds.): AIME 2015, LNAI 9105, pp. 307–316, 2015.
DOI: 10.1007/978-3-319-19551-3_39

for two reasons. The first reason is the sheer volume of medical publications. Not only the number of medical articles and the size of medical information are very large, but they are also updated very frequently. For example, PubMed[2] is a bibliographic database of citations and abstracts. Just in the PubMed, there are more than 24 million citations for biomedical literature from MEDLINE[3], life science journals, and online books. Just in 2013, more than 700,000 articles were added (amount to almost 2000 new entries each day of the year). The second reason is that updating a guideline is laborious and time-consuming. The update of guidelines usually abides by a strict schedule and takes an average of 2 years from the beginning of update to its finishing[6]. The long duration of the update process may cause the situation that a guideline might be out of date by the time it has been published. Indeed, in an evaluation of the need for updating systematic reviews, [11] found that almost one quarter of systematic reviews are likely out-of-date at two years post-publication. In the National Guideline Clearinghouse, guidelines are required to have been re-examined every three years, but [3] concluded that for their purposes that a three monthly literature search would be needed. So how to find new relevant evidences in realtime to support the guideline update becomes an important issue.

In order to solve those disadvantages, some approaches have been proposed that use information retrieval or machine learning technology to find relevant new evidence. Reinders et al.[9] describe a system to find relevant new evidence for guideline updates. The approach is based on MeSH terms and their TF-IDF weights, which results in the following disadvantages: i)the use of MeSH terms terms means that if a guideline statement does not use any MeSH term, there is no way to measure the relevance, ii)the use of TF-IDF weights means that the system has to gather all relevant sources, which is time-consuming, iii)the number of returned relevant articles is sometimes too large (sometimes over a few million), so that it is impossible for an expert to check if an evidence is really useful for the guideline update.

Similar to Reinders' method, Iruetaguena et al.[6] also developed an approach to find new evidences. That method is also based on gathering all relevant articles by searching the PubMed website, and then uses the Rosenfeld-Shiffman filtering algorithm to select the relevant articles. The experiment of that approach shows that the recall is excellent, but the precision is very low (10,000 articles contain only 7 goal articles) [9].

In this paper, we propose a method that uses a semantic distance measure to automatically find relevant new evidence to support guideline updates. The advantage of using semantic distance is that the relevance measure can be achieved via the co-occurrence of terms in a biomedical article, which can be easily obtained via a biomedical search engine such as PubMed, instead of gathering a large corpus for the analysis. We have conducted several experiments in finding new relevant evidence for guideline updates.

The contributions of this paper are: i)we propose a semantic distance measure for ranking terms which have been used in PubMed, ii)we show how this

---

[2] http://www.ncbi.nlm.nih.gov/pubmed
[3] http://www.nlm.nih.gov/bsd/pmresources.html

semantic distance measure can be used for finding relevant evidence in PubMed for updating a guideline, iii)we present several strategies based on this semantic distance to direct the search for such new evidences, iv) we report on the experiments and evaluation of our method for finding new and relevant evidences.

This paper is organized as follows: Section 2 presents the basic structure of guidelines and the procedure of guideline update. Section 3 proposes an approach based on semantic distance measure over terms, and describes several strategies which uses the semantic distance measure for finding new and relevant evidences for guidelines. Section 4 discusses several experiments of our method on the update of guidelines. Section 5 discusses future work and make the conclusions.

2   Guidelines and Guideline Updates

Evidence-based medical guidelines are based on published scientific research findings. Those findings are usually found in medical publications such as those in PubMed. Selected articles are evaluated by an expert for their research quality, and are graded for the degree to which they contribute evidence using a classification system[8].

A classification of research results in level of evidence is proposed in [8,7] and consists of the following five classes: Type A1: Systematic reviews(i.e. research on the effects of diagnostics on clinical outcomes in a prospectively monitored, well-defined patient group), or that comprise at least several A2 quality trials whose results are consistent; Type A2: High-quality randomised comparative clinical trials (randomised, double-blind controlled trials) of sufficient size and consistency; Type B: Randomised clinical trials of moderate quality or insufficient size, or other comparative trials (non-randomised, comparative cohort study, patient control study); Type C: Non-comparative trials, and Type D: Opinions of experts.

Based on this classification of evidence, we can classify the conclusions in the guidelines (sometimes called *guideline items*) with an evidence level. The following evidence levels on guideline items, are proposed in [7]: Level 1: Based on 1 systematic review (type A1) or at least 2 independent A2 reviews; Level 2: Based on at least 2 independent type B reviews; Level 3: Based on 1 type A2 or B research, or any level of C research, and Level 4: Opinions of experts.

Here is an example of a conclusion in a guideline in [7]:

```
Classification: Level 1
Statement:      The diagnostic reliability of ultrasound with
                an uncomplicated cyst is very high.
Evidence:       A1 Kerlikowske 2003
                B Boerner 1999, Thurfjell 2002, Vargas 2004
```

which consists of a conclusion classification 'Level 1', a guideline statement, and its evidence items with one item classified as A1 and three items classified as B (jointly justifying the Level 1 of this conclusion).

In order to check if there is any new evidence from a scientific paper which is relevant to the guideline statement, a natural way to proceed is to use the terms which appear in the guideline statement (in the example above: terms such as 'diagnostic', 'reliability', 'ultrasound', and 'uncomplicated cyst') to create a query to search over a biomedical search engine such as PubMed. In the experiments of this paper, we use Xerox's NLP tool to identify the terms from UMLS and SNOMED CT which appear in guideline statements[1], and then use these terms to construct a PubMed query to search for relevant evidence. A naive approach to create such a PubMed query is to construct the conjunction or disjunction of those terms. In [9], the following facts have been observed: i)conjunctive queries often result in no results at all (67% of all conjunctive queries), ii)disjunctive queries often result in too many results (on average over 800,000 results per query). The main problem of these simple approaches is that the semantic relevance of the terms is not well considered. We will use a semantic distance measure to create search queries in which more relevant terms are preferred to less relevant terms. In other words, the semantic distance measure provides us with a method to rank the terms in the search query.

Algorithm 1.1 describes the workflow of our semantic distance method to find new evidence for medical guidelines.

Algorithm 1.1. Workflow

Select a guideline item;
Obtain the terms from the item's statement;
Select a term ranking strategy based on semantic distances;
Select a PubMed query construction strategy;
repeat
    Construct a PubMed query based on the combination of ranked terms;
    Obtain the result (i.e., a PMID list[4]) of the PubMed query;
    Evaluate the query result;
until The result is satisfying

3   Semantic Distance as a Relevance Measure

In Algorithm 1.1 above, ranking the terms is a crucial step in the procedure, because it tells us which term is more important than others. In this paper, we propose a method that uses semantic distance as a relevance measure. The advantage of using semantic distance is that the relevance measure can be calculated simply via the co-occurrence of terms in a search engine such as PubMed. The semantic distance measure is based on the assumption that the more frequently two terms co-occur in the same paper, the more semantically related they are. This assumption is inspired by the Normalized Google Distance from [2]. The equation for our Normalized PubMed Distance (NPD) is as follows:

$$NPD(x,y) = \frac{max\{\log f(x), \log f(y)\} - \log f(x,y)}{\log M - min\{\log f(x), \log f(y)\}}$$

Where $f(x)$ is the number of PubMed hits for the search term x; $f(y)$ is the number of PubMed hits for the search term y; $f(x,y)$ is the number of PubMed hits for the search terms x and y; M is the number of PMIDs indexed in PubMed (where M=23,000,000 at the time of writing). $NPD(x,y)$ can be understood intuitively as the symmetric conditional probability of co-occurrence of x and y.

Using the Normalized PubMed Distance (NPD) value to measure the importance of term. Let G be a set of guideline statements and $Terms$ be the set of all terms. The function $T : G \rightarrow Powerset(Terms)$ assigns a set of terms to each guideline statement such that $T(g)$ is the set of terms which appear in the guideline statement g. For each guideline statement $g \in G$ and a term x in g, we can define the average distance of term $x \in g$, written $AD(x,g)$, as the average distance of x to other terms in g as follows:

$$AD(x,g) = \frac{\sum_{y \in T(g), y \neq x} NPD(x,y)}{|T(g)| - 1}$$

We define the *center term* $CT(g)$ as the term whose average distance to other terms (in the guideline statement g) is minimal:

$$CT(g) = arg_x\ min(AD(x,g))$$

We can now consider the following different strategies to do term ranking:

- *Average Distance Ranking*(ADR): this strategy ranks the terms by their average distance value.
- *Central Distance Ranking*(CDR): this strategy ranks the terms by their distance to the center term, where the central distance of a term x in a guideline statement g, written $CD(x,g)$, is defined as:

$$CD(x,g) = NPD(x, CT(g))$$

After we get the ranked terms according to one of these (or possibly other) strategies, we send the terms as keywords to query the PubMed website to get the relevant articles for guideline updates. However, if we send all the ranked terms to query the PubMed website, the query is maximally specific, which will often cause no results. On the other hand, if we send only the most important term to query the PubMed website, the query is too broad, and often leading to too many relevant articles[9]. We therefore propose the following strategies to select only some terms in the search procedure [5]:

- *Increment strategy*: we start from the single highest ranked term t_1, then adding the next important terms one by one ($t_2, ...$), until we get the first result that is of sufficient quality.
- *Decrement strategy*: we start from the conjunction of all ranked terms $[t_1, ..., t_n]$, then remove the least important terms one by one (first t_n, then t_{n-1}, etc), until we get the first result that is of sufficient quality.
- *Thorough strategy*: we consider all term combinations following the linear order composed by the term ranking (i.e. $[t_1]$, $[t_1, t_2]$, $[t_1, t_2, t_3]$, etc), and we select the best result among all of them.

---

[5] In the below, all t_i are terms, with t_1 the top-ranked term, and each t_i ranked higher than t_{i+1}.

Clearly, the thorough strategy is the most expensive, because it will always consider all queries n possible queries $[t_1, ..., t_k]$ of $k = 1, ..n$, but our experiments will show that this thorough strategy is still efficient enough to be feasible.

In order to check whether or not a result is satisfying, we need an evaluation function to measure how good the results are. We consider the following criteria for this evaluation.

- *Term Coverage Criterion*: the more terms from a guideline statement are used for the PubMed query, the more relevant the results are;
- *Evidence Coverage Criterion*: the more of the original evidence have been covered in the search, the more relevant the results are. This is based on the assumption that good search terms will not only uncover new (recent) evidence, but will also yield the evidence that was underlying the current version of the guideline. This assumption would break down for very radical revisions of the guideline, instead of more incremental updates, such as the ones we are targeting.
- *Bounded Number Criterion*: it is not effective to have too many results (for example, more than 10,000 papers). Furthermore, we are likely to miss a lot of evidence if there are too few results (for example, less than 10 papers). Thus, we set an upper bound and lower bound on the results. The former is called *the upper bounded number* P_u, whereas the latter is called *the lower bounded number* P_l.

Based on the three assumptions above, we design a heuristic function $h(i)$ to evaluate the search results at each step in the workflow processing above. The heuristic function $h(i)$ can be defined based on the three criteria above as follows:

$$h(i) = k_1 T(i)/T + k_2 E(i)/E + k_3 (P_u - P(i))/P_u$$

where T is the total number of terms in the guideline statement; $T(i)$ is the number of selected terms in this search i; E is the total number of the evidence items for the guideline statement; $E(i)$ is the number of the original evidence items which has been covered in this search i; P_u is the upper bounded number; $P(i)$ is the number of PMID's that result from this search i, if $P(i)$ is a number between P_u and P_l, and k_1, k_2, k_3 are the weights of the different criteria. It is easy to see that the first part of the heuristic function (e.g.,$k_1 T(i)/T$) measures the Term Coverage Criterion, the second part of the function (e.g., $k_2 E(i)/E$) measures the Evidence Coverage Criterion, whereas the third part of the function (e.g., $k_3 (P_u - P(i))/P_u$) measures the Bounded Number Criterion with the meaning that the fewer results are returned, the more preferred they are (if the result size is between P_u and P_l). We propose the following constraints on the heuristic function $h(i)$:

- Normalized: $k_1 + k_2 + k_3 = 1$, implying that the value of $h(i)$ will be between 0 and 1;
- Bounded: $k_3 = 0$ if $P(i) > P_u$ or $P(i) < P_l$, stating that result sizes which are larger than P_u or smaller than P_l are not preferred;
- Default: $k_1, k_2, k_3 = 1/3$, i.e. we can consider the three assumptions equally important by default.

 – Non-trivial: $k_1 = 0$ if $P(i) = 0$. Namely we are not concerned with results for which the number of found evidence items is zero.

Note that in the constraints above we set the weight k_3 for the third criterion to zero if the number of found evidence items $P(i)$ is smaller than the lower bounded number P_l. However, the value of the heuristic function may not be zero. Thus, the heuristic function still accepts those results for which the size of the found evidences is smaller than the lower bounded number. A similar argument holds for the case of the upper bounded number P_u. We consider the size constraints as a weak boundary condition. Of course, we can also introduce a strong condition in which we would not accept any result with a number of evidence items. The following constraint introduces such a strong bound:

 – Strongly Bounded: $k_1, k_2, k_3 = 0$ if $P(i) > P_u$ or $P(i) < P_l$.

4   Experiment and Results

We have conducted several experiments for finding new relevant evidence for a guideline update. For these experiments, we selected the Dutch Breast Cancer Guideline, with version 1.0 of 2004 and version 2.0 of 2012 as the test data. The 2004 version of this guideline covers only partially the content of the 2012 version. For our experiments we have therefore selected 16 conclusions which appear in both versions of the guidelines. The conclusions of both guidelines have been converted into RDF NTriple data, and loaded into SemanticCT, a semantically-enabled system for clinical trials[5]. SemanticCT is powered by LarKC, a semantic platform for scalable semantic data processing and reasoning[4]. We use the Xerox's NLP tools to detect the terms of UMLS and SNOMED CT which appear in guideline statements. We found that in the Dutch breast cancer guidelines, the average number of the terms in each guideline statement is 6(min=3, max=12). Thus, the computation of all the semantic distances among those small sizes of terms (which is quadratic in the number of terms) is not prohibitively expensive: even for 12 statements, these amounts to only 12*11=132 PubMed queries. Our first experiment is using Central Distance Ranking with the default weights for the three criteria (i.e, $k_1 = k_2 = k_3 = 1/3$), $P_u = 1000$ and $P_l = 25$. Among the 16 guideline items, the system can find goal evidence items for five of them ('goal evidence items' are evidence items do indeed appear in the 2012 updated version of the guideline). For some conclusion statements (for example 04_3_2), our method can find all of the goal evidence items. It is also nice to see that the number of suggested new evidence candidates is not too large (max=327) and not too low (min=9), with an average of 87. On the other hand, for many of the guideline conclusions, the system does not find any of the goal evidence items. The results of the searches with the Central Distance Ranking ($Pu = 1000$ and $Pl = 25$), and always using the thorough search strategy, are shown in Table 1.

   Our second experiment is similar to the first, but now uses the Average Distance Ranking instead. Among the 16 guideline items, the system can now find its goal evidence items for four guideline conclusions. Similarly, for some guideline conclusions(04_3_2) all of the goal evidence items have been found. It is also

Table 1. Found New Evidences with Central Distance Ranking(Experiment 1) and with Average Distance Ranking (Experiment 2) ($Pu = 1000$ and $Pl = 25$). FGE=Found Goal Evidence.

Guideline Item (2004)	Evidence Number (2004)	Evidence Number (2012)	Experiment 1			Experiment 2		
			Found New Evidence	FGE (2012)	FGE Percentage	Found New Evidence	FGE (2012)	FGE Percentage
04_1_1	4	5	69	1	20%	69	1	20%
04_1_2	2	2	60	1	50%	189	1	50%
04_1_3	2	4	327	3	75%	70	0	0%
04_3_1	12	4	89	0	0%	80	0	0%
04_3_2	2	2	62	2	100%	62	2	100%
04_3_3	1	2	27	0	0%	27	0	0%
04_3_5	2	2	39	0	0%	41	0	0%
04_3_6	3	8	159	3	37.5%	26	0	0%
04_3_7	4	2	52	0	0%	34	0	0%
04_4_1	6	5	219	0	0%	219	0	0%
04_4_2	6	5	42	0	0%	0	0	0%
04_5_1	3	3	77	0	0%	74	0	0%
04_6_1	3	5	62	0	0%	135	0	0%
04_6_2	2	3	89	0	0%	89	0	0%
04_7_1	2	2	9	0	0%	9	0	0%
04_8_1	2	2	15	0	0%	15	0	0%

nice to see that the number of suggested new evidence candidates is again not too large (max =219) and not too low (min=9), with an average of 77. The results of the searches with the Average Distance Ranking ($P_u = 1000$ and $P_l = 25$) are shown in Table 1.

From these two experiments, we can see that Central Distance Ranking strategy can find goal evidence items for more guideline conclusions. However, the system can find such goal evidence items for only five guideline items, although the number of suggested evidence candidates are reasonably good (e.g., on average 87). In order to increase the number of found goal evidence items, we can allow for larger sizes of search results. That can be achieved by a bigger weight of the evidence coverage criterion, i.e. k_2. Thus, our third experiment is using Central Distance Ranking with the weights $k_1 = 0.25, k_2 = 0.50, k_3 = 0.25$, and with upper and lower bound numbers unchanged at $P_u = 1000$ and $P_l = 25$. Among the 16 guideline items, our method can now find goal evidence items for 10 guideline items (up from 5). In other words, at least some goal evidence items can be found for 62.5% of guideline conclusions, and all goal evidence items are found for 25% of guideline conclusions. However, the total number of suggested new evidence candidates are larger than those in the previous two experiments (average=2824, max =19130, and min=9), and are perhaps too large. The results of this third experiment (CDR, $k_1 = 0.25, k_2 = 0.50, k_3 = 0.25, P_u = 1000$, $P_l = 25$) are shown in Table 2. Table 2 shows that for 10 out of 16 conclusions we can find some goal evidence items, and for 4 out of 16 conclusions we can find all of the goal evidence items; however, for 6 out of 16 conclusions we find 0 evidence and for 5 out of 10 we just find some of the goal evidence items. One of

Table 2. Experiment 3: Found New Evidences with Central Distance Ranking($k_1 = 0.25$, $k_2 = 0.5$, $k_3 = 0.25$, $P_u = 1000$, and $P_l = 25$)

GuidelineItemID (2004)	Evidence Number (2004)	Evidence Number (2012)	Found New Evidence	Found Goal Evidence (2012)	Found Goal Evidence Percentage
04_1_1	4	5	69	1	20%
04_1_2	2	2	60	1	50%
04_1_3	2	4	327	3	75%
04_3_1	12	4	89	0	0%
04_3_2	2	2	62	2	100%
04_3_3	1	2	27	0	0%
04_3_5	2	2	10654	2	100%
04_3_6	3	8	159	3	37.5%
04_3_7	4	2	10657	2	100%
04_4_1	6	5	2495	5	100%
04_4_2	6	5	1300	3	60%
04_5_1	3	3	19130	3	100%
04_6_1	3	5	62	0	0%
04_6_2	2	3	89	0	0%
04_7_1	2	2	9	0	0%
04_8_1	2	2	15	0	0%

the reasons for this low recall is that the number of suggested new evidence candidates is bounded. Another reason is different terminology is used in the guideline conclusions and in the evidence items (e.g. 'carcinoma' vs. 'cancer'). In future work, we will use medical ontologies to deal with the semantic relations among such terms. Finally, we have observed that the task can be done with a reasonably good performance: the minimal time cost is 2.15 minutes, the maximal time cost is 30.6 minutes, and the average time cost is 10.9 minutes per guideline statement in Experiment 3.

5   Conclusion and Future Work

The experiments above show that semantic distances can be used to find new relevant evidence for updating guideline conclusions. Even when these experiments were only initial variations with different ranking strategies and different weighted criteria, we could find at least some of the goal evidence items from the literature for 62.5% of the updated guideline conclusions.

From these experiments, we also see that the numbers of found goal evidence items would be increased if we increase the weight of the evidence coverage criterion (k_2) or if we increase the upper bound number of the search (P_u). However, both methods would lead to a large amount of suggested evidence candidates. That would imply time consuming work for a guideline designer to know which evidence candidates are really useful for the guideline update. Therefore, one of the future challenges is to reduce the large size of suggested evidence candidates and thereby improve the precision of the search results.

In the near future we will investigate the following methods for reducing the number of irrelevant (or less relevant) evidence candidates:

- Contextualised search. We can add some terms from the context to the search (for example, terms from the the title of the guideline section and subsection). It is quite clear that adding more terms in the search would reduce the sizes of suggested evidence items significantly.
- Search within a time period. Usually we are not interested in evidence items which have been published a long time ago, and we are more interested in recent evidence. Thus, adding the period limit (for example, search only for those papers that appeared in the last 10 years (2005-2015), or only papers which appeared since the last guideline update, would reduce the sizes of found evidences significantly as well.
- Search with higher levels of evidence. Usually we are not interested in those evidence candidates which have weaker evidence class.

Acknowledgments. This work is partially supported by the European Commission under the 7th framework programme EURECA Project.

References

1. Ait-Mokhtar, S., Bruijn, B.D., Hagege, C., Rupi, P.: Initial prototype for relation identification between concepts, D3.2. Technical report, EURECA Project (2013)
2. Cilibrasi, R., Vitanyi, P.M.B.: The google similarity distance. IEEE Trans. Knowledge and Data Engineering 19, 370–383 (2007)
3. Johnston, M.E., et al.: Keeping cancer guidelines current: results of a comprehensive prospective literature monitoring strategy for twenty clinical practice guidelines. International Journal of Technololgy Assessment in Health Care 19, 646–655 (2003)
4. Fensel, D., et al.: Towards LarKC: a platform for web-scale reasoning. In: Proceedings of the IEEE International Conference on Semantic Computing (ICSC 2008), IEEE Computer Society Press, CA (2008)
5. Huang, Z., ten Teije, A., van Harmelen, F.: SemanticCT: A semantically enabled clinical trial system. In: Singh, S., Murshed, N., Kropatsch, W.G. (eds.) ICAPR 2001. LNCS (LNAI), vol. 2013, pp. 11–25. Springer, Heidelberg (2001)
6. Iruetaguena, A., et al.: Automatic retrieval of current evidence to support update of bibliography in clinical guidelines. Expert Sys. with Apps. 40, 2081–2091 (2013)
7. NABON. Breast cancer, dutch guideline, version 2.0. Technical report, Integraal kankercentrum Netherland, Nationaal Borstkanker Overleg Nederland (2012)
8. NSRS. Guideline complex regional pain syndrome type i. Technical report, Netherlands Society of Rehabilitation Specialists (2006)
9. Reinders, R., ten Teije, A., Huang, Z.: Finding evidence for updates in medical guideline. In: Proceedings of HEALTHINF 2015, Lisbon (2014)
10. Shekelle, P.G., Woolf, S.H., Eccles, M., Grimshaw, J.: Developing guidelines. BMJ: British Medical Journal 318(7182), 593–596 (1999)
11. Shojania, K., Sampson, M., Ansari, M., Ji, J., Doucette, S., Moher, D.: How quickly do systematic reviews go out of date? a survival analysis. Annals of Internal Medicine 147, 224–233 (2007)

Analyzing Recommendations Interactions in Clinical Guidelines

Impact of Action Type Hierarchies and Causation Beliefs

Veruska Zamborlini[1,2(✉)], Marcos da Silveira[2], Cedric Pruski[2],
Annette ten Teije[1], and Frank van Harmelen[1]

[1] Department of Computer Science, VU University Amsterdam,
Amsterdam, The Netherlands
{v.carrettazamborlini,a.c.m.ten.teije,f.a.h.van.harmelen}@vu.nl
[2] Luxembourg Institute of Science and Technology - LIST, Luxembourg,
Luxembourg, Europe
{marcos.dasilveira,cedric.pruski}@list.lu

Abstract. Accounting for patients with multiple health conditions is a complex task that requires analysing potential interactions among recommendations meant to address each condition. Although some approaches have been proposed to address this issue, important features still require more investigation, such as (re)usability and scalability. To this end, this paper presents an approach that relies on reusable rules for detecting interactions among recommendations coming from various guidelines. It extends previously proposed models by introducing the notions of action type hierarchy and causation beliefs, and provides a systematic analysis of relevant interactions in the context of multimorbidity. Finally, the approach is assessed based on a case-study taken from the literature to highlight the added value of the approach.

Keywords: Clinical knowledge representation · Combining medical guidelines · Multimorbidity

1 Introduction

Accounting for patients with multiple health conditions is an important and complex task that requires analysing potential interactions among recommendations meant to address each condition. The need for supporting multimorbidity has called attention in the medical community [1]. A family of approaches [2,3,4,5,6] has emerged aiming to enhance the reasoning capabilities of computer systems to combine several clinical guidelines addressing multimorbidity. However, there are still important features that require more investigation, among which are (i) rules (re)usability - having generic rules to detect recommendation interactions, independent of specific conflicts or guidelines, and applicable in a (semi)automatic way; (ii) scalability - allowing the combination of "any" number

V. Zamborlini—Funded by CNPq (Brazilian National Council for Scientific and Technological Development) within the Science without Borders programme.

© Springer International Publishing Switzerland 2015
J.H. Holmes et al. (Eds.): AIME 2015, LNAI 9105, pp. 317–326, 2015.
DOI: 10.1007/978-3-319-19551-3_40

of CIGs (Computer Interpretable Guidelines), i.e. detecting interactions among any number of recommendations; (iii) knowledge reusability - allowing the reuse of existing clinical knowledge as well as providing reusable knowledge.

We started addressing the aforementioned features in our previous work [6,7,8]. While [6] focuses on providing a conceptual model covering core concepts underlying clinical recommendations, namely TMR (Transition-based Medical Recommendation), [7,8] focuses on extending it for detecting of Interactions (TMR4I) by providing reusable FOL (First Order Logic) rules to identify different types of recommendation interactions when guidelines need to be merged in a multimorbidity scenario. In addition, the aforementioned models are implemented using Semantic Web technologies and reusing available clinical knowledge sources. Although good results were obtained by applying the models to case studies taken from the literature, further research is required to apply them in more complex scenarios. The contribution is an analysis of the impact of introducing the notions of care action type hierarchies and causation beliefs when detecting interactions among the recommendations, from which formal rules are derived to enable automated detection. These notions improve the representation originally proposed for *Care Action* and *Transition Types*, favoring flexibility and re-usability of the model elements. Finally, an experimental assessment of the models is provided through a case study borrowed from the literature [2].

The remainder of this paper is structured as follows: Section 2 introduces the concepts used in this article. Section 3 presents the model and its components. Section 4 deals with our case study. Section 5 discusses our approach and future work while Section 6 presents conclusions.

2   Medical Recommendations and Interactions

This section presents some concepts and relations underlying clinical recommendations. They are further incorporated into the TMR models (c.f. Sect. 3). For instance, consider the following recommendation: "*Administering aspirin is recommended to decrease the body temperature; in addition it does not cause nauseas and it reduces blood coagulation*". In our approach it is addressed as a positive **recommendation** about the execution of the **care action type** *administer aspirin*, justified by the positive **causation belief** on the promotion of the **transition type** *decreasing the body temperature*[1]. Moreover, in the same recommendation two other beliefs are indicated: one negative belief *it does not cause nausea* and one positive belief *it reduces blood coagulation*. Those are addressed as "secondary" beliefs or **side-beliefs** associated to **sub-recommendations**, which are part of the main one.

By empirically analysing guidelines, we observed that different guidelines can have the same beliefs associated to main recommendation or sub-recommendation. For instance, *Aspirin reduces the blood coagulation* appears as main effect in

---

[1] The need for distinguishing action and action types is discussed in [6]. However, for sake of simplicity, hereafter we refer to both *care action types* and *transition types* as simply *care action* and *transition/effect*.

Diabetes Guideline, but as side-effect in the Osteoarthritis Guideline (see Sect. 4). We consider the "common-sense term" **side-effect** as being the positive (causation) side-belief. Negative causation beliefs in particular were only observed associated to sub-recommendations. For instance, the following recommendation is extracted (adapted) from the dutch Breast Cancer Guideline[2]: "*Breast reconstruction is recommended for improving the breast aesthetics and (additionally) it will NOT increase the risk of cancer recurrence*". The negative side-belief *does not increase the risk of cancer recurrence* is associated to the action *Breast Reconstruction* as a sub-recommendation in the context of the main one.

Moreover, care action types can be organised in **hierarchies** according to a "grouping criterion". For example, *pharmacotherapy* is an action type that groups (or subsumes) action types in which *pharmacological drugs* are administered, for instance, *administer NSAID*. The later in turn subsumes action types regarding the administration of *non-steroidal drugs* that have the *anti-inflammatory* effect, for instance, *administer Aspirin and Ibuprofen*. In this work, we are interested in the criteria related to promoted effects. For example, the *anti-inflammatory* effect associated to *administer NSAID* is also expected for its subsumed action types, e.g. *administer Aspirin and Ibuprofen*.

Different combinations of recommendations, beliefs, actions and transitions may give rise to a number of issues. A systematic approach is adopted to analyse **interactions** among recommendations. Tables 1 to 3 contain the part of this analysis that was considered relevant for the multimorbidity use-case, divided into three parts: (i) interactions involving beliefs, (ii) interactions among main recommendations and (iii) interactions involving sub-recommendations. Three main types of interactions, introduced in [7], are considered: **contradiction**, **repetition** (of action) and **alternative**. In addition, new ones are defined: **opposed beliefs** and **repeated side-effects**. The latter regards different actions promoting the same side-effect, i.e. if they are both prescribed, the repeated side-effects are potentially harmful. A color-code is adopted as an additional resource for distinguishing the interaction types, which reappears in Fig. 2. The following definitions are adopted:

- T is a set of *transition types* defined in the healthcare domain and concerns the transformation of a certain situation (type) into another.
  - Two transitions $t_i, t_j \in T$ are *inverse* if they produce opposite effects, denoted as $inv(t_i, t_j)$.
  - Two transitions $t_i, t_j \in T$ are *unrelated* if they are neither the same nor inverse, denoted as $t_i \not\cong t_j$.
- A is a set of *care action types* defined in the healthcare domain, which can be performed by healthcare agents with the aim of promoting a transition.
  - An action type a_i subsuming another action type a_j is a transitive relation denoted as $a_i > a_j$, where $a_i, a_j \in A$.
  - Two actions $a_i, a_j \in A$ are *unrelated* if they are neither the same nor subsuming one another, denoted as $a_i \not\cong a_j$.

---

[2] http://www.oncoline.nl/uploaded/docs/mammacarcinoom/Dutch%20Breast%20Cancer%20Guideline%202012.eps

- B^s is a set of *causation beliefs* about actions $a_i \in A$ promoting transitions $t_j \in T$ according to a source S. The source can be the clinical literature (clinical studies or guidelines) or clinical KBs. In other words, it maps pairs (action,transition) to belief values such that $B^s : A \times T \rightarrow \{positive, negative\}$. We adopt $b^s_{a_i,t_j} = positive$ as short notation for a certain $b_k \in B^s$.
- G is a set of CIGs, each of which is composed of clinical *recommendations*, while R is a set of recommendations extracted from CIGs.
  - Main recommendations composing a CIG are denoted as $r_n \lhd g_i$, where $g_i \in G$ and $r_n \in R^i \subset R$.
  - Sub-recommendations composing a main recommendation are denoted as $sr_m \lhd r_n$, where $r_n \in R$ and $sr_m \in R^n \subset R$.
  - Main recommendations are valued as positive (or negative) based on causation beliefs that justify recommending (or not) an action $a_i \in A$ in order to achieve (or avoid) a transition $t_j \in T$. It is denoted as $r_n \bullet b^S_{a_i,t_j} = \{positive, negative\}$, where $r_n \in R, b_{a_i,t_j} \in B^S$.
  - Sub-recommendations are associated to side-beliefs to indicate that the same action (a_i) can also promote (or not) other secondary transitions (t_k). It is denoted as $sr_m \circ b_{a_i,t_k}$, where $sr_m \in R, b_{a_i,t_k} \in B^S$. In this work we consider them as not relevant to influence the recommendation valuation as positive or negative.

To illustrate the analysis, we select the recommendation *Do administer aspirin to decrease the body temperature* and vary its components[3]. We first analyze the **interactions involving causation beliefs**, i.e. we verify if there is any incompatibility regarding the causation beliefs on which recommendations are based. Since clinical knowledge is not necessarily a general consensus, it is reasonable to consider that different guideline authors rely on different literature sources that can be contradictory about causality beliefs regarding a care action. For instance, opposed beliefs on the effects of G. biloba and CYP450 isoenzymes are highlighted by [9]. Table 1 presents an analysis considering two beliefs, fixing a positive one (b_{a_1,t_1}) as "(a_1) *administer aspirin does* (t_1) *decrease the body temperature*" and varying the other one (b_{a_2,t_2}). For example, in the first row, the other belief varies as either *Administer Aspirin* ($a_1 = a_2$) or *Administer NSAID* ($a_2 > a_1$) *increasing the body temperature*, which is the inverse effect stated by the first belief, thereby resulting in one opposing the other.

In the sequel we analyse **interactions among main recommendations**, i.e. we verify the possible interactions between positive and/or negative main recommendations. For each pair of main recommendations we analyse the relations between the care actions ($=, >, \not\cong$) against the relations between transitions ($=, inv, \not\cong$). For instance, consider two positive recommendations to unrelated actions (e.g. *Administer Aspirin* $\not\cong$ *Administer Ibuprofen*) that promote the same transition (*decrease the body temperature*). They are in an alternative interaction because one can be recommended in the place of the other to achieve the same

---

[3] It means that we also analyze "clinically irrelevant" sentences like *Do administer aspirin to increase the body temperature*.

Table 1. Interactions between recommendations based on a positive belief (b_{a_1,t_1} = positive), fixed as "(a_1) administer aspirin does (t_1) decrease the body temperature" and another belief (b_{a_2,t_2}) varying as described in the rows and columns.

	b_{a_2,t_2} = positive a_2 does (promote) t_2	
	$a_1 = a_2$ a_2: Administer Aspirin	$a_1 > a_2$ or $a_2 > a_1$ a_2: Administer NSAID
$inv(t_1, t_2)$ t_2: increase body temperature	√ Opposed beliefs	√ Opposed beliefs
	b_{a_2,t_2} = negative a_2 does not (promote) t_2	
$t_1 = t_2$ t_2: decrease body temperature	√ Opposed beliefs	√ Opposed beliefs

Table 2. Interactions between a positive main recommendation (b_{a_1,t_1} = positive), fixed as "do (a_1) adm. aspirin to (t_1) decrease the body temperature" and another main recommendation (r_2) varying as described in the rows and columns.

	$r_2 \bullet b_{a_2,t_2}$= positive Do a_2 to achieve t_2		
	$a_1 = a_2$ a_2: Adm. Aspirin	$a_1 > a_2$ or $a_2 > a_1$ a_2: Adm. NSAID	$a_1 \ncong a_2$ a_2: Adm. Ibuprofen
$t_1 = t_2$ t_2: decrease body temperature	√ Repetition	√ Repetition √ Alternative	√ Alternative
$inv(t_1, t_2)$ t_2: increase body temperature	√ Repetition √ Contradiction	√ Repetition √ Contradiction	√ Contradiction
$t_1 \ncong t_2$ t_2: heal inflammation	√ Repetition	√ Repetition	-
	$r_2 \bullet b_{a_2,t_2}$= negative Do not a_2 to avoid t_2		
$t_1 = t_2$ t_2: decrease body temperature	√ Contradiction	√ Contradiction	√ Contradiction
$inv(t_1, t_2)$ t_2: increase body temperature	√ Contradiction	√ Contradiction	√ Alternative
$t_1 \ncong t_2$ t_2: heal inflammation	√ Contradiction	√ Contradiction	-

transition. This and other cases are covered in Table 2. It presents the combination of two main recommendations: fixing a positive recommendation (r_1) while (i) varying another positive one (r_2) and then (ii) varying another negative one (r_2). The cells shaded gray regard the interactions originally addressed in our previous work [7].

We also analyse **interactions involving sub-recommendations**, i.e. we verify possible interactions between one sub-recommendation and another either positive, negative or sub-recommendations. For instance, considerthe recommendations *do (a_1) administer aspirin to heal the pain and additionally (t_1) decrease the body temperature* and *do not (a_2) administer ibuprofen to avoid (t_2)*

Table 3. Interactions between a sub-recommendation ($sr_1 \triangleleft r_1, sr_1 \circ b_{a_1,t_1}$), fixed as "*do ($a_1$) administer aspirin to heal the pain and additionally (t_1) decrease the body temperature*" and other recommendations varying as described in the rows and columns

	$r_2 \bullet b_{a_2,t_2} = $ **pos.** *Do administer Ibuprofen to t_2*	$r_2 \bullet b_{a_2,t_2} = $ **neg.** *Do not administer Ibuprofen to avoid t_2*	$sr_2 \triangleleft r_2, sr_2 \circ b_{a_2,t_2}$ *Do adm. Ibuprofen ... and, additionally, to t_2*
$t_1 = t_2$ *t_2: decrease body temperature*	√ **Alternative**	■ **Contradiction**	√ **Repeat. Side-Effects**
$inv(t_1, t_2)$ *t_2: increase body temperature*	■ **Contradiction**	√ **Alternative**	■ **Contradiction**

decreasing the body temperature. They are in a contradiction interaction, since the former would produce, as a side-effect, the undesired effect stated in the latter. This and other cases are presented in Table 3, where a sub-recommendation is fixed, while the other recommendations vary. We consider relations between transitions promoted by *unrelated* action types ($a_1 \not\cong a_2$), since the derivable interactions for related actions, as well as negative beliefs, are already addressed in the previous analysis.

Finally, some interaction types entail cumulative behaviour, which is an important aspect when combining two or more guidelines[7]. For example, recommending 4 times *Administer Aspirin* for different purposes should not be considered as 6 different interactions between each pair of recommendations, but one interaction among 4 recommendations, favouring the optimisation of recommendations or the avoidance of overdose. We consider that repetition and alternative interactions can accumulate when the same recommendation is related by interactions of the same type. In summary, *the additional interactions with respect to [7] are due to the introduction of action type hierarchies and causation beliefs*.

3   TMR Models and FOL Rules

The concepts and their relations discussed in section 2 are incorporated into the TMR models as presented in Fig. 1. The classes depicted in gray shading are the ones that remain unchanged with respect to our previous work. Only the main classes are represented in this diagram (more details in [7]).

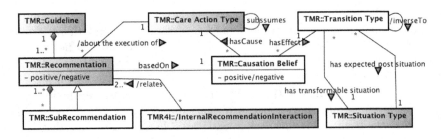

Fig. 1. UML class diagram for an excerpt of TMR and TMR4I Models

Table 4. FOL rules for detecting interactions

Contradiction	$\forall g, r1, r2, b1, b2, a1, a2, t1, t2($ Guideline(g) $\wedge$ r1 $\neq$ r2
$r_1 \bullet b_{a_1,t_1} = pos.$	$\wedge$ **PositiveRecommendation(r1)** $\wedge$ partOf(r1,g) $\wedge$ **basedOn(r1,b1)**
	$\wedge$ PositiveBelief(b1) $\wedge$ **hasCause(b1,a1)**
$r_2 \bullet b_{a_2,t_2} = neg.$	$\wedge$ **NegativeRecommendation(r2)** $\wedge$ partOf(r2,g) $\wedge$ **basedOn(r2,b2)**
	$\wedge$ PositiveBelief(b2) $\wedge$ **hasCause(b2,a2)**
$a_1 > a_2$	$\wedge$ CareActionType(a1) $\wedge$ CareActionType(a2) $\wedge$ **subsumes(a1, a2)**
	$\rightarrow \exists i($ **Contradiction(i)** $\wedge$ relates(i,r1) $\wedge$ relates(i,r2) $)$
Alternative	$\forall g, r1, r2, sr1, b1, b2, t1, t2($ Guideline(g) $\wedge$ r1 $\neq$ r2
	$\wedge$ Recommendation(r1) $\wedge$ partOf(r1,g)
$sr_1 \lhd r_1$	$\wedge$ **SubRecommendation(sr1)** $\wedge$ **partOf(sr1,r1)**
$sr_1 \circ b_{a_1,t_1}$	$\wedge$ PositiveBelief(b1) $\wedge$ **basedOn(sr1,b1)** $\wedge$ **hasEffect(b1,t1)**
$r_2 \bullet b_{a_2,t_2} = pos.$	$\wedge$ **PositiveRecommendation(r2)** $\wedge$ partOf(r2,g) $\wedge$ **basedOn(r2,b2)**
	$\wedge$ PositiveBelief(b2) $\wedge$ **hasEffect(b2,t2)**
$t_1 = t_2$	$\wedge$ Transition(t1) $\wedge$ Transition(t2) $\wedge$ **t1 = t2** $)$
	$\rightarrow \exists i($ **Alternative(i)** $\wedge$ relates(i,r1) $\wedge$ relates(i,sr2) $)$
Alternative	$\forall i1, i2, r1, r2, r3($ **Alternative(i1)** $\wedge$ **Alternative(i2)**
Cumulative rule	$\wedge$ relates(i1,r1) $\wedge$ relates(i1,r2) $\wedge$ relates(i2,r2) $\wedge$ relates(i2,r3) $\wedge$ r1 $\neq$ r3
	$\rightarrow$ **i1 = i2**

FOL Rules for detecting the interactions are defined according to the TMR models, derived from the analysis outlined in Tables 1 to 3. Table 4 presents three rules illustrating the formalisation derived from the analysis. The first column reuses the notation provided in Sect. 2 for reference and the second column contains the formulas, highlighting the clauses that refer to the mentioned notation. The first rule corresponds to the contradiction interaction defined in Table 2, column 2 (T2C2), i.e., the whole column is comprised in one rule, since it holds true regardless of the relations among the transitions. The second rule corresponds to the alternative interaction in table 3, line 1, column 1 (T3L1C1), while the third rule represents the cumulative behaviour for alternative interactions.

4   Multimorbidity Case Study

The approach is evaluated using a case study on combining three CIGs, Osteoarthritis (OA), Diabetes (DB) and Hypertension (HT), defined in [2]. We previously addressed it in [7] and compared it to the original experiment. In this section, the results are compared against our previous experiment.

Figure 2 illustrates the aforementioned case study according to the TMR models. The dotted box in the middle represents the merged-CIG for OA+HT+DB containing the recommendations inside (e.g. *avoid thrombi*). The rectangles surrounding the CIG represent the beliefs that transitions regarding a property are promoted by executing a care action type (e.g. *blood coagulation* does change from *normal to low* by *administering aspirin*). The care action type is represented in a dotted ellipse inside the believed transition. A positive (or negative) recommendation is indicated by a thick arrow labelled with "do" (or "do not"). The sub-recommendations are placed inside the main ones and connected to the respective belief by unlabelled thick arrows. Interactions are depicted by labelled thin arrows (**repetition**, **contradiction** and **alternative**) connecting the interacting recommendations.

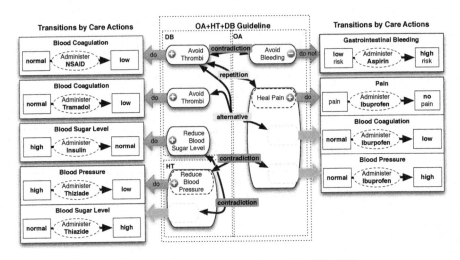

Fig. 2. Case Study for combining OA+HT+DB

In the left side of Fig. 2, three recommendations are taken from the DB CIG, for instance *Avoid Thrombi: Do administer NSAID (or Tramadol) to reduce the blood coagulation.* From the HT CIG just one main recommendation is considered *Reduce BP: Do administer thiziade to decrease the blood pressure,* which in turn has one side-effect to be taken into account: *it increases the blood sugar level.* In the right side, the negative recommendation from the OA CIG is *Avoid Bleeding: Do not administer aspirin to avoid increasing the risk of gastrointestinal bleeding.* The two recommendations in the top, briefly "*Do Administer NSAID*" and "*Do not Administer Aspirin*", have a contradiction interaction according to T2L6C2 in section 2. The other interactions and corresponding cells are: one repetition (T2L3C2), one alternative interaction (2x T2L1C3 + T3L1C1 accumulated) and two contradictions (2x T3L2C1).

Therefore, the previous experiment [7] is improved on the detection of inter-actions that hold due to subsumed action types, besides the ones involving sub-recommendations. For instance, the two side-effects involved in contradiction, namely *Increasing the blood sugar level* and *Increasing the blood pressure,* were represented as negative recommendations instead. However, it was not possible to detect the alternative interaction between *Administer Ibuprofen* and *Admin-ister Tramadol* due to the side-effect *decreasing blood coagulation,* since it would require having a positive recommendation to a side-effect, which makes no sense. In summary, the new approach allows for a more faithful representation of the recommendations and extends the ability to detect recommendation interactions.

5   Discussion

By extending the TMR models and rules with care action type hierarchy and cau-sation beliefs, a more **reusable** and **scalable** approach is provided for detecting recommendation interactions in the context of multimorbidity. The evaluation illustrates its applicability and the improvements achieved with respect to our previous experiment [7].

The FOL rules for detecting interactions, which can be derived from the analysis are **reusable**, i.e. independent of specific conflicts/interactions or guidelines. In other words, the very same rule can be applied to different CIGs and detect similar interactions, e.g. *do and do not perform a certain action*. In turn, related work would require two specific rules to define, for instance, *"give and do not give aspirin"* and *"give and do not give ibuprofen"* as interactions. Particularly, Wilk et al. [4] also provide FOL rules, although specific rules are still required for each possible conflict (they are not universally quantified). Piovesan et al. [5] also proposed guideline-independent algorithms based on an ontology to detect interactions, restricted to types "concordance" and "discordance". The use of intentions associated to actions for detecting "intention interactions" is close to what we do on verifying the transitions related to recommendations, although their approach is restricted to positive recommendations justified by positive causation beliefs. They also address action type hierarchy for detecting interactions, but restricted to drug administration. To the best of our knowledge, other related work does not address those issues in a broader sense. Finally, our approach is **scalable** in number of combined CIGs, since the rules, besides being reusable accross different CIGs, address the cumulative behavior of interactions (originally introduced and discussed in depth in [7]).

The formal account provided to the TMR models and rules allows an **implementation** relying on Semantic Web technologies, **reusing** existing biomedical linked open data (LOD), as we have done in previous work [8]. The TMR-based data were linked to Drugbank[4], complementing the knowledge originally provided within CIGs in order to detect external interactions, such as drug-drug interactions and alternative drugs. In future work, our current prototype [5] will be extended to benefit from other biomedical LOD, to detect external interactions, such as side-effects defined in Sider[6]. We advocate that providing means to reuse extensive biomedical background knowledge is an important ingredient for enhancing the ability to detect problems and alternatives that were not explicitly mentioned in CIGs, including very up-to-date information. To the best of our knowledge, related work does not address this feature in depth.

Finally, we also intend to investigate other use-cases beside multimorbidity together with relevant aspects that would influence them, namely temporal and qualitative aspects. We will particularly investigate whether the approach presented in [10] regarding temporal aspects is complementary to ours.

6   Conclusion

We introduce the notions of care action type hierarchy and causation beliefs to the TMR model, and provide a systematic analysis of recommendation

---

[4] http://www.drugbank.ca

[5] http://guidelines.hoekstra.ops.few.vu.nl

[6] http://sideeffects.embl.de

interactions that are relevant in the context of multimorbidity, while pursuing (re)usability and scalability. Our approach is evaluated in a realistic case-study on combining 3 CIGs. As future work we will implement the proposed models, and we will analyse the applicability of our approach to other use-cases (such as update or adaptation). We also plan to evaluate our approach in more complex scenarios with the support of a prototype.

References

1. Shekelle, P., Woolf, S., Grimshaw, J.M., Schünemann, H.J., Eccles, M.P.: Developing clinical practice guidelines: reviewing, reporting, and publishing guidelines; updating guidelines; and the emerging issues of enhancing guideline implementability and accounting for comorbid conditions in guideline development. Implementation Science: IS 7(1), 62 (2012)
2. Jafarpour, B.: Ontology Merging using Semantically-defined Merge Criteria and OWL Reasoning Services: Towards Execution-time Merging of Multiple Clinical Workflows to Handle Comorbidity. PhD thesis, Dalhousie University (2013)
3. López-Vallverdú, J.A., Riaño, D., Collado, A.: Rule-based combination of comorbid treatments for chronic diseases applied to hypertension, diabetes mellitus and heart failure. In: Lenz, R., Miksch, S., Peleg, M., Reichert, M., Riaño, D., ten Teije, A. (eds.) ProHealth 2012 and KR4HC 2012. LNCS (LNAI), vol. 7738, pp. 30–41. Springer, Heidelberg (2013)
4. Wilk, S., Michalowski, M., Tan, X., Michalowski, W.: Using First-Order Logic to Represent Clinical Practice Guidelines and to Mitigate Adverse Interactions. In: Miksch, S., Riano, D., ten Teije, A. (eds.) KR4HC 2014. LNCS, vol. 8903, pp. 45–61. Springer, Heidelberg (2014)
5. Piovesan, L., Molino, G., Terenziani, P.: An ontological knowledge and multiple abstraction level decision support system in healthcare. Decision Analytics 1(1), 8 (2014)
6. Zamborlini, V., da Silveira, M., Pruski, C., ten Teije, A., van Harmelen, F.: Towards a conceptual model for enhancing reasoning about clinical guidelines: A case-study on comorbidity. In: Miksch, S., Riano, D., ten Teije, A. (eds.) KR4HC 2014. LNCS, vol. 8903, pp. 29–44. Springer, Heidelberg (2014)
7. Zamborlini, V., Hoekstra, R., da Silveira, M., Pruski, C., ten Teije, A., van Harmelen, F.: A Conceptual Model for Detecting Interactions among Medical Recommendations in Clinical Guidelines. In: Janowicz, K., Schlobach, S., Lambrix, P., Hyvönen, E. (eds.) EKAW 2014. LNCS, vol. 8876, pp. 591–606. Springer, Heidelberg (2014)
8. Zamborlini, V., Hoekstra, R., da Silveira, M., Pruski, C., ten Teije, A., van Harmelen, F.: Inferring Recommendation Interactions in Clinical Guidelines: Case-studies on Multimorbidity. Semantic Web Journal (2015 - Invited submission as extension of [7], Under Revision, Open Acess, http://www.semantic-web-journal.net/content/inferring-recommendation-interactions-clinical-guidelines-case-studies-multimorbidity
9. Chavez, M.L., Jordan, M.A., Chavez, P.I.: Evidence-based drug–herbal interactions. Life Sciences 78(18), 2146–2157 (2006)
10. Piovesan, L., Anselma, L., Terenziani, P.: Temporal Detection of Guideline Interactions. In: Int. Conf. on Health Informatics (HEALTHINF), Lisbon (2015)

A General Approach to Represent and Query Now-Relative Medical Data in Relational Databases

Luca Anselma[1], Luca Piovesan[1(✉)], Abdul Sattar[2], Bela Stantic[2],
and Paolo Terenziani[3]

[1] Department of Computer Science, University of Turin, Italy
{anselma,piovesan}@di.unito.it
[2] Institute for Integrated and Intelligent Systems, Griffith University,
Queensland, Australia
{a.sattar,b.stantic}@griffith.edu.au
[3] DISIT, Institute of Computer Science, Università del Piemonte Orientale,
Alessandria, Italy
paolo.terenziani@unipmn.it

Abstract. Now-related temporal data play an important role in the medical context. Current relational temporal database (TDB) approaches are limited since (i) they (implicitly) assume that the span of time occurring between the time when facts change in the world and the time when the changes are recorded in the database is exactly known, and (ii) do not explicitly provide an extended relational algebra to query now-related data. We propose an approach that, widely adopting AI symbolic manipulation techniques, overcomes the above limitations.

Keywords: Temporal relational databases · Now-related data · Temporal algebra

1 Introduction

Most clinical data are naturally temporal. To be meaningfully interpreted, patients' symptoms, laboratory test results and, in general, all clinical data must be paired with the time in which they hold (called *valid time* henceforth). The research about temporal data has demonstrated that designing, querying and modifying time-varying *relational* tables requires a new set of techniques [1]. In the medical area, several TDB approaches have been devised. For instance, Chronus II [2] has provided an implementation of a subset of the "consensus" approach TSQL2 [3] (which is the basis of the recent SQL:2011 standard), and Das and Musen have focused on temporal indeterminacy [4]. In the recent years, we have extended such a basic core of results to face with the telic/atelic distinction [5], periodically repeated data [6], and proposal vetting [7], proposing the adoption of AI symbolic manipulation techniques in the TDB context. In this paper, we continue such a line of research, facing "now-related" data, to cope with data such as "*John is in the Intensive Care Unit (ICU henceforth) from January 10 to now*". We call valid-time "***now-related***" those facts (tuples) starting in the past and still *valid* until the current time, as in John's example. Such data are very frequent in the medical context, where specific

© Springer International Publishing Switzerland 2015
J.H. Holmes et al. (Eds.): AIME 2015, LNAI 9105, pp. 327–331, 2015.
DOI: 10.1007/978-3-319-19551-3_41

attention has to be devoted to patient symptoms, treatments, measurements *holding at the current time*. Recent TDB approaches have identified four different ways to implement "now" in a standard relational database, using (i) NULL, (ii) the smallest timestamp (MIN approach), (iii) the largest timestamp (MAX approach), or (iv) degenerate zero-point intervals (POINT approach) (see, e.g., [8]). However, such approaches have three main limitations: (1) they propose models to store data, but (except (iv)) no algebra to query them, (2) implicitly or explicitly follow the semantics by Clifford et al. [9], in which "now-related" tuples are interpreted assuming that the span of time occurring between (the time of) a change of the world and (the time of) the database update (henceforth called *latency*) is *exactly known*, and (3) they cannot cope with bounds on the future persistence of now-related facts. In this paper, we propose a new TDB approach overcoming the above limitations.

2   Now-related Facts and Latency of Updates

All TDB approaches are (explicitly or implicitly) based on Clifford et al.'s semantics [9]; most of them assume that all "current" data remain current unless they are modified, which corresponds to assuming latency equal to zero. This is a severe limitation, since *generalized relations* cannot be treated [10]. The effect of such an assumption can be shown on Example 2 below (asserted at time 14).

Example 2. John is hospitalized in ICU from January 10 to NOW.

On January 14 (the time of assertion), we are certain that John has been in ICU on January 10, 11, 12 and 13 (homogeneously with treatment of 'now' in transaction time in BCDM [11], we assume that NOW is excluded. Notice, however, that our approach is mostly independent of such a choice). Possibly, John may stay in ICU all January 14, and on the 15, and so on, but this is not certain. Then, let us look at the same information two days after, i.e., on January 16, supposing that no modification has been done in the TDB. Clearly, if latency were known, the fact that the TDB has not been changed would provide us an additional knowledge. For instance, if the latency is 0, we are certain that John was in ICU also on January 14 and 15; if latency is 1 (i.e., facts are recorded one day after they happen in the real world), we are only certain that John has been in ICU also on January 14. However, in the more general case in which latency is unknown (which is more realistic in several medical domains), the valid time of now-related tuples depends only on the time when the now-related fact is asserted (henceforth called *assertion time*), and it is independent of the value of NOW. Indeed, if latency is unknown, the fact that the TDB has not been changed until January 16 (or, in general, any time t greater than 14) does not provide any additional information. Maybe John has been dismissed on January 14, but this fact has not been recorded yet (e.g., due to a long-term strike of data entry clerks). In general, if no assumption can be made on when changes in the modeled world are recorded in the TDB the (intended) meaning of *"the fact f holds from t_{start} to NOW"*, *asserted at time t_a* (i.e., NOW=t_a when the fact is asserted) is that f holds at each time unit from *start* to t_a (excluded), and it will end sometime in the future (i.e., some time after t_a). In other words, the semantics of NOW (with unknown latency) involves *temporal indeterminacy in the future* with respect to the *assertion time* t_a (notice that assertion time may differ from the time of insertion of the fact in the DB –i.e., from *transaction time*– and is related with Combi and Montanari's *availability time* [12]). In the following, we provide a relational model covering such an intuition.

3   1NF Relational Data Model

In this section, we propose a compact *1NF representation* for now-related tuples, considering valid time, coping with unknown latency and with now-bounded tuples.

Definition: pn-tuple and pn-relation. Given a schema $(A_1, ..., A_n)$ where each A_i represents a non-temporal attribute on the domain D_i, a pn-relation r^{pn} is an instance of the schema $(A_1, ..., A_n | VTs, VTa, VTe)$ defined over the domain $D_1 \times ... \times D_n \times T^C \times T^C \times T^C$, where T^C is the domain of *chronons* [3]. For each instance of the schema, $VTs \leq VTa \leq VTe$. Each tuple $x = (a_1, ..., a_n | v_s, v_a, v_e) \in r^{pn}$ is termed a pn-tuple ("pn" stands for possibly now-related).

Intuitively speaking, and considering a valid-time now-related tuple, VTs represents the starting time of valid time, VTa the assertion time, and VTe the future bound for 'now' (the value c_{max} –the maximum possible time in T^C– is used in case no bound has to be modelled, see first row of Table 1). Example 3, at the granularity of days, can be expressed in our model as shown by the second row of Table 1. Notice that, in our representation, time intervals are closed to the left and open to the right.

Example 3. A patient that reaches the emergency department (henceforth ER) can be kept under observation for a maximum period of two days. Afterwards, (s)he must be moved to another ward. Tom was hospitalized in the ER on April 4. Such fact was asserted on day April 5.

Intuitively speaking, the second row of Table 1 represents the fact that we are certain that Tom is in the ER on April 4, and will possibly stay there one more day (until April 6, excluded). In our model, tuples that are not now-related can still be represented, using the convention introduced in Property 1.

Table 1. Pn-relation representation of Examples 2, 3 and 4

Patient	Ward	VTs	VTa	VTe
John	ICU	Jan 10	Jan 14	c_{max}
Tom	ER	Apr 4	Apr 5	Apr 6
Bill	Cardiac Surgery	Aug 16	Aug 31	Aug 31

Property 1: consistent extension (wrt TSQL2). Any not now-related tuple can be easily represented as a special case of the above representation, in which $VTa = VTe$.

Thus, pn-relations can include heterogeneous types of tuples, in the sense that any of them, independently of the others, may be now-related or not. For instance, Table 1 represents both the now-related facts of Examples 2 and 3 (first and second rows) and the not now-related fact that Bill has been hospitalized in the Cardiac Surgery ward from August 16 to 30 (third row).

4   Relational Algebra

Our representation models temporal indeterminacy in a compact and implicit way. The interval $[VTs, VTa)$ is the span of time in which the fact certainly occurs, while $[VTa, VTe)$ is the span of future time in which the fact might hold (resembling Das and Musen's *intervals of uncertainty* [4]). Thus, for instance, the first row of Table 1 is a *compact representation* of the fact that John is in ICU from 10 to 13, *or* from 10 to 14, *or* ... *or* from 10 to c_{max}. We provide a temporal extension to Codd's relational algebra operators in such a way that our operators *directly operate on our implicit 1NF representation*, but are **consistent** with such an underlying *semantics*. Additionally, our temporal relational operators are **reducible** to TSQL2 ones (which, in turn, are reducible to standard Codd's operators). Reducibility grants for the interoperability of our approach to TSQL2-based ones, and with standard DBMS. For the sake of brevity, only Cartesian product is reported. We follow the TSQL2 notation; x[X] represents the value of attribute X in the tuple x.

Definition (Cartesian product). Given two pn-relations r^{pn} and s^{pn} defined on the schemas R: $(A_1, ..., A_n | VTs, VTa, VTe)$ and S: $(B_1, ..., B_m | VTs, VTa, VTe)$ respectively (where $A_1, ..., A_n$ and $B_1, ..., B_m$ represent the non-temporal attributes), the Cartesian product $r^{pn} \times^{pn} s^{pn}$ has schema $(A_1, ..., A_n, B_1, ..., B_m | VTs, VTa, VTe)$ and is defined as follows:

$$r^{pn} \times^{pn} s^{pn} = \{x \setminus \exists x1 \in r^{pn} \wedge \exists x2 \in s^{pn} \wedge$$
$$x[A_1, ..., A_n] = x1[A_1, ..., A_n] \wedge x[B_1, ..., B_m] = x2[B_1, ..., B_m] \wedge$$
$$x[VTs] = max(x1[VTs], x2[VTs]) \wedge$$
$$x[VTa] = max(min(x1[VTa], x2[VTa]), x[VTs]) \wedge$$
$$x[VTe] = min(x1[VTe], x2[VTe]) \wedge x[VTs] < x[VTe]\}.$$

Cartesian product manages the non-temporal attributes $A_1, ..., A_n, B_1, ..., B_m$ in a standard (i.e., Codd's) way and it evaluates the intersection of the "certain" (i.e., [x1[Vts],x1[VTa]) ∩ [x2[Vts],x2[VTa])) and "possible" times of the paired tuples.

5   Conclusions and Future Work

Now-related temporal data play an important role in the medical context, where specific attention is devoted to patient symptoms, treatments, measurements holding at the current time. Current relational approaches to now-related data assume that the *"latency"* of updates is known and do not explicitly provide an extended relational algebra to query them (except the POINT approach [8]). We propose an approach that, adopting AI techniques, overcomes such limitations, and we analyze its properties (reducibility). In our future work, we aim at extending our approach to cope also with *transaction time*, considering also cases in which the *latency* of updates is *known*. Also, in this paper, we considered only the temporal indeterminacy derived from now-related tuples, and we want to extend it to deal with more general cases (as, e.g., in [9], where, notably, temporal indeterminacy is **not** used to cover the semantics of "now"). Finally, a major extension would consist in the addition of suitable AI-based mechanisms to deal with persistence. Indeed, in this paper, we suppose that no additional knowledge is available with respect to the facts in the TDB, so that each of them can persist from the assertion time to a future bound (or, if it is missing, forever). This resembles McCarthy's inertia principle [13], which was extended by McDermott [14] considering the typical lifetime of facts. Recent AI approaches have investigated a knowledge-based analysis of persistence. In particular, considering the medical domain, Shahar has studied persistence in the general context of data interpolation, considering both forward and backward persistence, and stressing the fact that it depends on the concepts, concepts' values, and even context [15].

Acknowledgments. The work was partially supported by Compagnia di San Paolo in the Ginseng project.

References

1. Das, A.K., Musen, M.A.: A foundational model of time for heterogeneous clinical databases. In: Proc. AMIA Annu. Fall Symp., pp. 106–110 (1997)
2. O'Connor, M.J., Tu, S.W., Musen, M.A.: The Chronus II temporal database mediator. In: Proc. AMIA Symp., pp. 567–571 (2002)
3. Snodgrass, R.T.: The TSQL2 temporal query language. Kluwer (1995)
4. Das, A.K., Musen, M.A.: A temporal query system for protocol-directed decision support. Methods Inf. Med. 33, 358–370 (1994)
5. Terenziani, P., Snodgrass, R.T., Bottrighi, A., Torchio, M., Molino, G.: Extending temporal databases to deal with telic/atelic medical data. Artif. Intell. Med. 39, 113–126 (2007)
6. Stantic, B., Terenziani, P., Governatori, G., Bottrighi, A., Sattar, A.: An implicit approach to deal with periodically repeated medical data. Artif. Intell. Med. 55, 149–162 (2012)
7. Anselma, L., Bottrighi, A., Montani, S., Terenziani, P.: Managing proposals and evaluations of updates to medical knowledge: theory and applications. J. Biomed. Inform. 46, 363–376 (2013)
8. Stantic, B., Sattar, A., Terenziani, P.: The POINT approach to represent now in bitemporal databases. Journal of Intelligent Information Systems 32, 297–323 (2008)
9. Clifford, J., Isakowitz, T., Dyreson, C., Jensen, C.S., Snodgrass, R.T.: On the Semantics of "Now" in Databases. ACM Transactions on Database Systems 22, 171–214 (1997)
10. Jensen, C.S., Snodgrass, R.: Temporal specialization and generalization. IEEE Transactions on Knowledge and Data Engineering 6, 954–974 (1994)
11. Jensen, C.S., Snodgrass, R.T.: Semantics of Time-Varying Information. Information Systems 21, 311–352 (1996)
12. Combi, C., Montanari, A.: Data Models with Multiple Temporal Dimensions: Completing the Picture. In: Dittrich, K.R., Geppert, A., Norrie, M. (eds.) CAiSE 2001. LNCS, vol. 2068, pp. 187–202. Springer, Heidelberg (2001)
13. McCarthy, J.: Applications of Circumscription to Formalizing Common-Sense Knowledge. Artif. Intell. 28, 89–116 (1986)
14. McDermott, D.V.: A Temporal Logic for Reasoning About Processes and Plans. Cognitive Science 6, 101–155 (1982)
15. Shahar, Y.: Knowledge-based temporal interpolation. J. Exp. Theor. Artif. Intell. 11, 123–144 (1999)

Temporal Conformance Analysis of Clinical Guidelines Execution

Matteo Spiotta[1,2(✉)], Paolo Terenziani[1],
and Daniele Theseider Dupré[1]

[1] DISIT, Sezione di Informatica, Università del Piemonte Orientale,
Alessandria, Italy
[2] Dipartimento di Informatica, Università di Torino, Turin, Italy
matteo.spiotta@gmail.com, paolo.terenziani@unipmn.it, dtd@di.unipmn.it

Abstract. Physicians often have to combine clinical guideline recommendations with their own basic medical knowledge to cope with specific patients in specific contexts. Both knowledge sources may include temporal constraints for the execution of actions. In this paper we approach the problem of compliance analysis with both sources of knowledge, pointing out discrepancies – including temporal ones – with respect to them, and where such discrepancies may be due to multiple and possibly conflicting recommendations.

1 Introduction

Clinical Guidelines (CGs) are developed in order to capture medical evidence and to put it into practice, and deal with "typical" classes of patients, since the CG developers cannot define all possible executions of a CG on any possible specific patient in any clinical condition. When treating "atypical" patients, physicians have to resort to their Basic Medical Knowledge.

The interplay between CG and BMK recommendations can be very complex. For instance, actions recommended by a CG could be prohibited by the BMK, or a CG could force some actions despite the BMK discourages them (see, e.g., [1]). Such a complexity significantly increases in case the temporal dimension is taken into account. Actions, in both CGs and BMK recommendations, have pre-conditions which temporally constrain them, and may be temporally constrained with each other. Also, CG and BMK recommendations must often be "merged" along time, and such a merge can lead to the violation of some temporal constraints in one of the knowledge sources.

In this paper, we extend [2] focusing on the *temporal* interplay between CGs and BMK from the viewpoint of *a posteriori* conformance analysis [3], intended as the adherence of an observed CG execution trace to both the CG and BMK. We do not provide any form of evaluation of how the interplay has been managed (i.e., whether the treatment was appropriate or not): we aim at identifying, in the trace, situations in which some recommendation (either in the CG or in

This research is partially supported by Compagnia di San Paolo.

© Springer International Publishing Switzerland 2015
J.H. Holmes et al. (Eds.): AIME 2015, LNAI 9105, pp. 332–336, 2015.
DOI: 10.1007/978-3-319-19551-3_42

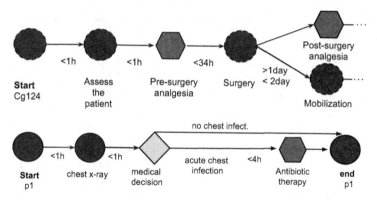

Fig. 1. Hip fracture CG (above) and chest infection plan (below). Circles are atomic actions, hexagonal nodes are composite actions, diamond nodes are decisions.

the BMK) has not been followed, and at providing potential justifications for non-conformance to one knowledge source based on another source.

2   The Framework and an Example Case

We present the framework on the clinical case of a patient hospitalized for a hip fracture. Conformance analysis is based on a log trace, a CG and a set of BMK rules. Fig. 1 shows an adapted excerpt of the hip fracture CG in [4], represented in GLARE [5], where temporal constraints can be provided: in particular, constraints that impose a minimum and maximum delay between the start/end points of actions and/or preconditions. In the example, surgery should be executed within 36 hours from patient admission, and mobilization should be started the day after surgery. The BMK may account both for additional actions and for cancellation or a different timing of actions prescribed by the CG. BMK rules considered in this paper are formed by a *trigger*, i.e., conditions on the patient and context that make the piece of knowledge relevant, and either a simple or composite action, which is suggested in the given conditions, or the suggestion to avoid or delay some action, in one of the following forms:

- *Avoid a*: states that action *a* should not be executed; we assume that such a statement is triggered by conditions that are not reversible;
- *Delay a while c*, i.e., *a* should not be performed as long as *c* holds;
- *Delay a for d*: suggests delaying action *a* for time *d*.

Knowledge involving suggested actions (**"do"** knowledge for short) is similar to exceptions in [6] and guideline-independent exceptions in [7], which may be triggered at any point of the CG execution. Both "do" knowledge and the one that suggests avoiding or delaying an action (**"do not"** knowledge for short) refine rules proposed in [2], taking into account the temporal dimension.

In our example the following BMK rules R1 and R2 are considered.

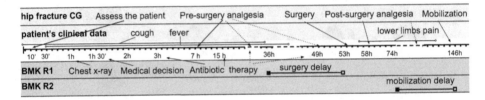

Fig. 2. Example case

(**R1**) For patients with high body temperature and cough, the presence of a chest infection has to be investigated through a chest x-ray, and, if present, treated with an antibiotic therapy (see figure 1; actually, in [4] acute chest infection is explicitly mentioned as one of the conditions to be checked and, if necessary, treated, to avoid delaying surgery too much; however, it is also mentioned that there are less common concerns which may require delaying surgery: we consider chest infection like one of these).

(**R2**) Mobilization has to be delayed for patients having pain in lower limbs.

The analysis is performed on a log trace, in this example containing only **patient data**, shown in fig. 2, and in general also **context data** (such as availability of personnel and resources). Patient data consists in *patient findings* (line 2) and *action log* (lines 1-3-4) containing the start and end points of the executed actions. We assume to have complete knowledge about log data.

3   Execution Model and Conformance Analysis

The control flow of the CG execution, or triggers in the BMK, may indicate that a given action has to be considered for execution (is a candidate). A candidate action could become active or discarded; if active, it could either be completed or aborted. In the following we only discuss the case of an action which is candidate by the CG, and its transition to the active or discarded state.

We assume that constraints on the time t_{act} when action a could become active are given with respect to the time t_{ca} when the action becomes candidate, or the start and end times of episodes of preconditions. We assume that at least the control flow provides a constraint $t_{act} \leq t_{ca} + n$ so that $t_{ca} + n$ is a deadline for starting the action in order to conform to the CG. The conformant execution can be characterized as follows:

1. The action should start at a time t_{act} such that all preconditions, with their temporal constraints, enable the action, if one such time exists.
2. Otherwise, when the first deadline is reached, the action should be discarded.

When case 2 occurs, i.e., an action is correctly discarded (according to a strict interpretation of the CG), we however point this out. Indeed, there might be valid medical alternatives, such as relaxing a constraint on a precondition, or the deadline. Analogously, for a non-conformance case where a deadline or a precondition is violated, it should be pointed out whether meeting all the recommendations was possible or not.

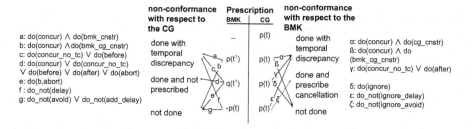

Fig. 3. Discrepancies and their justifications

We consider the following alterations to the guideline execution based on BMK. When a (possibly composite) action a in the *"do"* BMK knowledge is triggered, several options are considered (similarly to [7]): the execution of a and the CG proceeds concurrently (**concur** case); or they are both executed, but temporal constraints are not enforced (**concur_no_tc**) with the special cases where a is delayed after the end of the CG execution (**after**), and where a is executed before proceeding with the CG (**before**); as further alternatives, the BMK suggestion is ignored (**ignore**); or the execution of the CG is aborted and a is executed (**abort**). A special case occurs for the concurrent modality, in case the same action is candidate for both CG execution and the execution of the BMK action: temporal constraints from both the CG and BMK (**cg_bmk_constr**), or from either of them (**cg_constr, bmk_constr**), may be enforced.

When an action a is candidate, if a *"do not"* BMK rule *Avoid a* is triggered, either the action a is discarded (**avoid**), or the BMK rule is ignored (**ignore_avoid**). For the case *Delay a while c*, either the BMK rule is ignored (**ignore_delay**), or c is used as an additional precondition for a (**add_delay**), or it replaces preconditions for a (**delay**). For the case *Delay a for d*, either the BMK rule is ignored (**ignore_delay**), or it adds the constraint $t_{now} + d \leq t_{act}$ (**add_delay**), or replaces with it the constraints on t_{act} (**delay**).

Conformance analysis is performed in Answer Set Programming, similarly to [2]; the results are ways to interpret a log according to the CG model and its possible alterations described above, with a minimum number of non-conformances.

In the example (figure 2), actions *chest x-ray, medical decision, antibiotic therapy*, are justified by rule R1. The identified modality is **concur_no_tc**, which accounts for the delay of *hip surgery* beyond the CG recommendation. Rule R2 is triggered because of pain in lower limbs and it justifies the delay of *mobilization*.

The coverage of the approach is illustrated in figure 3, which lists cases where a discrepancy with one knowledge source may be justified by the other source. Different lines in the table correspond to different cases as regards current candidates from the CG and the BMK ($p(t)$ means that action p is candidate to start at time t). Arrows connect a line to a type of discrepancy with respect to the CG or the BMK, and labels below shortly describe the case. For example, in case the CG and the BMK propose the same action as candidate (2nd line), it may be the case (a) that the action is performed without conforming to the CG constraints (the exception runs in concurrent modality and only the BMK constraints are enforced), or (α) it is performed without conforming to the BMK constraints, or (b and/or β) it is not performed because all constraints are enforced, but they are never all true.

4   Conclusions

CGs do not include all knowledge that physicians have to take into account [1,8], since patient states and contexts of execution cannot always be foreseen. In this paper we propose an approach for analyzing temporal conformance of execution traces with respect to a richer form of medical knowledge, which may be used to justify deviations from a strict application of the guideline, both as regards extra actions for situations that are not foreseen (and whose treatment may alter the timing of guideline execution), and cancellation or delay of actions that are prescribed by the guideline, when there are reasons to do so. Given that we do not assume that all exceptions and interactions are modeled, and a temporally non-conformant execution of a guideline is always potentially justified by a concurrent treatment of a different problem, the final evaluation about the clinical correctness of justifications is left to physicians.

References

1. Bottrighi, A., Chesani, F., Mello, P., Montali, M., Montani, S., Terenziani, P.: Conformance checking of executed clinical guidelines in presence of basic medical knowledge. In: Daniel, F., Barkaoui, K., Dustdar, S. (eds.) BPM Workshops 2011, Part II. LNBIP, vol. 100, pp. 200–211. Springer, Heidelberg (2012)
2. Spiotta, M., Bottrighi, A., Giordano, L., Theseider Dupré, D.: Conformance analysis of the execution of clinical guidelines with basic medical knowledge and clinical terminology. In: Miksch, S., Riano, D., ten Teije, A. (eds.) KR4HC 2014. LNCS, vol. 8903, pp. 62–77. Springer, Heidelberg (2014)
3. Groot, P., Hommersom, A., Lucas, P.J.F., Merk, R., ten Teije, A., van Harmelen, F., Serban, R.: Using model checking for critiquing based on clinical guidelines. Artificial Intelligence in Medicine 46(1), 19–36 (2009)
4. British National Institute for Health and Care Excellence. Hip fracture: The management of hip fracture in adults, http://www.nice.org.uk/guidance/cg124
5. Terenziani, P., Molino, G., Torchio, M.: A modular approach for representing and executing clinical guidelines. Artif. Intell. in Medicine 23(3), 249–276 (2001)
6. Grando, A., Peleg, M., Glasspool, D.: A goal-oriented framework for specifying clinical guidelines and handling medical errors. Journal of Biomedical Informatics 43(2), 287–299 (2010)
7. Leonardi, G., Bottrighi, G., Galliani, G., Terenziani, G., Messina, G., Della Corte, G.: Exceptions handling within GLARE clinical guideline framework. In: AMIA 2012, American Medical Informatics Association Annual Symposium (2012)
8. Brandhorst, C.J., Sent, D., Stegwee, R.A., van Dijk, B.M.A.G.: Medintel: Decision support for general practitioners: A case study. In: Adlassnig, K.-P., Blobel, B., Mantas, J., Masic, I. (eds.) MIE. Studies in Health Technology and Informatics, vol. 150, pp. 688–692. IOS Press (2009)

Combining Decision Support System-Generated Recommendations with Interactive Guideline Visualization for Better Informed Decisions

Lucia Sacchi[1(✉)], Enea Parimbelli[1], Silvia Panzarasa[1], Natalia Viani[1], Elena Rizzo[1],
Carlo Napolitano[2], Roxana Ioana Budasu[2], and Silvana Quaglini[1]

[1] Department of Electrical, Computer and Biomedical Engineering,
University of Pavia, Pavia, Italy
[2] IRCCS Foundation S. Maugeri, Pavia, Italy
lucia.sacchi@unipv.it

Abstract. The main task of decision support systems based on computer-interpretable guidelines (CIG) is to send recommendations to physicians, combining patients' data with guideline knowledge. Another important task is providing physicians with explanations for such recommendations. For this purpose some systems may show, for every recommendation, the guideline path activated by the reasoner. However the fact that the physician does not have a global view of the guideline may represent a limitation. Indeed, there are instances (e.g. when the clinical presentation does not perfectly fit the guideline) in which the analysis of alternatives that were not activated by the system becomes warranted. Furthermore possibly valid alternatives could not be activated due to lack of data or wrong knowledge representation. This paper illustrates a CIG implementation that complements the two functionalities, i.e., sending punctual recommendations and allowing a meaningful navigation of the entire guideline. The training example concerns atrial fibrillation management.

Keywords: Decision support systems · Computer interpretable guidelines · Knowledge representation · Atrial fibrillation

1 Introduction

Physicians' willingness to use guideline-based computerized decision support systems (DSS) may be impaired by the intrinsic "rigidity" of DSSs [1]. As a matter of fact, the accuracy of their automatic suggestions strongly depends on two basic contributions, namely the patient's data, normally stored in the electronic health record (EHR), and the formalized medical knowledge, often encoded in the form of production rules. Moreover, a DSS inference engine often has to perform complex routings of tasks, such as parallel and cyclic paths, which require precise conditions, also based on temporal constraints. One of the main reasons for DSSs' incorrect delivery of recommendations is the lack of synchronization between the underlying inference engine and the process of EHR updating. The issue is complicated by the fact that data are

J.H. Holmes et al. (Eds.): AIME 2015, LNAI 9105, pp. 337–341, 2015.
DOI: 10.1007/978-3-319-19551-3_43

entered in the EHR by multiple users, who could be either DSS users or not, and are not all equally committed to enter data timely and knowingly. Other problems could arise at knowledge acquisition time, such as misunderstandings between medical experts and knowledge engineers, or misinterpretation of the guideline (GL) text, resulting in inaccurate knowledge representation. Having these information in mind it becomes clear that DSS users might benefit from instruments that allow to verify the correctness of the delivered recommendations, thus gaining confidence in the use of the instrument. The issue of gaining insights into the received recommendations is not new. Few years after their introduction, expert systems in medicine found useful to include explanation facilities to improve physicians' confidence and compliance [2]. In general, the explanation consists in showing to the user not only the process outcomes but also the patient's data together with all the matching rules . However, this approach only provides a partial solution, since the physician can see only the specific GL path that was activated, whereas a more general view is lacking. As a matter of fact, an alternative path could have not been activated simply for lack of data or, even worse, for wrong knowledge representation.

In this paper we illustrate a solution proposed within the MobiGuide project, where a DSS has been implemented relying on the latest GLs for atrial fibrillation (AF) [3]. The system includes an intuitive graphical user interface (GUI) that allows cardiologists both to obtain the specific DSS recommendations for AF patients and to visualize the entire GL. The opportunity to explore the GL is augmented by specific functionalities that allow users to better understand the received DSS recommendations and consider possible alternative, evidence-based decisions.

2   Methods

When knowledge engineers and physicians collaborate to formalize a textual GL into a computer-interpretable one, they usually adopt a simple formal flowchart representation, which represents an intermediate step toward GL computerization [4]. Once the computerization process is finalized, the flowchart is never used again, since it is replaced by the final computer-interpretable formalism which, although generally relying on a graphical approach, can actually be much more complex [5]. In this paper, we argue that physicians could continue to benefit from the former, simpler representation even at DSS running time, and we propose a method for exploiting such representation.

We first interviewed physicians with a user-oriented approach to understand their requirements for DSS use in clinical practice. From the interviews it emerged that physicians tend to be skeptics with a system that only delivers recommendations. On the other hand, they appreciate a system able to provide a sort of "second opinion", therefore confirming or contradicting their hypotheses, possibly together with a scientific explanation for that judgment. On the basis of these observations, we report some of the use-cases that could be useful to implement.

- Use-case #1 *For this patient I would prescribe drug D1, while the DSS suggested drug D2. Which GL sections do recommend D1?*

- Use-case #2 *I know that this patient is eligible for section S of the GL. Which are all the drugs recommended in that section?*
- Use-case #3 *I know that there are critical decisions to be taken with some of my patients. Can the DSS help me in the shared decision making process?*
- Use-case #4 *I know this patient is eligible for the section S of the GL. Which are all the diagnostic procedures that probably I have to book for him?*
- Use-case #5 *My hospital administration is undergoing a spending review. Which are the treatment options with similar outcomes but different costs?*

Thus, physicians are looking for a tool that is a DSS and an educational support at the same time, and that carries additional information rather than strictly medical content.

In this short paper, we do not focus on the technological solutions, but on the methodological ones. Our graphical representations of the GL are produced with Microsoft Visio, the same tool used during the meetings with cardiologists for the knowledge elicitation process. First of all, a tree-like index of the graph was derived, reflecting the main structure of the GL in terms of tasks/subtasks, and parallel/sequence routings. This is the top-level GL navigation tool for the physician. According to the requirement analysis, three main sets characterize the GL sections, namely the set of diagnostic recommendations, the set of therapeutic recommendations, and the set of recommendations that mention shared decision making.

Each section is composed by a set of tasks organized in a flowchart, and each task is characterized by a set of attributes. We used a subset of the GEM (Guideline Element Model) elements [6]. Those attributes can be used by the physician in two complementary ways, i.e. to visualize all the tasks, within a GL section, that show a certain value for a specific attribute, or to visualize all the values that a certain attribute can take within a GL section. The *action cost* element deserves a short insight. The direct cost related to a task is a useful information (e.g., the price of a drug), but it may be insufficient to estimate medium- or long-term costs (e.g., the cost of a drug side effects). Thus, the cost attribute may also contain links to cost/effectiveness models. Finally, as well motivated in [7], it is important to "... ensure no restrictions are placed on staff's access to online resources that contain relevant research evidence". Thus, every section and every task of the graphical representation is linked with the corresponding original GL text.

3   Results

In the MobiGuide project, the DSS is fully integrated with the caregiver GUI, where doctors manage patients' data and receive recommendations. At any time, and particularly after receiving a recommendation from the DSS, the physician may access an interactive representation of the GL, as shown in Figure 1. Each index item is labeled with T, D, or SDM, indicating that the specific section contains therapeutic, diagnostic, or shared-decision processes [8], respectively. Figure 1 shows the list of tasks, classified into *drugs* and *procedures*, which can be obtained by clicking on one of the "T" buttons. Similarly, after clicking on a specific "D" button, the diagnostic tasks related to the considered section are displayed, again classified according to their type (ematochemical, image, signal, etc.). Through the "Search" button (middle top) the physician may select a drug or procedure name and see all the GL sections containing it. Moreover, clicking an index item triggers the opening of the corresponding extended flowchart, as shown in Fig. 2. Green diamonds represent physicians' choices, which are proposed along with the underlying recommendation's class and level of scientific evidence (top-left color and letter), and the related cost (bottom-right).

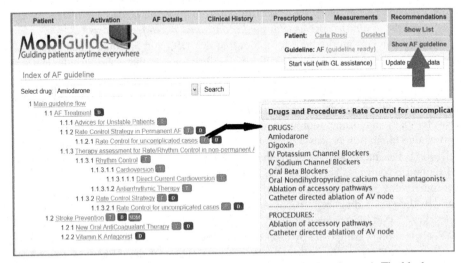

Fig. 1. The GL navigation tool, accessible from the caregiver GUI (red arrow). The black arrow stands for the visualization of all the therapeutic options treated in a certain GL section.

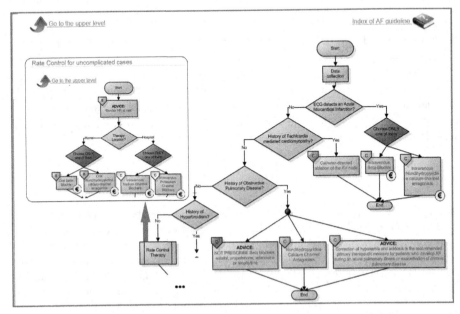

Fig. 2. Visualization of the flowchart. Double-edge rectangles may be expanded (brown arrow).

Importantly, red color indicates an action to be avoided. Double click on a recommendation allows to retrieve the corresponding GL text. In case of a shared decision making recommendation, the system may provide with decision aids for patients, such as simple description of the decision problem, with *pro and cons* for every option.

4   Discussion and Conclusion

This work is intended to provide a proof of concept for the exploitation of an augmented flowchart representation of a GL during interaction with a dynamic DSS. Our claim is that enriching the simple flowchart, which was developed in collaboration with physicians during the very first GL formalization phase, with the features that are most appreciated by physicians as aids for their decision processes, may increase their confidence in the decision itself. The next step will be the validation of our approach within the pilot study of the project, which will be performed on 15 AF patients. The system actually shows some limitations, among which the synchronization of the DSS and the flowchart in front of an update of the clinical GL, and lack of integration of coding systems to better characterize the flowchart elements.

References

1. Ash, J.S., Sittig, D.F., Campbell, E.M., Guappone, K.P., Dykstra, R.H.: Some Unintended Consequences of Clinical Decision Support Systems. In: AMIA Annu. Symp. Proc. 2007, pp. 26–30 (2007)
2. Sotos, J.G.: MYCIN and NEOMYCIN: two approaches to generating explanations in rule-based expert systems. Aviat. Space Environ. Med. 61(10), 950–954 (1990)
3. American College of Cardiology Foundation/American Heart Association Task Force: 2011 ACCF/AHA/HRS focused updates incorporated into the ACC/AHA/ESC 2006 guidelines for the management of patients with atrial fibrillation: a report of the American College of Cardiology Foundation/American Heart Association Task Force on practice guidelines. Circulation123(10), e269-e367 (2011)
4. Ciccarese, P., Caffi, E., Quaglini, S., Stefanelli, M.: Architectures and tools for innovative Health Information Systems: the Guide Project. Int. J. Med. Inform. 74(7-8), 553–562 (2005)
5. Peleg, M., Tu, S., Bury, J., Ciccarese, P., Fox, J., Greenes, R.A., Hall, R., Johnson, P.D., Jones, N., Kumar, A., Miksch, S., Quaglini, S., Seyfang, A., Shortliffe, E.H., Stefanelli, M.: Comparing computer-interpretable guideline models: a case-study approach. J. Am. Med. Inform. Assoc. 10(1), 52–68 (2003)
6. Hajizadeh, N., Kashyap, N., Michel, G., Shiffman, R.N.: GEM at 10: a decade's experience with the Guideline Elements Model. In: AMIA Annu. Symp. Proc., pp. 520–528 (2011)
7. Ellen, M.E., Léon, G., Bouchard, G., Ouimet, M., Grimshaw, J.M., Lavis, J.N.: Barriers, facilitators and views about next steps to implementing supports for evidence-informed decision-making in health systems: a qualitative study Implement Sci. 9(1), 179 (2014)
8. Sacchi, L., Rubrichi, S., Rognoni, C., Panzarasa, S., Parimbelli, E., Mazzanti, A., Napolitano, C., Priori, S.G., Quaglini, S.: From decision to shared-decision: Introducing patients' preferences into clinical decision analysis. Artif. Intell. Med. (November 2014)

Author Index

Printed in the United States
By Bookmasters